THERAPEUTIC MASSAGE

A SCIENTIFIC APPROACH

ROSS TURCHANINOV, MD

Edited by K. Gray

Published in the United States by Aesculapis Books

AESCULAPIUS BOOKS
18420 N 46 Str
Phoenix AZ, 85032

ISBN: 0-9675868-1-X

Manufactured in the United States of America

Second Edition: December 2012

9 8 7 6 5 4 3 2 1

CONTENTS

II. PRESSURE AND MECHANISMS OF THE THERAPEUTIC EFFECT OF MASSAGE THERAPY

III. PATHOPHYSIOLOGY OF PAIN. THE PAIN-ANALYZING SYSTEM AND ITS CORRECT ACTIVATION BY MASSAGE THERAPY

IV. THE HAND AS A THERAPEUTIC TOOL. THE CONTACT AREAS OF THE HAND

V. THERAPEUTIC MASSAGE TECHNIQUES

EFFLEURAGE

FRICTION

KNEADING

VIBRATION

PERCUSSION

COMPRESSION

PASSIVE STRETCHING

INTRODUCTION

In approximately 2590 BC the Chinese emperor and also talented physician Huang Ti wrote the oldest medical textbook: The *Yellow Emperor's Classic of Internal Medicine.* This is the first written evidence of the use of massage for medical purposes (Goats, 1994). Millenniums have passed by and great civilizations are gone but massage survived all historical turmoils and now is one of the oldest medical procedures which is still important in our modern world.

Despite the recent positive changes, at this point the medical aspects of massage therapy do not have significant value for the American Medical Community. As correctly pointed out by T. Field, (1998) "Massage therapy disappeared from the American medical scene at approximately the time of the pharmaceutical revolution of the 1940s". Kamenetz, (1985) identified 3 main causes of the disappearance of massage from the American medical field in 20th century: the pharmaceutical industry; development of new machines for physical therapy; and dehumanization of the relationship between medical practitioners and patients.

During the last decade especially, under the influence of New Age philosophy, the status of massage therapy in the USA and some other Western countries slowly changed and more and more physicians and hospitals started to incorporate massage into the routine medical practice. This process is now well documented in several statistical studies.

In 1998 Falkenbach, et al., published the results of a survey of 199 students of Frankfurt University Medical School which has included the course of medical massage in its curriculum since 1987. 66% of students studied medical massage to be better able to (later) prescribe massage; 23% of students planned to practice massage as a medical doctor; 75% of students wanted to improve their palpatory skills. A similar interest in complementary therapies, especially massage and acupuncture, was expressed by 800 students from 2 medical universities of Melbourne, Australia (Hopper and Cohen, 1998).

Verhoef and Page (1998) examined the knowledge, opinions and referral behavior of 300 family physicians in Alberta province of Canada. The authors used a method of random, cross-sectional mailed survey. 68% of physicians reported minimal or no knowledge of massage therapy; 55% agreed that massage therapy includes ideas and methods from which traditional health care could benefit; 22% strongly agreed that massage therapy stimulates the body's natural healing powers; 71% had referred patients to massage therapists.

In several statistical studies conducted by Eisenberg, et al., (1993 and 1998) and published in the *New England Journal of Medicine* and *Journal of American Medical Association*, the authors examined the patterns of use, costs and prevalence of methods of alternative medicine in the USA. They found that in 1997 Americans spent $ 21.2 billion on alternative medicine with approximately $12.2 billion paid out-of pocket. Massage therapy ranked second in popularity after chiropractic care.

The comparison of obtained data allowed the authors to conclude that alternative medicine has increased dramatically and the probability of visiting an unconventional medical practitioner increased from 36.3% in 1991 to 46.3% in 1997. The number of visits to all alternative therapy practitioners was 38.6% higher than to all primary care physicians in the USA in 1997. This information reveals the strong positive tendency of patients to utilize alternative therapy. However I strongly believe that the ideal structure of modern medicine is the merging of so called traditional and alternative approaches. They shouldn't compete with each other because they are sides of the same coin. I think that patients will get enormous benefits from this integration.

To present the Western approach to the medical massage treatment I wrote the textbook *Medical Massage*, Volume I and II. These manuscripts were published by Aesculapius Books. In these books the different methods of medical massage were described as well as their application in cases of disorders of the central and peripheral nervous system, musculoskeletal system and various abnormalities of inner organs.

Classical or therapeutic massage was also discussed as one of the possible methods of treatment in every case where it can be applied. However I think that matter of therapeutic massage is very important and it deserves separate publication.

In this book, readers will not find any information about spiritual aspects of therapeutic massage. This equally important part of massage treatment is already well described in the modern American massage literature. We will look on therapeutic massage as a science. I saw as my goal the detailed representation of modern scientific approaches to the theory and practice of therapeutic massage treatment.

I don't want readers to conclude that I consider massage therapy as some kind of medical panacea. My personal position on this matter is as follows: Massage is an integral part of traditional medicine which should be considered as an important and sometimes even critical component of the patient's entire treatment (e.g., in cases of numerous somatic disorders) conducted by different medical professionals.

I hope that this book will be extremely helpful for students in physical therapy or massage therapy schools as well as for every beginning massage practitioner. I also hope that doctors, experienced physical therapists and massage practitioners will find a lot of new and usable information.

I want to express my deep appreciation to Mrs. K. Beacham, LMT and Mr. S. Tsechanov, LMT for their help in the preparation of this book.

Dr. Ross Turchaninov

I. PHYSIOLOGICAL AND THERAPEUTIC EFFECT OF MASSAGE ON THE SYSTEMS AND ORGANS OF THE HUMAN BODY

Massage can be used as a preventive therapy or, for medical purposes, as a powerful method of treatment for numerous disorders. Recognition of the massage' medical value by the American medical community will bring great benefits to patients. It will also restore the real significance of massage therapy as a profession while building up massage therapists' self-confidence as well as their personal income. Massage therapists are able to speed up this process by working with doctors to show and explain to them the possibilities of massage therapy offers. To do this the practitioner has to talk with doctors in the same language, using the same terminology, and be able to convince the well educated but frequently skeptical professionals. This chapter helps readers accomplish that.

Chapter I is a review of the most significant books and articles concerning the physiological and therapeutic effects of massage treatment from as early as the middle of the 19th century to present day. All references which are discussed here were written by medical, osteopathic, chiropractic, and physical therapy scientists; published by prestigious medical journals and publishing companies throughout the Western world.

For this purpose, the statistical results of experimental and clinical studies from the most important (in the author's opinion) books and articles are included. Each section of this chapter can then be paired with the references it is based on (see list of references), forming an independent brochure which the practitioner can distribute among local physicians to build up referral base. This will help massage practitioners establish necessary connections with other medical professionals. We also hope that other health practitioners will find a lot of new and usable information in these chapters.

The reader will also notice that this chapter is not just a general review of references. We tried to present the information from the discussed sources with the authors' conclusions and recommendations to increase the value of the review. Thus, we encourage the reader to go over this chapter carefully because it is filled with a great deal of practical information. You will find a lot of important practical tips which can be immediately put into work. It will make your treatment more efficient and your patients more satisfied.

The statement that "massage affects all organs and systems of the human body," is very general. Many studies were done to analyze the physiological effects of massage on the healthy body as well as clinical studies of medical massage treatments were conducted to determine its therapeutic impact on different somatic and visceral disorders. Let us review the most valuable information which the world's leading scientists found during decades of experimental and clinical studies.

A. NERVOUS SYSTEM

The nervous system is the main coordinator of all body functions. The nervous system maintains the functions of all organs and systems within the physiological limits and properly adjusts them to any changes in the internal (i.e. homeostasis) or external environment. To effectively coordinate the body functions the nervous system executes 3 basic functions: sensory, integrative and motor.

a. Sensory Function

Sensory function or afferent (ascending) input is the generation, processing and transmission of sensory signals from peripheral receptors to the central nervous system.

b. Integrative Function

Integrative function is the analysis of different sensory inputs to produce the optimal motor response; the storage of information in short and long term memory; decision making ability.

c. Motor Function

Motor function or efferent (descending) output is the generation, processing, and transmission of motor signals to the somatic and visceral structures where peripheral receptors were originally stimulated. This function is carried out by voluntary or involuntary (i.e. reflex) mechanisms.

Massage affects the peripheral and central nervous system as well. The therapeutic impact of massage is produced by direct and reflex ways (Sherbak, 1936; Kohlrausch, 1955; Shterngertz and Belaya, 1992; Aksenova, 1997). The **direct** therapeutic impact produces various local changes in the massaged tissues. The therapeutic impact which is produced by **reflex way** has a more complicated mechanism. It based on **viscero-somatic** or **soma-somatic** relations between different structures and organs of the human body. As it was stated by Dr. J. Weiss (1952) “The reflex value of massage is probably the most important of all”.

To find more information about reflex zones formation and treatment options we suggest to visit **www.scienceofmassage.com** website or refer to *Medical Massage* Volume I textbook.

1. CENTRAL NERVOUS SYSTEM

The therapeutic impact of massage on the central nervous system has not been explored enough but the results of some studies have been published. In 1965 Andreeva, and Belaya, conducted a clinical study of massage’s effect on the cortex of patients with the **cervical** and **lumbosacral spondylosis**. All patients had different degrees of symptoms of intervertebral disk herniation with spinal nerve roots’ irritation or compression.

The authors examined the effect of massage therapy using electroencephalography (EEG) to record and analyze the electric activity of the brain before and after the massage session. The patients showed significant improvement and normalization of the brain’s electrical activity during and after the massage treatment. The EEG before the massage treatment displayed the significant desynchronizing of **alpha-waves** and a 50% reduction of evoked response to the visual (bright light) and auditory (loud noise) stimuli. After the massage treatment the same patients showed normalization of the amplitude of alpha-waves from 25mV until normal level of 50 mV. The evoked responses were also improved or completely restored to the normal magnitude.

The authors found that these positive changes occurred only in the hemisphere opposite to the massaged side if the massage was performed on one side. At the same time, the patients who had symptoms of sympathetic trunk involvement showed positive changes on the EEG recorded from the same hemisphere as the massage side.

Jacob, (1960) discussed the analgesic effect of massage, correctly pointing out that massage strokes create massive sensory input to the central nervous system. These stimuli are transmitted through the large myelinated nerve fibers and they in some degree block the sensory impulses which arrive via the smaller nerve fibers usually transmitted pain stimuli.

In 1973 Dubrovsky, reported results of an interesting clinical study. The author examined the vasomotor effect of massage strokes on patients under **general anesthesia** by conducting capillaroscopy and testing skin temperature. The author did not find any significant changes of peripheral blood circulation after applying massage strokes on patients under general anesthesia. As soon as the general anesthesia was over the massage strokes in the same area produced local hyperemia, the increasing of local temperature and the opening of reserve capillaries. Thus, author concluded that the central nervous system plays a critical role in local circulation.

In 1977 Ebner with cooperation of Dr. McKechnie, conducted a clinical study on 30 patients in the Psychiatry Unit at Bangour Village Hospital in Scotland. The authors examined the effect of **connective tissue massage** on patients who suffer from sleep disturbances, migraine, depression, emotional blocks, general tension and exaggeration of relatively minor physical problems. The first signs of improvement were detected after 3-5 sessions with relief or complete disappearance of pathological symptoms at the end of treatment. Similar results were reported earlier by Teirich-Luebe, (1960) and later by McKechnie, et al., (1983).

Barr and Taslitz, (1970) studied the effect of back massage on the **autonomic nervous system** of 10 healthy females. The authors measured the arterial blood pressure, the heart rate, the respiration rate, the galvanic skin response, the skin temperature, the body temperature (oral measurement), and the pupil diameter before, during and after 20 minutes of back massage.

Data collected during this study showed the significance of the physiological impact of massage on the autonomic nervous system. Systolic blood pressure initially decreased from 109.8 mmHg to 105.9 mmHg and later during massage slightly increased from 105.9 mmHg to 107.9 mm Hg, but stayed lower than in a control study; the diastolic blood pressure decreased from 62.1 mmHg to 59.2 mmHg; the heart rate slightly increased from 72.7 beat/min to 73.7 beat/min; the galvanic skin response showed a decrease in skin resistance caused by stimulation of sweat glands (drop in skin resistance in the control group was 1.7 kOhm while after the massage this parameter decreased on 41.6 kOhm); peripheral skin temperature varied differently through the body but it was slightly higher on the posterior aspect then on the anterior aspect of the same part of the body; pupil diameter increased during massage from 4.7 mm to 5.5 mm; and the respiration rate decreased from 17.3 mm to 17.0 mm. Thus, the impact of back massage on the autonomic nervous system had mixed effects because along with the stimulation of the sympathetic nervous system the parasympathetic nervous system was stimulated as well (decreasing systolic and diastolic pressure).

In 1982 Longworth, studied the psychophysiological effects of slow stroke back massage on 32 healthy females. As a sign of the relaxation and reduced anxiety the author tested generalized muscle tension by electromyography (EMG), heart rate, systolic and diastolic pressure, galvanic skin response and finger temperature. Thus, the author tried to find out if the level of anxiety and can be lowered through **subcortical habituation** to tactile stimulation.

The results displayed immediately (after 3 minutes) lowered systolic blood pressure (from 105 mm Hg to 98 mmHg), heart rate (from 76 beat/min to 70 beat/min), EMG (from 2.80 mV to 1.90 mV) and raised the diastolic blood pressure (from 57 mmHg to 60 mmHg), increased the skin temperature (from 88 to 89.8 degrees F) and increased the galvanic skin response (from 380 - 10 Ohms to 550 -10 Ohms) i.e., decreasing the skin's electric resistance. The patients also felt relaxed, less anxious and more emotionally stable. Thus, the author recommended slow back massage for persons with high psychoemotional arousal and anxiety as well as for cardiac and hypertensive patients. Practically the same results were reported by Fakouri and Jones (1987). Ebner, (1985) also registered the reduction of skin electric resistance after connective tissue massage.

McGary, (1984) recommended massage as a part of treatment of patients with **epilepsy**. The author thinks that massage stimulates the autonomic nervous system and helps to overcome the imbalance between it and the central nervous system.

One of the most methodologically complete studies of the **psychological effect** of massage treatment on athletes was completed in 1988 by Weinberg, et al. The authors tested 183 students who studied physical education. They were randomly assigned to different sports activities in combination with rest (control group) or massage therapy (tested group). The results were examined by several psychological tests: Profile of Mood States (POMS); State Anxiety Inventory; Thayer's Adjective Checklist. Because of large tested groups and accurate statistical analysis, the authors concluded that massage therapy has profound effects on the athlete's psychological state.

After massage students showed a significant decrease in: tension (up to 5.2 scores); depression (up to 3.7 scores); anger (up 2.3 scores); fatigue (up to 3.7 scores); and confusion (up to 2 scores).

Leone and Kukulka, (1988) examined the effect of continuous and intermittent pressure on the Achilles tendon on the excitability of alpha-motoneurons, i.e. the level of muscle relaxation in 8 patients who had suffered stroke. The effect of compression was estimated by evaluation of amplitude of the **H-reflex**.

This test indirectly estimates the alpha-motoneurons' excitability in the anterior horns of the spinal cord and changes along the spinal reflex pathways. The results showed that both permanent and intermittent pressure decrease the amplitude of H-reflex from the soleus muscle with its following relaxation. However the significant inhibition of H-reflex in 45 seconds after cessation of pressure application was detected only in a group of patients where intermittent pressure was applied. The authors recommended the intermittent application of pressure on the tendons of hemiparetic patients as an effective method of the relaxation of hypertonically changed muscles.

In 1989 Shterngertz, studied the effect of massage in the areas of neck and shoulders on the brain electrical activity of children with **cerebral palsy**. The patients with cerebral palsy showed different degrees of alpha-waves desynchronization. Patients whose cerebral palsy was clinically more severe had more significant abnormalities in the electrical activity of the brain. Their electroencephalograms displayed an increased frequency (more than 12 Hz) and amplitude (more than 50 mV) of the alpha-waves as well as abnormal changes in the normal sinusoidal wave pattern. The author reported positive improvement in all analyzed parameters. The patients with a more severe clinical picture of cerebral palsy showed more dramatic positive changes.

Dossetor, et al. (1991) reported very interesting results in one case study. A 14 year old girl was diagnosed with **Cornelia de Lange Syndrome** at the age of 4. This psychiatric disorder is associated with self-injury behavior. In the described case the patient had an extremely severe case of this syndrome. The patient beat her face and eyes, hit face against the door, door-knobs or floor, cut herself and picked at her fresh wounds. The child also had numerous surgeries to heal wounds. Later, the patient started to hurt nurses in the hospital. She was the most difficult and aggressive patient in an entire hospital for retarded children. To protect her and others, she was wearing a protective helmet, with a visor for her eyes, splints for her arms and legs, and bandages to prevent picking at wounds. The patient was under permanent sedation to control her self-injury behavior. Any possible methods of treatment developed by modern medicine failed for 10 years.

At the age of 14 she was for the first time introduced to massage therapy by the nurse. After the first session she enjoyed it and was relaxed. As a last hope the massage treatment was performed daily or even 2 times per day. From week to week she started to feel better and better. She was allowed to take her helmet and splints off for 30 minutes per day after 3 weeks of treatment. If the patient had attacks of self-injury behavior, additional massage treatment was immediately applied and it restored normal behavior. The patient's episodes of aggression got shorter and became less frequent and her mood improved dramatically. After 6 months of treatment she was off any medication for the first time in 10 years! These improvements were stable for 18 months prior to the article's publication with sporadic mild relapses which were easily controlled. The authors found that massage is an extremely useful adjunct to the treatment of such severe psychiatric disorders.

Sullivan, et al., (1991) examined the effect of massage in the **inhibitory regime** on alpha-motoneuron excitability in 16 healthy individuals by measuring changes in the amplitude of

H-reflex. The test was applied on the triceps surae and hamstring muscles before, during and after massage (mostly slow petrissage). All subjects in the experimental group showed significant reduction of the amplitude of H-reflex (1.95 mV) compared to the control group (2.23 mV). The authors estimated this reduction as a sign of general lowering of excitability in the alpha motoneuron pool in the lower motor centers of the spinal cord with the following reduction of muscle reflex activity and muscular relaxation. The authors also pointed out the specificity of neuromuscular response to the inhibitory massage treatment. In other words, massage techniques when applied to one particular muscle mostly decreased the excitability of the motoneurons of this particular muscle without significant involvement of other groups of motoneurons. This opens clinical perspectives for inhibitory massage therapy for patients with hyperactive muscle reflexes.

Other authors also supported the idea of decreasing the excitability of alpha-motoneurons by massage treatment in the inhibitory regime. Morelli, et al., (1991) reported the reduction of H-reflex amplitude by 71% after manual massage. Goldberg, et al. in 1992 and 1994 studies examined the effect of massage on H-reflex amplitude. As mentioned above this test indirectly estimates the alpha-motoneurons' excitability in the spinal cord and changes along the spinal reflex pathways. All authors agree on the matter of applied pressure: it shouldn't activate pain receptors.

In a 1992 study the authors estimated the effect of light kneading massage (manual pressure 1.25 kPa) and strong kneading (manual pressure 2.50 kPa) on H-reflex amplitude in 20 healthy subjects. The authors founded that massage with strong pressure produced a 49% reduction in H-reflex amplitude compared to the control group, and massage with light pressure produced a 39% reduction. Another finding is the carryover effect of strong massage (i.e. reduction of H-reflex amplitude) which was detected during 10 seconds after cessation of massage strokes. There was no carryover effect after massage with light pressure. The authors concluded that inhibition of alpha-motoneurons' activity in the spinal cord recorded during massage is caused by the inhibition of both cutaneous and muscle mechanoreceptors.

In a 1994 study the same authors examined the effect of massage in the inhibitory regime on patients who had previous spinal cord injuries with subsequent development of **hyperreflexia** and muscular tension. The authors estimated the effect of massage (kneading) by measuring the amplitude of the H-reflex. In all patients the amplitude of the H-reflex was heightened after the spinal cord injury. In the control group the amplitude of H-reflex ranged between 3.48 mV and 3.79 mV, but the amplitude of the H-reflex in the clinical group during the massage treatment was reduced up to 27% (1.59 mV). Thus, the authors showed that massage in the inhibitory regime is able to reduce the excitability of the motoneurons in the spinal cord. This is a very important matter for patients after spinal cord injury. Emphasizing the clinical perspectives of massage treatment for these patients, the authors correctly pointed that:

> "... **no other currently used physical modality** appears to be consistently effective in reducing motoneuron excitability in a neurologically impaired sample...".

Wittlinger, H and G. (1992) consider lymph drainage massage as an important type of stress reduction treatment. Because this type of massage treatment has strong **sympatholytic** effect, the authors see it as powerful breaker of a vicious stress cycle.

Field, et al., (1996) examined the effect of chair massage therapy on the anxiety level, EEG pattern and math performance of 50 healthy adults. 26 subjects from the experimental group got a 15 minute chair massage 2 times per week during 5 weeks study. 24 subjects from the control group conducted general relaxation. The authors reported an increase in **delta-waves** in both groups. This is a clear indication of relaxation. However, the patterns of alpha- and beta-waves were significantly different in both groups as well. In the experimental group the authors registered a significant decrease in alpha- and beta-waves which is indication of alertness. In the control group an increase of both waves was registered which suggested drowsiness. These findings were additionally supported by the results of math tests performed after massage or relaxation sessions. The subjects from experimental group completed the math tasks more quickly with fewer mistakes. The authors concluded that tactile and pressure stimulation

> "...enhances parasympathetic activity (elevated vagal tone) which is characteristic of a more relaxed, alert state during which cognitive performance improves".

Malaquin-Pavan, (1997) conducted a long detailed research of the effect of massage on 4 patients with a severe form of **Alzheimer's dementia**. The massage treatment was conducted 2 times per week for 30 minutes for 6 months or 51 sessions per patient in total. The following responses were registered after treatments (% is to total number of all sessions): signs of physical relaxation - 52%; different manners to communicate with researcher - 23%; sleepiness - 42%; stop or decrease of the abnormal behavior - 70%. The author concluded that massage increases the possibility of nursing care for this difficult category of patients. It helps "... to take in charge every day an elderly demented patient".

Aksenova and Romanova, (1998) conducted a clinical study of the effect of segment-reflex massage in combination with muscle stretching on 80 patients with chronic **gastric ulcers** during a period of reactivation. The authors examined and compared the activity of the sympathetic and parasympathetic divisions of the nervous system before and after the segment-reflex massage session. They examined the correlation between electroencephalography, pulse rate and respiration rate using 16 different mathematical and statistical parameters. After the segment-reflex massage, the clinical and mathematical analysis showed credible evidence of stimulation of the parasympathetic nervous system and suppression activity of the sympathetic nervous system in 83% of patients. The suppression of the sympathetic nervous system or sympatholytic effect plays an important role in the general success of gastric ulcer treatment.

Richards, (1998) examined the effect of 6 minutes of back massage on the sleep of 69 critically ill patients. A control group received a 7.5 minute audio taped relaxation session. The author used polysonography and estimated the sleep efficiency index. The patients in the clinical group slept on average 1 hour longer compared to patients in the control group and their sleep efficiency index was 14.7% higher. Besides this, the patients in the control group spent in average of 35 minutes in **REM-sleep** compare to 25 minutes in the control group. The author concluded that:

> "... back massage is alternative or adjunct to pharmacological treatment and is clinically effective nursing intervention for promotion of sleep".

Turner, et al. (1999) examined the effect of massage, positive and negative emotions on the level of plasma **oxytocin** in 25 normally cycling women. The hypothalamic neurohormone oxytocin is responsible for numerous functions in the female body: initiating labor, regulation of lactation and maternal behavior. This hormone is also strongly connected with a building the human's close relationships.

Authors found that relaxation massage is responsible for the elevation of oxytocin level during 30 minutes after the end of massage with the peak of up to 5.2 pg/ml in 5 minutes. The positive emotions did not produce any increasing of oxytocin level in the blood but negative emotions decreased level of oxytocin up to 4.2 pg/ml. Women who demonstrated increased level of oxytocin had a lower level of anxiety, and more positive emotions especially in close relationships.

Craig et al., (2006) examined the effects of **neuromuscular therapy** in 36 patients with **Parkinson's disease**. The authors found a significant and sustained improvement in motor skills ($P <$ or $= 0.0001$) with the most notable changes being in the tremor scores.

Garner et al., (2008) examined the impact of massage therapy on anxiety, stress, hostility, and the aggression level in young adult patients in the psychiatric inpatient unit. Daily 20-minute massages significantly improved hostility ($p = 0.007$) of the patients with a simultaneous decrease in anxiety, heart rate, and cortisol level. The authors concluded that massage therapy has a unique impact on psychiatric patients because it has immediate beneficial effects and may be a useful de-escalating tool to help acutely hospitalize psychiatric patients.

Moraska and Chandler, (2009) examined the effect of massage therapy on the level of anxiety and depression in 18 patients with **tension-type chronic headaches**. The authors detected statistically significant improvements during the application of all tests especially in the group where massage was regularly performed for 3 weeks.

Posadzki and Parekh-Bhurke (2011) based on their review of modern scientific data concluded that massage therapy is a critically important part of **holistic psychotherapy** where the integrative approach to the treatment of depressed patients is the most effective approach to the therapy.

Manella and Backus (2011) reported a case study when the authors treated a patient with a partial **spinal cord injury** using a specially designed massage protocol. The authors registered an improvement in gait speed, stride length, and swing as well as stance phase percentages.

Oliveira et al., (2012) examined the effect of massage therapy on insomnia, anxiety, and depression of 44 **menopausal women**. Therapeutic massage was tested against a control group where passive movements were performed. Women from the clinical group who received therapeutic massage exhibited a significant improvement in all measured parameters with the level of significance fixed at $p \leq 0.05$.

2. PERIPHERAL NERVOUS SYSTEM

The sensory receptors in the skin, connective tissue structures, skeletal muscles and periosteum are the initial link in the complex chain of events activated in the nervous system by massage therapy. Every type of receptor has its own **level of adaptation**. The adaptation of the receptors is their ability to produce an **action potentials** during and after actual exposure to the original stimuli.

For example, pressure receptors called Ruffini nerve endings, which detect pressure are slowly adapting receptors, and vibration receptors called Pacinian corpuscles, are quickly adapting receptors. This means humans feel pressure longer than vibration if both are applied to the same area in different time. In other words, the adaptation of the receptor is its failure to maintain action potentials' production after exposure to the original stimuli. By knowing the level of adaptation for every type of peripheral receptors, the therapist can deliver a stimulating or inhibiting impact on the nervous system. Table 1 presents the sensory receptors in the skin and their level of adaptation.

TABLE 1. SENSORY RECEPTORS IN THE SKIN

Receptors	Type of Sensory Perception	Adaptation
1. Free nerve endings	Pain	Slow
2. Meissner corpuscles	Touch	Quick
3. Merkel disks	Touch	Slow
4. Ruffini nerve endings	Pressure	Slow
5. Pacinian corpuscles	Vibration	Quick
6. Thermoreceptors	Hot and Cold	Slow

For example, the practitioner has to apply, withdraw and immediately reapply vibration stimuli to the massaged area to constantly activate the vibration receptors. At the same time, to inhibit Pacinian corpuscles, the practitioner has to apply and maintain constant vibration stimuli in the same area. This is a basic principle of the **inhibitory regime** of massage therapy (Turin, 1992). For more information about the inhibitory regime of massage treatment, see below in Chapter II.

Livingston, (1948) discussed the treatment of 33 veterans of WW II at the Oakland Naval Hospital who suffered from nerve trauma and later developed **causalgia**. Causalgia is caused by partial injury of the nerve trunk. This syndrome is a combination of severe burning pain, dystrophic changes in the skin and bones and different vasomotor reactions (glossy skin, edema, hyperthermia, cyanosis, etc.).

Because of the intensive pain the patients were unable to use the affected limb and even the simple touch generated the severe burning pain. The author examined the effectiveness of different types of surgical and non-surgical treatment available at that time. He considered gentle underwater massage and manipulations (and later the same treatment out of water when the patients were able to tolerate the operator's touch) as one of the most valuable methods of treatment for patients with causalgia. The author assumed that this type of therapy initiates an inflow of sensory impulses which reset the regulatory centers in the spinal cord to produce "normal" motor output to the affected limb.

Fulton and Barron, (1955) registered the vasodilation and increased blood circulation in the lower abdominal area alter massage along pathway of the sciatic nerve.

In 1960 Granovsky conducted an experimental study on dogs. The author examined the effect of massage on the regeneration of nervous tissue after partial **neurotomia** (i.e. surgical interruption) of the sciatic nerve. The histological evaluation of samples show that regeneration of the nerve tissue in the place of neurotomia was significantly quicker in the group of dogs which got regular massage treatment. The author also discovered that regeneration was mostly stimulated during first 10-15 treatments. Further application of massage therapy did not show significant improvement of nerve tissue regeneration. This is the exact time limit which is usually recommended for the course of medical massage treatment.

In an experimental study on animals Stoma (1964) detected that vibration stimuli increased the velocity of conduction of nervous impulses on the same side of the body as well as on the opposite one.

Sterngertz (1960) and later Mogutaev (1980) reported an increase of the cutaneous temperature of 1-2 C degrees as well as the excitability of skeletal muscles (detected by electromyography) in the extremity **opposite** to the massaged one.

For the successful inhibitory treatment Sister Elizabeth (1966) recommended rhythmic effleurage strokes by flatly placed palms from the parietal area of the head to the sacral region with the speed about 60 strokes per minute. The desirable inhibitory effect on the autonomic nervous system can be reached after at least 3 minutes of application.

In 1966 Professor Belaya studied the effect of massage therapy on the electric activity of major nerves. The author reported a significant increase in the nerves' electric activity. The major intensification (60-100 mkV) was registered when friction technique was applied to the areas of emerging cutaneous branches of tested nerve under the skin.

Borisov, (1984) also reported an increase of nerve conduction velocity through the reflex arc after vibration massage was performed along the pathways of major nerves.

Professor Kreimer, (1988) conducted long clinical study in the Neurology Department of Tomsk Medical School on 339 patients with residual neurological problems (pain, numbness, paraesthesia, muscle tension, muscle weakness) caused by **lumbo-sacral spondylosis**. The first group (161 patients) was treated using vibration massage on special points which were detected by the author during previous experimental and clinical studies. The second group (118 patients) was treated by vibration massage on acupuncture points. The third group (60 patients) was treated by general vibration massage on the lumbo-sacral area. Positive dynamics with a reduction or complete elimination of residual neurological symptoms was detected in 92% patients of 1st group, in 89.9% patients of the 2nd group, and 60% patients of the 3rd group.

Jabre (1994) successfully used light repetitive friction along ulnar nerve in cases of paraesthesia to stimulate metabolism in the affected nerve and decrease inflammation.

Cunningham et al., (2011) used a repetitive application of effleurage and petrissage on patients with chemotherapy-induced peripheral neuropathy. At the end of the treatment course the authors registered an almost complete resolution of the tingling and numbness associated with neuropathy and the restoration of skin temperature which indicted the restoration of blood circulation.

B. CARDIOVASCULAR SYSTEM

The main function of cardiovascular system is maintenance of the blood circulation throughout the body. Blood delivers oxygen to the cells and removes carbon dioxide and waste products from the cells. At the same time, the cardiovascular system participates in the regulation of body temperature.

Different methods and techniques of massage have different impacts on the cardiovascular system. Massage affects the cardiac function, especially heart rate, by using viscero-somatic nervous reflex pathways or by direct effect via enhancing peripheral vasodilation and increasing peripheral circulation.

The viscero-somatic reflexes are a key concept of the medical massage treatment of inner organ disorders including cardiac pathology. In the areas of Glezer/Dalicho zones the segment-reflex massage is the most effective method of medical massage treatment of myocardial ischemic disorders: angina pectoris or rehabilitation after myocardial infarction (Glezer and Dalicho, 1955; Belaya, 1974; Kordez et al., 1983; Kunichev, 1985; Shterngertz and Belaya, 1992).

The periostal massage is very important method of the treatment of cardiac arrhythmias (Vogler and Krauss, 1953, 1975; Vasichkin, 1991). The periostal massage on the ribs decrease the tachycardia on 15-20 beats /min and helps to reduce arrhythmias (Belaya, 1983).

1. CARDIAC AND CEREBRAL CIRCULATION

Even in 1899 Dr. Edgecombe and Dr. Bain reported that petrissage strokes caused an immediate transient increase in the blood pressure followed by its decrease.

Abrams, (1918) and later Kramarenko, (1953); Birukov, (1988) reported increasing heart rate during intensive friction and percussion in the area of spinous process of C7 vertebra. At the same time, slow friction and kneading with medium pressure between the scapulas in combination with shaking of the thorax produced bradycardia and a decrease in blood pressure. The same **cardiac reflex** is produced by using similar massage techniques on the head, especially in the occipital and temporal areas, on the upper neck and on both shoulders and upper extremities. Both systolic and diastolic pressure decreased by 15-20 mmHg (Moshkov, 1950; 1982).

In an article published in 1939 Jacobson summarized the results of 18 years of study of the dependency between arterial blood pressure and tension in the skeletal muscles. The author proved beyond a doubt that tension in the skeletal muscles is responsible for the increasing of peripheral vascular resistance and rising the arterial blood pressure in patients with primary hypertension. Just by relaxing the patient's skeletal muscles, the author obtained a decrease in systolic pressure of up to 17.3 mmHg and diastolic pressure of up to 9.3 mmHg.

Moshkov, (1950); Belaya, (1974); Fokin, (1997) clinically observed a significant decrease in arterial blood pressure and heart rate (i.e. bradycardia) after **abdominal massage**. Experimental proof of these data was obtained through experimental work by Kurosawa, (1995). The author examined the effect of abdominal massage on the blood pressure and heart rate in 28 anesthetized rats. After 1 minute of massage on the ventral/lateral sides of the abdomen blood pressure decreased by 50 mmHg and the heart rate slowed by 25 beats/min. If massage strokes were performed only on the lateral surface of the abdomen blood pressure decreased by 30 mmHg and heart rate slowed by 19 beats/min.

All collected data allowed the authors to conclude that massage strokes activated visceral afferent flow with the following inhibition of efferent sympathetic activity of the autonomic nervous system. The significantly different responses from massage of ventral and lateral parts of the abdomen were interpreted by the author as relating to the various densities of somatosensory receptors in the both areas.

Pugachev, (1965) analyzed the ECGs of athletes and patients with different forms of arrhythmia during the vibration strokes in the area of the shoulders and heart. The author reported the increasing speed of **atrio-ventricular conductance**, the increase of arterial blood pressure and the restoration of cardiac rhythm after the course of vibration massage treatment.

Akhmedzhanov, (1981) examined the role of **pericardiac massage** in the rehabilitation of patients who had myocardial infarctions 5-12 months before. The authors estimated the effect of the combination of pericardiac massage and traditional physical therapy on the process of rehabilitation. The method of pericardiac massage was originally developed in the Yalta Scientific Research Institute of Physiotherapy and includes the sequential massage of all cardiac reflex zones. It starts from the more distant (from the heart) **cardiac zones** and slowly, from session to session, involves all of them into the treatment.

The authors conducted the clinical study on 135 patients who were separated in 2 groups. In the first group the 16 sessions of pericardic massage were conducted daily before physical therapy treatment (bicycle training exercises). Thus, authors used the peripheral and cardiac vasodilation effect of pericardic massage as a preparation for physical therapy. In the second group the patients underwent the physical therapy only.

The results were measured clinically, by lab tests (level of heparin in the blood and catecholamines in the urine) and by ECG including the exercise tolerance test. 50% patients in the first group showed significant positive clinical changes compared to 32.6% in the second group. The positive changes on the ECG (ST segment and T wave) were comparable in both groups: 31.4% in the first group and 24.1% in the second group. Only patients in the first group showed an increase in heparin blood levels and urine excretion of cathecholamines. Heparin is a natural anticoagulant and its level is extremely important for every patient after a myocardial infarction. However the authors considered the **adaptogenic role** of pericardiac massage in the tolerance of increasing physical exercises as the most important benefit of the combination of massage and physical therapy. Thus, pericardiac massage, when conducted before physical therapy, allows the patients to quickly adapt to every new level of physical exercises and it speeds up the whole rehabilitation program and increases its effectiveness.

Curtis, (1994) described the case of restoration of **cardiac rhythm** by massage. The patient was a 57 year old male who had 2 previous attacks of atrial fibrillation caused by stress. In both cases sinus rhythm was restored in the ER only after intravenous drug intervention. In the described case of his 3rd attack, the patient had a very erratic pulse, fluctuating between 96 and 140 beats/min and shallow, rapid breathing. The author used massage of the back and anterior surface of the thorax on the left side. The patient was positioned on his right side. During the long effleurage strokes along and across the lower angle of the left scapula the patient noticed a worsening of atrial fibrillation. However the sinus rhythm was completely restored after several minutes of massage around the left nipple and strokes along 8-10 ribs directed to the vertebral column. As the author quoted the patient: "It's like a switch". While Curtis suggested further clinical study of this matter she correctly pointed out that this procedure has thousand years of medical history and it is safe and simple.

Ezov, (1994) conducted a clinical study on 100 patients with insufficient cerebral blood circulation caused by cervical spondylosis accompanied by hypertension and **cerebral atherosclerosis.** The author tested the effect of segment-reflex massage with following chiropractic adjustments (first group) and classic therapeutic massage (second group). The results were examined: clinically; by monitoring of arterial pressure; by reoencephalography; and by lab tests (cholesterol, b-lipoproteins, epinephrine, and serontonin excretion). Table 2 summarizes the results of this study.

TABLE 2. Results of Ezov's Study (1994)

Results	Ist Group (50 patients)	2nd Group (50 patients)
1. Clinical symptoms: pain, dizziness, sleep disorders, etc.		
a. complete elimination of symptoms	48%	16%
b. no stable improvement	44%	68%
c. no improvement	8%	16%
2. Normalization of blood pressure	56%	24%

The patients in both groups also showed comparable insignificant decrease of their cholesterol level (in average of 1.0 mmol/L). However, the decrease of B-lipoproteins in the first group was much more impressive from 76.9$\pm$6.8 to 56.8$\pm$0.9. The same parameter in the second group changed from 70.1$\pm$1.81 to 62.6$\pm$1.7.

The author pointed out the importance of appropriate massage therapy, especially segment-reflex massage, before the every chiropractic treatment. The right combination of these two medical procedures as dramatic impact on the health of patients with insufficient cerebral blood circulation caused by cervical spondylosis and complicated by hypertension and cerebral atherosclerosis.

Guan Zheng and Zheng Guiqiu (1995) reported the results of the treatment of 50 patients with angina pectoris by a combination of traditional therapeutic massage manipulations (effleurage, friction, shaking, compression) and acupressure massage. The major areas for traditional massage treatment recommended by the authors are as follows: spinous process of the 5th thoracic vertebra; cervical and thoracic paravertebral areas with the strokes directed up and down; transverse strokes through both shoulders and the thorax in the direction from left to right and from right to left; both arms and hands; each finger separately. All strokes have to be performed at the frequency of the heart rate, i.e. 70-75 strokes per minute. After this treatment in combination with acupressure massage the authors obtained stable remission of angina pectoris symptoms (palpitation, pain, etc.) in 57% of patients.

The authors also detected a significant drop in the ration of a/E-O value from 14.68$\pm$4.57% to 11.31$\pm$4.52%. Changes in this parameter are a clear indication of a drop in the left ventricular diastolic end pressure. Another finding was the reduction of the ratio PEP/LVET from 40.06$\pm$8.75% to 34.96$\pm$6.20%. This parameter reflects the left ventricular functions between actual ventricular contractions. All these data demonstrated the improvement in the left ventricular function after the massage treatment. However, the authors pointed out that this type of treatment is effective only for patients with the earlier studies of coronary heart disease to relieve symptoms and improve the left heart functions.

Gusarova, et al., (1998) conducted a clinical study on 41 patients after **transient ischemic attacks** (TIA) in the vertebral-basilar arterial system. TIAs are neurological abnormalities caused by the transient insufficiency of cerebral blood circulation. The authors examined and compared the effect of acupressure massage and therapeutic massage. All patients were separated into 3 groups: the first group was treated with classical therapeutic massage in the sequence scalp - neck - shoulders; the second group was treated with the same massage procedure but in the opposite sequence: shoulders - neck - scalp; the third group was treated with acupressure massage according to the recommendations of Peking Institute of Traditional Chinese Medicine.

The results were estimated by reoencephalography. The best results were obtained in the third group of patients. Blood circulation in the vertebral-basilar arterial system increased up to 20.8% on the right side and up to 20.5% on the left side. The patients in the second group showed moderate vasodilation in the vertebral-basilar arterial system. The patients in the first group did not show any improvement and in almost half of the cases even a slight increase in arterial vasoconstriction was detected. Thus, the authors recommended acupressure massage as the most effective method of treating patients alter a TIA. At the same time the authors warned about the importance of the correct sequence of therapeutic massage treatment. Every treatment of patients after a TIA must start with shoulder and neck area first to prevent reflex cerebral vasoconstriction.

Ouchi et al., (2006) studied the cerebral blood flow during the application of massage on the subjects in prone position. The authors detected an increase in blood flow in the parietal cortex (precuneus) which was also accompanied by a decrease in heart rate. This finding allowed the authors to conclude that the increased blood flow triggered by massage, affects the parasympathetic division of the autonomic nervous system.

Kim et al., (2009) examined the effect of manual **lymph drainage massage** on the cardiac autonomic tone of 32 healthy male subjects. Based on the data collected by bipolar electrocardiography and measuring the pressure-pain threshold, the authors concluded that lymph drainage massage was effective in decreasing the actively of the autonomic nervous system.

2. PERIPHERAL ARTERIO-VENOUS CIRCULATION

Peripheral vasodilation can be local or general (reflex). Local vasodilation is produced in the massaged area and it is a direct, mechanical result of massage strokes. General peripheral vasodilation occurs in the areas of the body which were not massaged at all and has reflex character.

a. Local Vasodilation

The first experimental study of local vasodilation after massage was conducted as early as 1876 by German scientist Dr. Von Mosengeil. The author injected India ink into the knee joint of rabbits and then massaged whole leg with special attention to the knee. He found that all the ink drained from the joint into periarticular tissues. Dr. Von Mosengeil was the first author who considered the increase of the skin temperature up to 3 degrees C as a result of peripheral vasodilation.

Another important finding was later reported by another German author, Dr. F. Pick. He was the first scientist who studied the impact of different massage techniques on **venous circulation**. Dr. Pick inserted a cannula into femoral vein of dogs, applied different massage techniques and measured the flow of venous blood. The author found that effleurage increases venous blood flow in the massaged extremity only during its application. As soon as operator stopped the effleurage strokes the blood flow returned to normal.

Kneading and percussion techniques also increased venous circulation but this effect was maintained for a longer period of time after strokes had been stopped. The author came to a very important practical conclusion: effleurage increases blood circulation by mechanical stimulation while kneading and percussion increase blood circulation through reflex vasodilation in the massaged tissues as well. Dr. Pick's works had significant influence on the technical development of the modern medical massage therapy.

In 1929 Dr. Krogh conducted an experimental study of the effect of massage treatment on blood circulation in the skeletal muscles of frogs and mammals. The results of the study showed that the amount of opened capillaries in a 1 mm cross section of the skeletal muscle increased from 31 to 1400; the general capillary surface in 1 cm increased from 2 to 200; the coefficient of the capillary capacity increased from 0.02 to 2.80.

Wakim et al. (1949) from the Mayo Clinic in Minnesota examined the effect of slow stroking and kneading (modification of Hoffa's technique) versus vigorous, stimulating massage on blood circulation in the extremities of: healthy adults (lst group of 48 subjects) and patients with **flaccid palsy** (2nd group of 7 subjects). The technique of vigorous, stimulating massage was performed by the physician (one of the authors) who studied medical massage in the Europe. Blood flow was examined using plethysmography.

The average increase in blood circulation after stimulating massage in the 1st group was 57% in upper extremities and 42% in lower extremities. For the patients from the 2nd group this value was 103% on lower extremities. Treatment by Hoffa's technique produced an average increase in blood circulation in the upper extremities of only 4% and an average decrease of blood flow in the lower extremities by 4%. However, Hoffa's technique increased blood flow in the patients from the 2nd group by 22% on average.

The authors concluded that vigorous medical massage had a remarkable stimulating effect on blood circulation. However, the tissues of patients with flaccid or spastic palsy are very sensitive to strong massage strokes. In such cases the more gentle approach of Hoffa's technique is favorable despite only moderate stimulation of blood circulation.

Ebel and Wisham, (1952) reported an increase in skin temperature of up to 6 degrees with a maximum time period of 12 minutes alter the massage of the posterior leg due to local peripheral vasodilation. At the same time they didn't register a significant increase blood flow through the massaged muscles. The authors also detected a moderate (0.5 degree) short-lived (4-5 minutes) rise of the skin temperature of the opposite non-massaged leg during 2-3 minutes after the end of treatment. This peripheral vasodilation was considered by the authors as a sign of the **reflex vasomotor effect** of massage treatment.

Verbov, (1966) reported a 140% increase in general capillary capacity in the skeletal muscles after the massage treatment.

Hansen, et al. (1973) studied the effect of massage, short wave diathermy and ultrasound upon the disappearance rate of radioisotope Xe-133 from muscle and subcutaneous tissue in the human leg. The higher disappearance rate was detected after massage treatment and was caused by the vasodilation and an increase in blood circulation.

Birukov and Peysachov (1979) used plethysmography to study blood circulation in the forearm of skiers after massage treatment. The authors found that increased blood circulation in the forearm is caused by vasodilation in the arterioles but not venous dilation. Thus, the authors made a following practical recommendation for sports massage: the massage practitioner has to start the massage on the more proximally located area of an extremity and gradually move to the more distal parts.

Golosova (1983) conducted a clinical study on 71 patients with cervical spondylosis. The author examined the effect of local electrical vibration in the areas of **trigger points**. Besides the analgesic effect of the treatment all patients who had increased arterial pressure showed its normalization after 1-2 sessions. Arterial blood pressure remained normal during the whole course of treatment (15-20 daily massages). The author recommended the use of no more than 4 trigger point areas in the skeletal muscles during the one session.

Dubrovsky and Dubrovsky, (1995) reported increased the blood circulation in the skeletal muscles from 4.2±0.01 ml/100/min to 63±0.01 ml/100/min after massage. The significant increase in blood circulation was still detected in 3 hours after the massage treatment. The authors also examined venous circulation in the leg using the phlebography (i.e. contrast material injection with the following X-ray examination). After 15 minutes of massage treatment no contrast material was detected in the venous circulation of the leg.

Besides the mechanical effect on the soft tissues in the massaged area LeRoy (1941) and later Jacobs (1960) pointed to the so called **axon reflex**. Afferent (sensory) nervous fibers which deliver information to the central nervous system give direct branches or collaterals to the nearby vascular structures, i.e. form the pathways for the axon reflex. As soon as sensory receptors in the skin and connective tissue are activated by massage strokes they form and send afferent nervous impulses. Before reaching the central nervous system these impulses are delivered to the vascular structures in the skin and skeletal muscles using the existing collaterals of the axon reflex. One has to remember that the first reaction of vascular structures is vasoconstriction; as soon as the impulses are perceived as harmless, and repeated over the same area, local vasodilation is produced. Thus, massage on the every new area has to be prolonged to achieve the appropriate therapeutic effect.

Castro-Sánchez et al., (2009) evaluated the impact of connective tissue massage on peripheral blood circulation and symptoms of **intermittent claudication** in 98 patients with type 2 diabetes. The authors measured the peripheral arterial circulation using the following criteria: differential segmental arterial pressure, heart rate, skin temperature, oxygen saturation and skin blood flow. All measurements were taken before and 30 minutes after each session and six months and one year after the 15-week treatment course. Such a long study showed that in the group of patients who received connective tissue massage its positive impact on peripheral circulation was registered even one year after the initial treatment. The authors concluded that connective tissue massage improves peripheral blood circulation in patients with type 2 diabetes but it also slows the development of Peripheral Arterial Disease.

b. General (Reflex) Vasodilation

General or reflex vasodilation is a result of several factors: the viscero-somatic reflexes; the vasomotor reflexes; the releasing of vasoactive substances; and the central inhibition of vasoconstriction.

Viscero-somatic reflexes

The viscero-somatic reflexes are afferent-efferent neural pathways which are formed between the visceral (inner organs) and somatic (parts of the body) structures innervated by the same spinal nerves from the same segments of the spinal cord. Thus, by the activating proprioreceptors in the massaged area the practitioner is able to deliver the therapeutic impact to the affected inner organ. The conception of viscero-somatic reflexes is the basis for any reflex massage treatment (e.g. segment-reflex massage, connective tissue massage, etc.)

Ebner, (1956) reported an increase in blood circulation in the intra-abdominal area and skin temperature on the lower extremities after connective massage in the **connective tissue zones** which are located in the lumbo-sacral area. The same results were obtained earlier by Snow, (1917) after vibration strokes in the areas around the spinous process of I and II lumbar vertebra.

Vasomotor reflexes

Vasomotor reflexes are responsible for peripheral vasoconstriction or vasodilation in arterioles. The vasomotor center which controls these reflexes is located in the medulla oblongata. Vasomotor reflexes are mostly controlled by the sympathetic division of the autonomic nervous system. In normal physiological conditions arterioles throughout the body are under about 50% of maximal vasoconstriction (Bullock et al. 1984). Thus, when we discuss the matter of vasodilation we should refer mostly to the activity of vasoconstrictor tone. Peripheral vasodilation is the direct sequence of the decreasing tone of physiological vasoconstriction.

The first study of viscero-motor reflexes was conducted by Prof. Zabludovsky in 1913. He registered by the plethysmograph increased blood flow in the forearm opposite to the massaged one as well as on the lower extremities of the same subject.

Cuthbertson, (1933) reported increasing of general body temperature by 2-3 C degrees after massage treatment. Ebel, and Wisham, (1952) detected a moderate (0.5 degree) short-lived (4-5 minutes) rising of the skin temperature of the opposite non-massaged leg 2-3 minutes after the end of massage treatment. This peripheral vasodilation was considered by authors as a sign of reflex vasomotor effect of massage treatment.

Belaya, (1974) and later Dubrovsky and Dubrovsky, (1995) also reported increased blood circulation detected by oscillography on the extremity opposite to the massaged one.

Shterngertz, (1985) conducted a clinical study on children with cerebral palsy. He found that after massage the local temperature of the skin increased by 2-6 degrees C. At the same time the skin's termoasymmetry, which was detected in all patients before massage, disappeared.

One of the possible mechanisms of general peripheral vasodilation is the stimulation of the parasympathetic nervous system with the following decrease of activity of the sympathetic nervous system and inhibition of vasoconstriction (Kohlrausch, 1955; Barr and Taslitz, 1970).

Chernigovsky, (1980) offered the interesting theory of the mechanism of general peripheral vasodilation produced by massage strokes. He considered the capillary network as a reflex zone for the entire cardiovascular system. Massage strokes in one area produce local vasodilation. At the same time whole capillary network immediately reacts with vasodilation causes a decrease in the peripheral vascular resistance. At the same time, the cardiac blood circulation also improves. Thus, the reflex stimulating impact of massage strokes affects the whole capillary network. The author estimated the local and general vasodilation as two sides of one physiological event caused by the massage treatment.

Airapetov, (1985) used oscillography to examine the effect of medical massage on blood circulation in the legs of patients with **tromboangiitis obliterans**. The author reported the decreasing of spasms in the arterial network of the lower extremities after massage treatment, improving and even restoration (in the earliest stages of pathology) arterial circulation.

Vasoactive substances

The vasoactive substances are produced in the body and have pressor or depressor effect. They affect cardiac function as well as changes in the peripheral vascular resistance (vasoconstriction or vasodilation).

Massage strokes, especially deep friction and compression, release vasoactive substances (i.e. histamine and kinins) from cells into the blood circulation as well as locally (LeRoy, 1941; Mennell, 1945; Kuprivan, 1995). **Histamine** vasodilates arterioles and capillaries and increase the capillary permeability (Jacob, 1960).

Kutz, et al. (1978) reported that the excretion of histamine in the urine increased up to 129% after a session of lymph drainage massage. The authors also found that blood level of **serotonin** decreased by 22% and blood level of serotonin's metabolite 5-HIAA decreased by 21% after lymph drainage massage treatment. Serotonin has strong pressor effect and significantly increases peripheral vascular resistance.

Ezov, (1994) also detected an increase serotonin urine excretion after segment-reflex massage treatment of patients with insufficient cerebral circulation caused by cervical spondylosis. Other important vasoactive substances are kinins: **bradykinin** and **kalidin**. They are also peptides which are formed from inactive precursors called kininogens (Ganong, 1993).

Yang et al., (2009) in the experimental study examined the mechanisms of the vasodilatory effect of massage therapy. The mechanical impact of massage therapy on soft tissue elicits a direct pressure on all cells (e.g. fibroblasts, mast cells, etc.) as a result of their mechanical compression. Additionally, the practitioner uses indirect or secondary mechanical impact which triggers the increase in interstitial pressure within the deep layers of the massaged tissues.

The authors of this study re-created the application of direct pressure on the mast cells isolated on the cell dish and examined their histamine release function. Mast cells are major histamine production factories. The study design (on the cell dish) allowed the authors to exclude any nervous system or hormonal and metabolic influences on the production and release of histamine.

The authors found that the immediate response of the mast cells to the application of simple mechanical pressure was an immediate increase in Ca $^{+2}$ concentration which was followed by a release of histamine. As it was concluded by the authors:

> "Histamine is a well-known mediator of microvascular tissue dilation, and these results may have an important impact on understanding the mechanism involved in massage therapy."

Central inhibition of vasoconstriction

As we already discussed above, the vasomotor center is located in the medulla oblongata. The cerebral cortex in turn controls the vasomotor center. The descending afferent nervous tracts reach the vasomotor center through the **hypothalamus**. Permanent stress, strong emotions and sexual excitement stimulate the vasomotor center with subsequent changes in heart rate and peripheral vascular resistance. Thus, any type of stress-reducing treatment diminishes the stimulating impact from the cerebral cortex to the hypothalamus and finally to the vasomotor center. As a result the heart rate decreased and peripheral vascular resistance diminished.

After 15 years of experimental and clinical studies Jacobson, (1939) concluded that the central inhibition of the vasomotor center is one of the main mechanisms of general stress reduction and skeletal muscles relaxation. These two effects play key roles in the treatment of patients with primary hypertension and can be used as a method of preventive therapy to unload the cardio-vascular system.

Jacobs, (1960) also considered the mechanism of central inhibition of vasomotor center with the following vasodilation as a part of general relaxation after a stress—reducing and therapeutic massage.

Petermans and Zicot, (1994) studied the effect of exercises and massage on the effectiveness of **musculo-venous pump** using photoplethysmograph. The authors compared two groups of volunteers: young adults and healthy elderly adults. After active and passive movements in the ankle joint venous refilling time and venous drainage was significantly lower in the group of elderly volunteers compared to young adults (see Table 3; 1st Study). However after massage therapy on the posterior leg of the same patients the tested parameters in the group of elderly subjects became practically same as in the young adult group (see Table 3; 2nd Group). Thus, the authors concluded that massage significantly improves the effectiveness of musculo-venous pump and reduces the venous stasis in the elderly adults.

TABLE 3. Results of Petermas and Zicot's Study (1994)

Tested Parameter	Exercise (1st Study)		Massage (2nd Study)	
Group	Young	Elderly	Young	Elderly
1. Venous Refilling Time	35.9 sec	16.1 sec	37 sec	30.6 sec
2. Venous Drainage	4.98%	2.97%	4.03%	3.8%

3. EFFECT OF MASSAGE ON BLOOD PARAMETERS

Kovacs, (1945) detected an increased **erythrocyte count** of up to 50% in the arterial vessels of the skin. Wood, (1974) also found an increased concentration of **hemoglobin** and erythrocyte count after massage treatment. The same findings were reported later by Dubrovsky, (1990).

Jungmarm, (1971) for the first time registered the acute reduction of the hematocrit after connective tissue massage. A hematocrit test reflects the blood's fluidity.

Van Hove, (1978) examined the effect of massage therapy on venous circulation in patients with **para-** or **tetraplegia**. One of the most serious and sometimes life-treating complications after acute spinal cord injuries is **thrombophlebitis** with following pulmonary embolization. As a result of flaccid palsy caused by the spinal cord injury, the "muscle pump" does not participate in the lymph and venous blood drainage. This reduction of blood flow causes profound changes in the coagulation system of the blood. The unfavorable combination of reduced blood flow and increased activity of the blood coagulation system creates optimal conditions for the development of thrombophlebitis. The more life-threating complication of thrombophlebitis for para- or tetraplegic patients is pulmonary embolization.

The author conducted a clinical study on 41 patients with complete para- or tetraplegias to find the right combination of conservative modalities which can prevent the development of thrombophlebitis. 15 patients were randomly assigned to a control group (Group A) and 26 patients to the clinical group (Group B). On Group A, pharmaceutical prevention, passive mobilization, respiration therapy and nursing were performed. In Group B the patients additionally were treated with massage and elastic stocking compression. Massage was applied 2 times per day on both lower extremities in the direction of lymph and venous blood drainage. In both groups treatment started on the first day after trauma. In the Group A 40% of patients (6 patients) developed acute thrombophlebitis and two of them had pulmonary embolization. In Group B no evidence of thrombophlebitis or pulmonary embolization was found.

Arko, et al. (1983) examined the effect of a 1-hour whole body massage on 17 different blood parameters. They found increased serum total protein and significantly increased potassium concentration (**hyperkalemia**) as well as activity of the serum enzymes creatine kinase (CK) and lactate dehydrogenase (LDH). These parameters started to rise immediately after the massage treatment and reached their highest level in 24 hours.

CK is an enzyme which catalyzes ATP production from phosphocreatine when the level of the ATP in muscles drops during vigorous exercise. Thus, the activity of CK reflects the level of metabolism in the skeletal muscles.

LDH is a complex enzyme which is composed of five isoenzymes, LDH 1-5, and also participates in normal cellular metabolism. In this study the authors found that values of isoenzymes LDH 4 and LDH 5 increased most. This finding suggests that permeability of the muscle cells' membranes was increased. The same mechanism is responsible for an increased amount of potassium in serum. The authors pointed out that exactly the same changes in the blood composition occurred after vigorous exercise.

Lastly, potassium is powerful vasodilator itself. Thus, hyperkalemia is an additional mechanism of peripheral vasodilation which is employed by the massage. The same increase of activity CK and LDH after the massage was reported by Bork, et al. (1978) and Dudina, (1983).

Dumev, et al. (1983) detected an increased amount of granulocytes (especially neutrophils, lymphocytes and monocytes) in the blood after 20 minutes of back therapeutic massage in 15 healthy individuals. This increase was detected during the first 30 minutes after the massage with subsequent slow restoration of the normal values. The authors concluded that therapeutic massage is able to activate the self defence mechanisms of the human body and stimulate the immune system.

Ernst, et al. (1987) studied the changes in blood fluidity after massage of skeletal muscles on 12 healthy volunteers and 10 patients with **ankylosing spondylitis**. The authors examined the 5 main parameters of blood viscosity before and immediately after the treatment in both groups. In the group of healthy volunteers the authors found significant reduction in native blood viscosity (from 11.3 mPa-s to 10.0 mPa-s), hematocrit (from 48.3% to 46.5%) and plasma viscosity (from 1.23 mPa-s to 1.19 mPa-s). The red cell filtrability and red cell aggregation did not changed significantly. The same results were obtained in the group of patients with ankylosing spondylitis but changes reached their peak after a series of 6 massages. Thus, the authors pointed out so called "**autohemodelution**", i.e. the increasing of blood fluidity, without infusing plasma expanders. The authors provided the following explanation of this massage-induced phenomenon. Vessels with stagnant flow are filled with cell-free interstitial fluid of low viscosity. The massage treatment decreases the sympathetic tone and this fluid is admitted into circulation, causing a general decrease in blood viscosity. Because of this sympatholytic effect of massage Buhring, (1985) recommended massage therapy for the treatment of peripheral vascular disorders.

Kaada and Torsteinbo, (1989) detected a 16% increase in plasma **endorphin** concentration after connective tissue massage. The authors considered the increased endorphin level as a main mechanism of reducing depression and anxiety and improving general well being after massage. At the same time this effect can be the one of possible causes of the analgesic effect of massage therapy. This response was similar to the data collected after 20-30 minutes of manual acupressure.

Makarova, et al. (1998) reported the stimulating effect of segment-reflex massage on the fibrinolytic system and simultaneous inhibition of the blood coagulation system. The clinical study was conducted on 74 women with **chronic salpingo-oophoritis** (i.e. chronic inflammation of fallopian tubes and ovaries). After the segment-reflex massage on the lumbo-sacral area the authors detected significant increases in the plasma fibrinolytic activity from $25.5 \pm 3.9\%$ until $33.8 \pm 2.8\%$.

Shor-Posner, et al., (2006) studied the impact of massage therapy on young children infected with **HIV-1**. In the clinical group, massage was used while in the control group, children received friendly visits twice weekly for 12 weeks. Blood was examined for determinations of CD4, CD8, and CD56 cell counts during 3 months after the initial treatment.

The authors found that in the control group subjects exhibited a decline in CD4 cell count (>30%, $p = 0.03$) while in the clinical group, subjects were stable or showed immune system improvement. However, the main surprise observed by the authors was a significant increase in CD4+ CD25+ cells in the 12-weeks after the initial treatment course ($p = 0.04$).

C. LYMPHATIC SYSTEM

The lymphatic system has three major functions: draining and cleaning of the interstitial fluid as well as returning it into venous circulation; immune defense of the body through the cellular and humoral immunity; transport of the dietary lipids and lipid-soluble vitamins from the intestine to the blood. Massage has a critical influence on the lymphatic system, especially on the drainage.

1. EXPERIMENTAL STUDIES

The first report on the stimulating impact of massage and active exercises on the lymph flow came as early as 1876 in the works of German physician Von Mosengeil. He injected India ink into the lymph vessel of a dog's leg and after massage treatment detected the ink in the abdominal lymph nodes. This occurred more quickly in the experimental group compared to the control group without massage. Later Lassar, (1877) confirmed Von Mosengeil's results by draining the lymph trunk and collecting the lymph after the massage. These first experimental findings found their theoretical explanation in the works of Starling (1894). He is the author of famous **Starling's law** of the heart and the first scientist who accurately described the now called Starling's forces which determine the rate of filtration at any point along a capillary.

Drinker, and Yoffey, (1941) pointed to massage as a valuable method of stimulation of lymph flow. The effectiveness of lymph drainage increases if there are 10-15 short breaks in massage treatment which give time for the lymph to fill up lymphatic sacks and vessels.

Ladd, et al. (1952) studied the effect of massage (lst group), passive movements (2nd group) and electric stimulation of muscles (3rd group) on lymph flow in a dog's foreleg. Animals in all 3 groups showed increased lymph drainage but the therapeutic impact of massage treatment had the greatest effect.

Elkins, et al. (1953) examined the effect of heat (infrared irradiation, short wave diathermy and microwave diathermy), passive and active exercises and massage techniques on the **flow of lymph**. The study was conducted on dogs with a surgically drained thoracic duct. The results did not show significant increases in lymph flow after heat procedures. The largest increase in lymph flow was registered after the application of stroking and kneading massage techniques (44-55 cc/ 10 min). The passive exercises also showed significant lymph flow increase (43-48 cc/ 10 min) and active exercises on the treadmill showed moderate increase (8cc/10 min). Thus, the authors recommended massage with breaks of passive exercises as a best combination for the stimulation of lymph drainage. It gives the time for the lymph sacks to be filled with the new portion of lymph.

Potapov, and Abisheva, (1989) examined the effect of massage on the formation and transport of lymph. In this study on 14 dogs the authors surgically drained the afferent lymph vessel on the animal's leg to obtain lymph before the popliteal lymph nodes. On the other leg of the same animal the efferent lymph vessel was drained to obtain the lymph after the popliteal lymph nodes. The authors measured the lymph flow and amount of lymphocytes in the lymph before and after 15 minutes of massage (a combination of kneading, vibration, and shaking techniques). The lymph flow increased in more than 2 times in both afferent (from 0.0038 ± 0.0004 ml/min- kg to 0.0087 ± 0.0009 ml/min- kg) and efferent (from 0.0042 ± 0.003 ml/min-kg to 0.0098 ± 0.0008 ml/min -kg) lymph vessels. The authors also registered an increased count of lymphocytes after the massage, especially in the lymph obtained from the efferent lymphatic vessel (from 2130 ± 250 cells/l mkl of lymph to 3860 ± 390 cells/l mkl of lymph). The authors agreed with Petrov, et al. (1981) who earlier concluded that massage increases the amount of lymphocytes in the lymph by activating their production and excretion from the lymph node. These studies experimentally proved the massage's stimulating effect on the immune system.

Mortimer, et al. (1990) studied the effect of massage on the lymph flow in the skin of 2 female large white pigs (one experimental and one control animal). The lymph flow was measured by radioisotope (99m Tc-colloid) clearance technique. After massage on the flank side the lymph flow was 0.37 ± 0.03 h versus 0.69 ± 0.05 h in the control animal. The authors also detected increased lymph flow on the flank opposite to the massaged one in the experimental animal 0.69 ± 0.05 h versus 1.43 ± 0.12 h in the opposite flank of the control animal. Thus, the authors came to the following conclusion: the increased lymph flow on the flank opposite to the massaged one is clear evidence of the spinal-reflex effect of massage therapy.

2. CLINICAL STUDIES

Swedborg, (1980) examined the effect of massage, isometric exercises and an elastic sleeve on upper extremity edema after **mastectomy** in 39 breast cancer patients. During the first week of treatment the volume of edema decreased by 11-13%. However, to maintain this effect, the author recommended the constant usage of an elastic sleeve. Significant reduction of postmastectomy edema on 20 patients after manual lymph drainage massage was also reported later by Zanola, et al. (1984).

In a series of publications Jemmon, et al. (1988 and 1989) showed convincing data about the strong correlation between stress and concentration of the secretory **immunoglobulin A** (lg A) in the patients' saliva. Ig A is one of the major defense mechanism of the humoral immunity especially for respiratory infections. The authors concluded that stress and anxiety dramatically decrease the concentration of salivary Ig A. From this data Groer, et al. (1994) examined the effect of massage on the concentration and rate of secretion Ig A in the patients' saliva. The study was conducted on 32 subjects between 44 and 77 years old. The control group included 14 subjects and the experimental group included 18 subjects. The clinical group received 10 minutes back massage and the control group received the general relaxation during the same 10 minutes. In both groups the saliva samples were collected before and after the procedures. The concentration of Ig A in the experimental group rose from 28.2 mg/dl before treatment until 45.5 mg/dl after the treatment. The rate of Ig A secretion increased from 13.7 mg/min to 23.7 mg/min. The same tests conducted on the control group showed insignificant increase of these parameters (concentration: 24.9 mg/dl before and 29.1 mg/dl after relaxation; rate of secretion: 10.6 mg/min before and 15.4 mg/min after relaxation). The authors concluded that massage reduces stress with the following increasing of Ig A concentration in the saliva. Thus, massage supports the body's defense mechanisms which are important for every patients from the risk group (elderly patients, patients with chronic pulmonary disorders, etc.) and especially for the immunocompromised subjects.

Dubrovsky, (1995) examined lymph circulation in the leg after massage, using the injection of radioisotope Tc- 131. Immediately after the massage session all radioisotope material was detected in the lymph nodes in the abdominal cavity. In the control group without the massage, radioisotope material was detected in the popliteal and inguinal lymph nodes alter the same period of time.

Ironson, et al. (1996) conducted an important clinical study of the effect of massage on the **immune system**. The subjects of this study were 20 HIV '+'(clinical group) and 9 HIV '-' (control group) gay men. Each of them got a daily massage for 1 month. The authors examined the acute effect after the first massage session and final effect after the whole course of the treatment. Alter the single session patients reported decreased anxiety and their cortisol level in saliva dropped significantly (from 38.79 to 27.32). After the whole course of treatment the authors reported many important results. All subjects showed a significant drop in stress hormones level: decrease of the urinary level of **cortisol** (from 44.9 to 23.51); lesser decrease in the concentration of **epinephrine** (from 6.30 to 3.43) and **norepinephrine** (from 31.19 to 26.45). However, the authors obtained more dramatic results after the examination of the immune system.

The major finding is the increasing amount of the natural killer cells from 24.43 to 33.29 as well as the increased activity of CD8 cells from 751.77 to 821.46. As is known, the **HIV virus** attacks the immune system, especially CD4 cells, with their following decrease which makes the disease progress. The number of natural killers also decreases but it happens during the advanced stages of AIDS. Thus, the increased concentration of natural killer cells after the massage treatment supports the defense function of the immune system damaged by the decreasing population of CD4 cells. The authors also pointed out on another important benefit of increased number and activity of natural killers caused by the massage: anti-cancer effect. As is known, AIDS patients suffer from different forms of cancer as a complication to the immune system's failure and natural killer cells are major figthers against cancer cells.

In a series of experimental and clinical studies Eliska and Eliskova, (1995) examined the possible mechanisms of massage's stimulating effect on lymph drainage. The study included 3 experiments: on the hind paw of a dog with **experimental lymphedema**; on the foot of healthy adults; and on the foot of patients with postthrombotic venous edema. Massage strokes were performed with a pressure of 70-100 mmHg and with a frequency of 25 strokes per minute for 1, 3, 5, and 10 minutes. After careful examination of the obtained results, the authors concluded that increased lymph drainage was the result of combination of several factors: changing the endothelial lining of the initial lymphatic vessels; translocation of edematous fluid into lymph vessels by increased interstitial pressure produced by massage strokes; opening of the junctions and the creation of artificial cracks into vessels' walls by external pressure with subsequent increasing drainage of edematous fluid from interstitium into lumen of lymphatic vessels.

Kuznetsov, et al. (1998) reported temporary increase of the lymphocyte count in the blood with subsequent decrease of **T-lymphocytes** up to 23% and **B-lymphocytes** up to 35% after a course of deep therapeutic massage. These results are matched with the previous findings of Dumev, et al. (1983); Kuznik, et al. (1989); and Mayanvsky, (1991). All the authors agreed that the decrease of T and B lymphocytes was caused by their migration into tissues and lymph nodes in the massaged area. Besides this the deep tissue massage can produce stress related reactions which are also responsible for the redistribution of lymphocytes.

3. VODDER'S LYMPH DRAINAGE MASSAGE

Lymph drainage massage has critical impact on the whole lymphatic system. This medical massage procedure in form of Vodder's Lymph Drainage Massage is the one of the most effective methods of treatment of peripheral edema.

The effect of lymph drainage massage on the patients with peripheral edemas was examined by Kuhnke, (1975) in a clinical study. The author reported increased edematous fluid reabsorbtion and a 200-400% acceleration of urine flow alter a session of lymph drainage massage.

Kutz, et al. (1978) studied the effect of lymph drainage massage on the urinary excretion of neurohormones and minerals in 29 patients with **chronic lymphedema**. The control group included 10 healthy individuals. The authors founded increased excretion of adrenaline of up to 50%; noradrenaline up to 19%; histamine up to 129%. At the same time urinary excretion of 17-OH was down by 31%; serotonin by 22%; and 5-HIAA by 21%.

The authors concluded that an increased concentration of the catecholamines in the blood is a sign of intensification of the blood circulation; the destruction of serotonin and its metabolite 5-HIAA partly blocks the nociceptors and decreases the peripheral vascular resistance by producing arteriolar dilatation; the increasing concentration of 17-OH is sign of additional releasing glucocorticoid hormones from the adrenal gland. Finally, patients who suffered from chronic lymphedema caused by the increased concentration of histamine showed significant improvement and in some cases complete recovery after the course of lymph drainage massage. This effect is caused by increased urine excretion of histamine and a decrease in its concentration in the patient's body.

Kaaja and Tiula, (1989) used lymph drainage massage for the treatment of the **nephrotic syndrome** during pregnancy. This pathological condition causes general edema, blood dilution with following **hypoalbuminemia** which in turn leads to retarded development of the fetus. The authors registered increases of diuresis up to 2 liters after just one session. They also detected considerable increases in the excretion of sodium. This process plays important role in reducing general edema. The authors think that in most cases 2-4 weekly massage sessions of 1-1.5 hours duration are enough to control edemas caused by the nephrotic syndrome.

Asdonk, (1981) examined the effect of manual lymph drainage in combination with exercises on patients with protein-rich edema caused by insufficiency of venous drainage. The author concluded that the best results were obtained when the treatment session was conducted in three stages. The **first stage** is the stimulation of lymph vasomotor activity on the area proximal to the edema. It should be done by fast, energetic massage strokes in the direction of the lymph flow. The strokes start from the upper border of edema and conducted in the proximal direction. The **second stage** is the manual lymph drainage from the edematous area. The slow lymph draining strokes are directed from the more distal segments of the affected extremity until edema is reduced. The **third stage** involves secondary treatment. After the edema is reduced in size the practitioner can easily detect all soft tissue abnormalities caused by long-lasting edema, i.e. trigger points, fasciitis, contractures of aponeurosis. etc. The practitioner should work on all these areas to restore the normal relations between all somatic components.

Wittlinger and Wittlinger, (1992) consider lymph drainage massage as an important indispensable part of the treatment of patients with lymphostatic and lymphodynamic edemas. This type of massage not only increases drainage of the lymph but also creates new anastomoses between different lymph capillary networks.

Casley-Smith, et al., (1998) discussed the procedure and results of the treatment of postrnastectomy lymphedema of the arm by the **Casley-Smith's Method**. The author additionally improved the original Vodder's lymph drainage massage by including some original techniques, skin care, and compression in the form of bandaging or garments after the treatment and exercise. In the Adelaide Lymphedema Clinic in Australia the author achieved an average of 64% of lymphedema reduction during the 1 month course of treatment. For everyone who is interested in the new developments of manual lymph drainage I highly recommend this article published by *Cancer.*

Weiss, (1998) reported the case of successful treatment of severe leg edema and wounds resulting from complex tibiofibular fracture and numerous surgeries. The patient also had several unsuccessful wound related surgeries during one year after initial trauma. The author used lymph drainage massage in the combination with compressive bandaging and exercise. At the end of 10 weeks of treatment, edema had reduced by 80.9%, one wound had healed and a second one had reduced by 93%.

Ekici et al., (2009) compared the effectiveness of lymph drainage massage *vs* connective tissue massage on fifty women with primary **fibromyalgia**. The authors found that both modalities showed improvements in terms of pain, health status, and quality of life but these parameters were much stronger in the group treated with lymph drainage massage especially in regards to morning tenderness and level of anxiety.

Bongi et al., (2011) examined the impact of lymph drainage massage on 35 patients who suffered from **scleroderma** in the edematous stage. In the group treated with lymph drainage massage, patients showed a significant decrease of hand edema ($P < 0.001$) compared to the control.

D. MUSCULAR SYSTEM

Skeletal muscle is the body's most abundant tissue. More than 600 skeletal muscles form approximately 48% of the body mass (April, 1990). About 80% of all muscle mass is located in the upper and lower extremities.

The skeletal muscles have extremely rich nervous and vasculatory support. Afferent sensory innervation is provided by nociceptors (i.e. pain receptors), Pacinian corpuscles (Sommer, 1940), muscle spindle receptors and Golgi tendon organ receptors. Efferent motor innervation is supplied by alpha-motor neurons which deliver commands from the anterior horns of the spinal cord to the neuro-muscular junctions to generate muscle contractions. Because of the large total mass, muscles even at rest consume about 20% of total resting O_2 consumption. During exercise the skeletal muscles extract about 80% of the O_2 from the arterial blood (Bullock, 1984). To serve this purpose the amount of the capillaries in 1 mm of skeletal muscle can vary from 41 at rest to 1400 after exercises or massage treatment (Krogh, 1927).

1. EXPERIMENTAL AND CLINICAL STUDIES

Massage was used for the treatment of muscle pain and tension in ancient Egypt and China thousand of years ago. The first scientific approach to massage treatment of the hypertonic muscular abnormalities started back in 19th century. German physician Dr. Helleday (1876) considered deep friction massage as the more effective method of treatment for patients with muscle rheumatism. Later, Professor Zabludovsky (1913) made the same recommendations. He also for the first time clinically proved the restorative effect of massage on fatigued muscles.

Dr. Williams and Dr. Elkins, at the Mayo Clinic of Rochester (1942) conducted a clinical study on 22 patients with the severe headaches caused by tension in the head and cervical muscles. The authors called this clinical condition "**myalgia of the head**". For treatment the authors used different sources of heat (infra-red rays, short wave diathermy, hot packs and paraffin); massage; and a combination of heat and massage. After analyzing the clinical results the authors concluded that massage is the most effective treatment of myalgia of the head. All patients showed signs of significant relief or a complete elimination of pathological symptoms in 1 week after the massage or combination of massage and heat treatment. The patients with only heat therapy did not show signs of significant relief. In the authors' opinion massage is especially effective during the acute stage when all other methods of treatment (including the drug therapy) failed. The authors recommended 10 minutes of massage treatment every day for 1-3 weeks. In their opinion, the more effective technique is deep friction. The session has to start with effleurage and kneading and later friction has to be the main part of the treatment.

Prof. Sarkisov-Sirasini conducted many experimental and clinical studies of the effect of massage on the skeletal muscles. In 1957 he compiled the results of his works in the classical textbook *Sports Massage*. This book contains well of important clinical information for the practitioners.

For example, he studied the effect of massage on the athletes' performance by electromyography. During breaks in sports competitions, for the quick restoration of contractile response of overloaded muscles, massage has to be performed on the muscles which played a supportive role in the movements the athlete used the most instead of the most overloaded ones. However the key point is that the massaged muscles must belong to the same **myotome** as the overloaded muscles and also include muscles from two neighboring myotomes. In this case the athlete's performance during the competition will maximally improve. Prof. Sarkisov-Sirasini also developed unique techniques of kneading which he called "passive exercises for muscles". We will review this subject below.

Jacobs, (1960) described the vicious cycle of somatic pain as sustained reflex muscle contraction - deep pain - reflex muscle contraction. The author considered massage, especially the kneading, as a major breaker of this vicious cycle and a powerful method of central inhibition of the motor cortex which control the tensed muscles. Krusen, et al. (1965) had the same opinion.

Bierman, (1960) examined the influence of 30 minutes of vibration massage on trunk flexion on 152 healthy individuals by estimating the "finger to floor test". After the treatment an average gain of 2.30 inches was registered as compared to an average gain of 0.28 inch in the same individuals when acting as controls.

Nordschow and Bierman, (1962) studied the effect of Swedish massage and Hoffa techniques on trunk flexion in 25 healthy individuals. The massage was performed on the back muscles and posterior group of the thigh muscles. The results were also examined by applying the "finger to floor test" before and after massage treatment. The authors registered a significant increase in ability to flex the trunk and hips after massage. The mean gain consisted of 1.35 inch.

The authors agreed with Bemhaup et al. (1953) who experimentally proved that relaxation of skeletal muscles is accompanied by the decreasing of excitability of the sympathetic part of hypothalamus. As a result of this, the hypothalamus diminishes its discharge to the cortex with subsequent inhibition of the motor areas of cerebral cortex and a decrease of efferent motor discharge.

Vasiliev, (1961) examined the effect of massage on lactate concentration after heavy exercises. The author reported increased lactate elimination from the muscle tissue caused by vasodilation and increased blood circulation. Simultaneously a significant decrease of lactic acid concentration in the blood was detected after massage compare to the control group. The author attributed this drop to stimulation of lactate transformation to piruvate in the liver with the following production ATP and restoration of energy resources.

Sirotkina, (1964) in a clinical study examined the effect of massage on patients with spastic and flaccid palsy. The author clinically proved that different massage techniques impact the muscles and nervous system of patients with these disorders differently. In the case of **spastic palsy**, gentle kneading, light, slow friction, and stretching inhibit the nervous system and reduce muscle spasms.

In cases of **flaccid palsy**, fast massage stimulation techniques with light to moderate pressure are able to restore muscular tone and increase muscular strength. Similar results were reported later by Myamoto and Okamoto, (1975) after vibration massage treatment.

Dembo, (1973) applied 50 seconds of massage on wrestlers during breaks in competitions and examined the results. After massage treatment the strength of hand flexors increased on 3.2 kg but in the control group after just general rest the same parameter increased by only 0.4 kg.

Fokin, (1997) estimated the increasing of muscular strength to be 3-7 times after the correct application of massage.

Belaya, et al. (1978) studied by electromyography the effect of massage on the skeletal muscles of patients with cervical and lumbo-sacral **radiculopathy** as a complication of spondylosis. In the clinical group the amplitude of the originally decreased electric potentials increased on 30-160 mcV compared to the control group. The authors registered the increase of this parameter on the massaged extremity as well as on the opposite one. Another reported result is the rising of muscle tone registered by myotonometer in the clinical group by 5-15 points compare to the control group.

Prudden, (1980); Popelansky, (1981); Travell and Simmons, (1983) considered manual compression as a valuable method of treatment of trigger points in the skeletal muscles. The creation of **ischemic compression** in the area of trigger points causes reflex vasodilation and the opening of reserve capillaries with following elimination of the trigger points. However, all authors emphasized that several session are needed. Otherwise the trigger point will transfer in "sleeping condition" instead of its elimination and can be easily reactivated.

Danneskiold-Samsoe, et al. (1982) examined the **myoglobine** plasma concentration in 13 patients with regional muscle tension and somatic pain before and after massage. Myoglobine is a macroprotein which is located in the muscle tissue and delivers the 0_2. The plasma concentration of myoglobine increased after the first session, reaching a peak value (up to 133 mg/L) within 3 hours after the massage session. The authors also founded that after a 7th session of treatment the increase of the plasma myoglobine concentration was insignificant (up to 7 mg/L). This period matched with the patients' clinical recovery. Thus, the authors scientifically proved the empirically found optimal duration of massage treatment in cases of somatic pathology to be 5-7 sessions.

Bogorodinsky, et al. (1975); Yumashev and Furman, (1984); Limansky, et al. (1988) used massage for the reducing spasms, muscle contractures and protective muscle tension on patients with neurological complications of intervertebral disk herniations caused by advanced stage of **cervical** and **lumbo-sacral spondylosis**. The authors suggested 20-30 minutes of massage therapy daily. All authors recommended massage therapy as an important method of preparation of patients for spinal surgery as well as a critical element of their rehabilitation in postsurgical period.

Vakulenko, (1980) recommended deep reflex massage in combination with others methods of physiotherapy to prevent the progress of spondylosis and decrease the possibility of neurological complications.

Cosman, et al. (1984) examined the effect of massage therapy on the hamstring muscles in 34 healthy volunteers. The authors detected an increasing of the hip flexion by 10.65 degrees immediately after massage treatment.

Kreimer, (1988) clinically examined the effect of vibration massage on 186 children with **cerebral palsy**. The author used vibration massage on special points throughout the body according to his previous discovery. All patients showed signs of decreasing spasticity (examined by electromyography); up to 10-25 degrees increased range of the motions in the joints; correction of the balance between the flexors and extensors (improvement of gait, self-serving, breathing); decreasing irritability and anxiety. Prof. Kreimer's method of treatment of children with the cerebral palsy is successfully used in hundreds of hospitals in republics of the former Soviet Union.

Turin, (1992) considered the stimulation of **acetylcholine** formation as the main cause of intensifying the contractile ability of muscles after the stimulating massage. The increase of acetylcholine's concentration in the neuromuscular junctions speeds up the transmission of the action potentials.

Chaitov, (1986) significantly improved the therapeutic procedure of **neuromuscular therapy** originally developed by S. Lief in the 1930s. The author combined the classical neuromuscular approach, massage techniques and muscle energy techniques to achieve optimal therapeutic impact for the patients with the different somatic dysfunctions.

Mitz, (1997) recommended massage for the treatment of **fasciitis** following a face lift. About 1.4% all face lift plastic surgeries are complicated by fasciitis on one or both side of the face and neck. It can be seen as firm retraction of the skin and subcutaneous tissue. This part of the face becomes painful to touch and emotionless. This pathological condition has also a strong psychosomatic link. Thus, the authors recommended the following conservative treatment: face massage in the combination with psychological help. This treatment is highly effective for these patients but sometimes takes a long period of time (e.g. in one case almost 1 year).

Blackman, et al. (1998) examined the effect of massage treatment on 7 athletes with chronic **anterior compartment syndrome** in the sports medicine clinic in Melboume. This pathological condition frequently affect professional athletes with pain and tension on the anterior surface of the leg especially during the dorsiflexion of the foot. Even light pressure on the leg muscles of the anterior compartment causes pain. The authors conducted a 5 week course of massage with 2 sessions during, the 1st week and 1 session per week after that with total of 6 sessions. Between treatments, athletes performed 2 daily regular stretching sessions. After the end of treatment the authors detected significant ($p = 0.016$) increase in work performed in dorsiflexion to pain onset.

Buonocore, et al. (1998) conducted the clinical study of effect a combination of massage and kinesiotherapy on 13 out - patients with **thoracic outlet syndrome**. After the course of conservative treatment all pathological symptoms disappeared in all patients. The authors concluded that massage treatment is a highly effective medical procedure and all cases of thoracic outlet syndrome should be treated by the massage first. Only in cases of failure this type of treatment other options should be considered i.e. injections, surgery etc.

In earlier clinical study on this matter conducted by Kotwica, et al. (1976) in the medical resort of Swieradow in Poland authors examined effect of massage and radon baths on 50 patients with anterior scalene muscle syndrome. In 38 cases complete recovery was obtained, in 6 cases the intensity on pains was significantly reduced and in 6 cases no positive dynamic was registered.

In 1984 Li, reported that massage and gentle, gradual stretching helped 205 patients with the **frozen shoulder**. The author registered the complete recovery with the total restoration of affected functions in 71.2% of patients.

Gam, et al. (1998) examined the therapeutic effect of 2 types of ultrasound, massage and exercises on 58 patients with **myofascial trigger-points**. The authors found that ultrasound did not relieve pain or decrease the number of active trigger points while massage and exercise program did reduce pain and the number of active myofascial trigger points. The authors followed the patients for 6 months. 64% of patients considered massage and exercises treatment as effective.

2. MASSAGE AND ATHLETE'S RECOVERY

I want to separately discuss the relation between massage and recovery from supramaximal exercises. This is a very important matter for everyone who is involved in sports and sports medicine and sports massage. Is massage able to speed up the athlete's recovery or does it not? The position of Russian scientists on this matter was clear from the early 1950s: when it was conducted properly, massage played a critical role in the athlete's recovery and in reducing muscle soreness (Sarkisov-Sirasini 1957; Krilov, et al. 1985; Kunichev 1985; Burovik, et al. 1989; Dubrovsky, and Dubrovsky, 1995).

The tremendous success of Soviet athletes in different types of sports competitions is a practical outcome of this basic concept of Russian sports massage. Soviet scientists formulated this concept during decades of practical application of sports massage.

The possibility of speeding up the athlete's recovery by massage captured the attention of West European and American scientists who work in the field of sports medicine. However, authors of numerous studies in different countries mostly concluded that massage does not have any significant impact on the process of recovery after maximal exercises (Drews, et al., 1990; Cafarelli, et al., 1990; Rodenberg, et al., 1994; Tiidus, et al., 1995; Gupta, et al., 1996; Jonhagen et al., 2004; Wiltshire et al., 2010, etc.). All these studies were conducted by very responsible scientists and published in respected professional journals. Thus, everyone who became familiar with this matter deserves the clear answer to the question: Who is right? After analysis of Western European and American sources I concluded that the problem suffered from significant misunderstanding and misrepresentation. First of all, Russian scientists always pointed out the importance of four equally important components of restorative massage after vigorous exercises: time of the treatment, duration of the treatment, massage techniques and applied pressure. Failure to include even one of them will ruin all efforts:

a. Time of the Treatment

All authors agreed that massage has to be started around **1.5-2 hours** after vigorous exercises. Not earlier and not later.

b. Duration of the Treatment

The massage session has to last from **30-40 minutes to 1 hour**. During this time the massage therapist works on the athlete's whole body with special attention to the muscle groups which were overloaded during the exercises or competition.

c. Massage Techniques

It is best to use the combination of effleurage, kneading, permanent vibration, compression, stretching and long range shaking. However, 40-50% of massage time has to be spent on **kneading**. With the proper execution of this technique the operator is able to alternate stimulation and relaxation of the massaged muscles. Thus, kneading is the best tool for restoring muscular strength (see details below in Chapter IV).

d. Pressure

The applied pressure has to be significant but **without** the activation of the pain analyzing system. The threshold of pain varies on different parts of the body or even within the borders of the same massaged segment. Thus, the pressure has to be continually adjusted.

All Western articles which reported the failure of massage therapy to speed up the process of recovery were united by one striking similarity. Despite a truly scientific approach to the evaluation of obtained data, the experimental protocol of each study failed to observe at least two elements: the time of treatment and its duration (see Table 4).

TABLE 4.

Authors	Time of the Treatment	Duration
1. Cafarell, et al., 1990	immediately after exercise	4 min
2. Drews, 1990	immediately after exercise	30 min
3. Wenos, et al, 1990	48 hours after exercise	N/A
4. Rodenberg, et al., 1994	15 minute after exercise	15 min
5. Tiidus, 1995	48 hours after exercise	10 min
6. Gupta, 1996	48 hours after exercise	10 min
7. Jonhagen S., et a., 2004	immediately after exercise	8 min
8. Wiltshire et al., 2010	immediately after exercise	during first 10 minutes

However, one important study on this matter I think put everything in the correct perspective. In this study, a group of authors (Smith, et al., 1994) from two scientific centers in North Carolina and Virginia proved the clinical value of the observational discovery of Russian scientists. The authors examined the effect of massage on delayed onset of muscle soreness, creatine kinase and neutrophil count.

First of all, the authors adjusted their experimental protocol according to the practical recommendations of Russian authors. Secondly, they took as a basis the theoretic concept which was formulated earlier by Cannon, et al. (1990) who considered that vigorous exercises damage muscle tissue with the following development of **aseptic inflammation** and **interstitial edema**. The body reacts to these events by sending neutrophils into the affected area for the major clean up. Neutrophils emerge into tissues and start their cleaning job (i.e., **phagocytosis**) to remove the waste products developed as a result of the muscle injury and inflammation. The increased concentration of neutrophils also attracts the other types of phagocytic cells: **macrophages**. In the process of cleaning (i.e., phagocytosis), catabolic enzymes are released from neutrophils and they additionally damage already injured muscle fibers.

Two major facts indirectly support this theory: temporary reduction of neutrophil count in the blood since they are leaving blood stream to assist in phagocytosis and increased concentration of creatine kinase in the blood. Thus, authors expected to find the margination of neutrophils along the vascular walls at the site of muscle injury and their following emigration into soft tissues. The authors expected the neutrophils' margination to occur 2 hours after the end of vigorous exercise.

From these theoretical speculations, the authors examined the **neutrophil count** and level of **creatine kinase** according to the previously discussed recommendations of Russian scientists. The study was conducted on 14 healthy subjects who performed eccentric contraction of forearm flexors and extensors. In the experimental group (1st group) sports massage was performed and in the control group (2nd group) lotion was applied. The subjects from the 1st group reported a peak of soreness value of 4.6 $\pm$ 0.7 points after 24 hours and the subjects from the 2nd group estimated their soreness value as 5.9 $\pm$ 0.5 points. Neutrophil count in the 1st group before the massage treatment was 3367 $\pm$ 505 cells/mm^3 and after the period of 24 hours it was 3883 $\pm$ 543 cells/mm^3 or 15.3 % elevation. In the 2nd group these parameters were 4066 $\pm$ 626 cells/mm^3 and 4267 $\pm$ 649 cells/mm^3 respectively or 4.9% elevation.

The smaller elevation of neutrophil count in the blood of subjects from the 2nd group is a clear evidence of the neutrophils' migration from the blood to the injured site. The authors also detected elevation of creatine kinase level in the 2nd group (from original 83.3 $\pm$ 9.0 U/L until 1917 $\pm$ 1023 U/L after 96 hours). In the 1st group no elevation was detected until 72 hours and its peak (1083 in 476 U/L) was registered at 120 hours.

I'll quote the authors' conclusions because of their importance:

> "During acute inflammation. blood flow slows as vessels dilate in an area of injury. When this occurs, the white blood cells, including neutrophils, are displaced from the central, axial zone of blood flow to the peripheral, plasmatic zone and subsequently marginate along the vessel walls. Since vigorous massage appears to increase blood flow through the vascular bed, we theorized that this increased flow rate in the area of microtrauma could prevent the typical outward displacement of neutrophils. In addition, we speculated that the mechanical action of vigorous massage could shear marginated cells from vessel walls and thus hinder emigration of cells from the circulation into tissues spaces."
>
> and
>
> "... control group exhibiting a more rapid and steeper increase CK (i.e., creatine kinase) values than the massage group." and "... vigorous sports massage rendered hours after termination of unaccustomed eccentric exercise reduces the intensity of delayed onset muscle soreness and reduces serum creatine kinase levels."

Crane et al., (2012) published the results of another important study which supports the findings of Smith, et al. They examined the effect of massage on the quadriceps muscle of 11 young males after exercise-induced muscle damage. The authors found that massage reduces inflammation and promotes mitochondrial biogenesis in muscle tissue damaged by eccentric exercise.

E. SKELETAL SYSTEM

The skeletal system includes bones, joints, periosteum, endosteum, cartilage and bone marrow. The human skeleton consists of 206 bones. Bone is a 50% calcified connective tissue with another 50% divided equally between water and the protein matrix.

The skeletal system has the following functions: form and support the body's framework as well as protect inner organs; the bones are levers of the biomechanical system which produces motions; the bones are reservoirs of Ca and P; the bone marrow is the site of hemopoesis and lipid storage.

Therapeutic massage generally affects the skeletal system by producing vasodilation in the soft tissues around the joints. The friction technique has an analgesic effect on patients who have pain in the joints caused by osteoarthritis (Kunichev, 1985; Dubrovsky, and Dubrovsky, 1995). For these patients, "intrajoint" massage therapy also is an important part of treatment (Shterngetz and Belaya, 1992).

The periostal massage is the only method of medical massage treatment specially designed for disorders of the skeletal system as well as some inner organ pathologies. The periostal massage delivers the therapeutic impact directly and by reflex way (Vogler and Krauss, 1953; 1975). Regular therapeutic and periostal massage treatment helps to prevent the further development of degenerative changes in the joint.

The effect of massage on the skeletal system was among the first scientific studies to establish the credibility of massage treatment. In 1889 Dr. Gurevich employed hystological methods to study the effect of massage on fracture healing in experimental animals. The author reported the stimulation of callus formation up to 20% in the experimental group compared to the control group of massage.

French physician J. Lucas-Championniere (1889) has to be credited as the first who applied massage as an important method of fracture healing. He called his method "early management of fractures" because the actual treatment started immediately after the fracture was detected and progressed through the whole period of callus formation with different types and combinations of rhythmic massage strokes. The author recommended gentle stroking and eflleurage at the site of the injury to reduce pain and swelling. With fracture healing in progress more and more energetic strokes were employed.

In 1908 Prof. Turner, one of the founders of the Russian orthopedic school, offered percussion as a method of stimulation the fracture reunion and callus formation in the area of delayed union or **psedoarthrosis**. Later, the similar treatment was also recommended by Kramarenko, (1953).

Verbov, (1966) conducted a clinical study on this matter and proved its high effectiveness by analyzing X-ray pictures of clinical and control groups of patients. The author suggested percussion by fingertips or a little wooden hammer as well as light manual vibration on the periostal areas of fractured bones after surgery to stimulate callus formation. The same clinical recommendations were made later by Vasichkin, (1991), Turin, (1992), and Fokin, (1997).

Zavadina, (1978) conducted a clinical study on 100 patients with **lumbo-sacral spondylosis**. 40% of these patients had different degrees of neurological symptoms. The author compared the effectiveness of classical therapeutic massage and segment-reflex massage by employing clinical evaluation, the examination of peripheral arterial circulation and electromyography. The results of this study allowed the author to recommend therapeutic massage only in cases when all neurological symptoms are eliminated. On the opposite side, patients with lumbo-sacral spondylosis complicated by the peripheral neurological disorders showed positive changes, mostly after segment-reflex massage.

Karmanov, and Belaya, (1985) conducted a clinical study on 106 patients with osteoarthritis of knee and hip joints. The authors compared the effectiveness of therapeutic massage (lst group of 53 patients) and segment-reflex massage (2nd group of 53 patients) treatment. The results were examined clinically, by electromyography and reovasography. Clinically, in the 1st group after only the 1st session, the patients felt some relief: warm feelings in the massaged area; reduced pain for

0.5-1.5 hours after treatment; some improvement in the ROM. The patients in the 2nd group after the 1st session felt great improvement of the clinical picture: warm feelings of circulation spread through whole body; pain relief was detected for at least 5 hours after treatment; significant restoration of the range of motion occurred. Reovasography tests (1.95 $\pm$ 0.15 normal value) revealed the restoration of the initially reduced level of blood circulation in the lower extremities. The patients in the both groups showed improvement of blood circulation in the lower extremities but changes in the 2nd group were more profound: 1.14 $\pm$ 0.10 before segment-reflex massage treatment and 1.61 $\pm$ 0.07 alter it. The electromyography test also showed increased electrical potentials in the skeletal muscles of the lower extremities. The electrical potentials were increased in average on 38.75 mcV in the 1st group and on 49.38 mcV in the 2nd group. From these data the authors concluded that the therapeutic effect of segment-reflex massage is significantly higher.

Children with cerebral palsy have significant delay in bone growth in the affected extremities. If the extremities are affected, the body looks disproportional, but in the case of one side pathology the bone growth delay causes severe problems for the patient's gait and vertebral column.

At the same time, children with severe forms of **cerebral palsy** show signs of delayed cranial bone growth. This is an additional factor which negatively affects the patient's mental development. Shterngertz, (1989) successfully used regular massage treatment during the patients' childhood to stimulate growth of the long and cranial bones. In case of delayed long bones development the author trained the parents to use slow, strong effleurage and friction strokes in the areas of epiphyseal plates (i.e. growth plates). In cases of delayed cranial bone development percussion by fingertips was performed regularly along cranial sutures.

Troisier, (1991) examined the effect of different types of conservative treatment of **tennis elbow** (i.e., lateral humeral epicondylitis). The author evaluated results of cervical manipulations (58 cases), deep transverse massage on the tendon below the lateral epicondyle (131 cases) and corticoid injections (257 cases). The cervical manipulations gave only temporary relief in all examined cases; injections of coiticoids gave full immediate pain relief in all cases but had very high rate of recurrences - 66.7%; deep transverse massage gave excellent, stable results in 63% of patients with moderate pain relief for the rest of patients. The authors concluded that surgical procedure (i.e., tenotomy) can be only an alternative method of treatment on patients with high rates of recurrences.

Field, et al. (1997) examined the effect of massage therapy on 20 patients with juvenile **rheumatoid arthritis**. The parents performed daily 15 minutes massage for 30 days in the following sequence: face; stomach; legs; arms; lower; upper back. The immediate effects after the massage treatment included diminishing anxiety in child and parents and reduced levels of stress hormone (salivary cortisol).

The longer term effect were confirmed by the primary physicians and formulated as: general pain relief, decreased numbers of trigger points, restoration of child's activity and reduced stiffness in the affected joints. The authors emphasized the pain-reducing power of massage therapy and its cost-effective effect for children with juvenile rheumatoid arthritis.

Nagrale et al., (2009) examined the efficacy of cross fiber friction (Cyriax's friction) on 60 subjects with **lateral epicondylitis** (Tennis Elbow) compared to the physical therapy treatment which consisted of phonophoresis with supervised exercise. The authors concluded that the efficacy of cross fiber friction well surpassed ($p<0.05$) the results obtained in the control group.

Perlman et al., (2012) in a randomized clinical study on 125 subjects with knee **osteoarthritis** identified the optimal dose of massage within an 8-week treatment course. The authors concluded that one weekly 60 minute massage session is an optimal dose of massage treatment to help patients with osteoarthritis.

F. RESPIRATORY SYSTEM

The main function of the respiratory system is gas exchange. In the lungs the venous blood releases carbon dioxide and becomes oxygenated. Besides this the respiratory system is responsible for numerous important functions: the filtration, moisturizing and warming the inhaled air in the upper airways; the maintenance of normal body pH (i.e. acid-base balance); activation hormone angiotensine I; inactivation serotonin and norepinephrine; speech; smell description; controlling the body temperature and removing waste products in the vaporized form.

1. EXPERIMENTAL STUDIES

Massage has various effects on the respiratory system. The first experimental studies were conducted at the end of 19th and beginning 20th centuries. In 1904 Dr. Eccles stated that massage strokes, especially percussion, increased the respiratory rate.

Emelyanova, (1968) conducted an experimental study on dogs to estimate massage's influence on the respiratory rate. The largest increase in respiratory rate was detected after stimulating massage techniques (i.e. percussion, vibration, shaking) were applied to the thoracic cage, especially along intercostal spaces.

Komarova, (1969) studied the effect of massage therapy on pulmonary function in healthy adults. The author registered increased maximal voluntary ventilation of up to 24.2% after massage treatment. The maximal voluntary ventilation (MVV) is the largest volume of air that can be moved into and out of the lungs during 1 minute by voluntary effort.

Barr and Taslitz, (1970) registered increased pulmonary ventilation after 20 minutes of back massage on 10 healthy females. The authors explained this event by stimulation of the sympathetic part of the autonomic nervous system. It causes reflex bronchodilation and allows passage of an increased volume of air in the lungs.

Chopra, et al. (1977) conducted an experimental study on anesthetized dogs to examine the effect of hydration, massage and postural drainage on the tracheal transport velocity (TTV). The authors measured TTV using a gamma scintillation camera. They placed the protein microspheres labeled with radioisotope Tc-99m at the lower end of the trachea and registered the speed of microspheres movement up to the larynx by tracheal ciliary activity. These measurements were conducted before and after applied physical factors. The experimental study showed that TTV increased: after hydration up to 4.91 mm/min; after postural drainage up to 7.7 mm/min; after 10 minutes of manual percussion and vibration up to 8.2 mm/min; after a combination of massage strokes and postural drainage up to 9.5 mm/min. Thus, the increasing of TTV under the influence of physical factors creates optimal conditions for the cleaning of the bronchial tree and drainage of sputum from the lungs of patients with pulmonary pathology. The best combination of physical factors is manual percussion and vibration over the thoracic cage and postural drainage.

Turin, (1992) reported up to 20% increased respiration rate after massage. The author offered the following explanation of this stimulation. Massage activates the local metabolism in the massaged area and as a result the increased amount of CO_2 is produced in the massaged tissues and carried by the blood. The increase of the partial CO_2 pressure in the blood activates central and peripheral chemoreceptors. They send information about changes in the blood chemistry to the respiratory center located in the brain steam. As soon as these stimuli reached the respiratory center, the respiration rate increases by reflex as a compensatory reaction.

Dubrovsky, (1995) studied the changes in pulmonary ventilation after massage treatment using pulmonography. The author reported increases in pulmonary function not only by stimulation of the respiration rate but also by the opening of reserve alveoli and involving them in respiration.

2. CLINICAL STUDIES

Massage has a significant therapeutic impact on patients with different pulmonary disorders. Dr. Stabrovsky (1887) was among the first authors who used massage to stimulate the sputum drainage from the lungs of patients with chronic bronchitis.

Sister Elizabeth (1966) recommended deep pressure and friction around the spinous process of T1-T2 vertebrae to suppress **cough**. She also used sensory stimulation to improve the breathing of patients with **emphysema**. The author recommended putting the patient in all-fours position and working on the areas between lower rib cage and iliac crests. Another important area for sensory stimulation of these patients is the external abdominal obliques muscle when the patient is in the supine position with both lower extremities elevated to 60 degrees.

Clark, et al. (1973) studied the effect of chest percussion and vibration on static and dynamic volumes as well as the amount and rheological parameters of the sputum in 23 patients with chronic bronchitis, bronchiectasis and cystic fibrosis. All patients had different degrees of airway obstruction. The results of this clinical study showed that **airway resistance** significantly decreased and drainage of sputum from the bronchial tree accelerated. These results allowed authors to conclude that physiotherapy and massage help bronchial clearance and thereby improve the lungs' function in patients with pulmonary disorders.

The Merck Manual (1992) also recommends the **vibropercussion** (slapping, cupping) on the thoracic cage up to 30 minutes 1-2 times per day to accelerate sputum drainage. The indications for this treatment are: macroatelectasis; bronchiectasis; cystic fibrosis; lung abscess; chronic obstructive pulmonary disease; pulmonary fibrosis; elder patients and patients with neuromuscular diseases.

Pham, et al. (1973) studied the respiratory function and rheological status of bronchial secretions collected before and after chest vibration and percussion on 38 patients with **chronic bronchitis**. The authors founded that after treatment the sputum was significantly less viscous; arterial PO_2 and alveolar-arterial PO_2 difference improved. Practically the same results were reported later by Cyrapet, (1985). All authors agreed that reducing the viscosity of sputum was one of the key components of effective treatment of patients with chronic bronchitis.

In a clinical study of 64 patients with **chronic pneumonia**, Kuznetsov, (1978) examined the effect of asymmetric segment-reflex massage on the respiratory functions and pharmacological effect of bronchodilator drugs. The author is a creator of **asymmetric segment-reflex massage** which is especially designed for the treatment of pulmonary disorders.

All patients were separated into two groups: the first group was treated with the bronchodilator and antibacterial drugs and the second group was treated with a combination of the same drug therapy and asymmetric segment-reflex massage. The results of the treatment were examined by the testing of 7 ventilatory parameters: respiratory rate; tidal volume; vital capacity; timed vital capacity; reserve volumes; respiratory minute volume; maximal voluntary ventilation. In the second group all tests showed significant improvement compared to the first group. The patients in both groups showed moderate hyperventilation. This clinical improvement in the first group was caused by the increasing of respiratory rate and the depth of respiration. In the second group the hyperventilation was caused by the increasing depth of respiration with the simultaneous decreasing of respiratory rate by 6 per minute. Thus, in the second group the same level of hyperventilation was achieved by more economic work of respiratory muscles and diaphragm. Finally, the author detected that in the second group the same effect bronchodilator drug (theophylline) was obtained quicker compared to the first group.

Dr. Kuznetsov offered the following explanation of this phenomenon. Massage, especially asymmetric segment-reflex massage, normalizes the acid-base balance affected by the pulmonary disorders. With the normal acid-base balance the bronchodilator drugs quickly penetrate into the bronchial tree causing the relaxation of smooth muscles with following bronchodilation. Similar results were reported earlier by Moshkov, (1977).

In another clinical study, Kuznetsov and Kuznetsova, (1981) examined and compared the effect of therapeutic and asymmetric segment-reflex massage on patients with **chronic pneumonia** and **bronchitis**. The study was conducted on 67 patients who were separated into two groups. In the first group (32 patients) a daily 15 minute classical therapeutic massage was performed on the thoracic cage. In the second group (35 patients) a 30 minutes asymmetric segment-reflex massage was performed 2 times per week. The authors examined the effect of both methods by the evaluating activity of the sympathetico-adrenal system. For this purpose, the urine excretion of epinephrine, norepinephrine as well as their precursors dopamine and DOPA was tested (7 different parameters).

The authors registered the following changes: in the first group after 5-6 sessions of therapeutic massage the excretion of norepinephrine decreased from 3.37 $\pm$ 1.0 ngr/ml to 0.81 $\pm$ 0.3 ngr/ml and the excretion of DOPA did not change; in the second group after 2-3 sessions of asymmetric segment-reflex massage the excretion of norepinephrine increased from 4.12 $\pm$ 0.91 ngr/ml to 34.3 $\pm$ 3.4 ngr/ml.

After careful evaluation of these and other parameters the authors made important practical recommendations for the treatment of respiratory disorders by massage. Therapeutic massage inhibits the sympathetico-adrenal system (decreasing epinephrine and norepinephrine excretion) but preserves its potential (unchanged level of DOPA). Asymmetric segment-reflex massage stimulates the activity of sympathetic-adrenal system (increasing epinephrine and norepinephrine excretion) and what is more important increases its reserve potential (the increasing of the DOPA excretion). Thus, therapeutic massage has to be applied to every **relapse** case of chronic respiratory disorders. In these patients the activity of the sympathetic-adrenal system increased and made the clinical picture significantly worse. Therapeutic massage is able to inhibit the sympathetic-adrenal system.

When the patients have **long lasting** chronic respiratory pathology during the period of remission, the asymmetric segment-reflex massage is a major therapeutic priority because it has a stimulating effect on the sympathetic-adrenal system which usually shows signs of inhibition. The regular application of this type of massage treatment prevents the acute reactivations of chronic pulmonary disorders. The two methods do not compete with each other but should be combined during the treatment of each case of pulmonary disorders.

Fedorovsky, et al. (1982) conducted a clinical study on 60 patients after the **upper abdominal surgeries** (cholecystectomy and partial gastrectomy). After these types of surgery older patients usually have various respiratory problems: the restriction of diaphragm and thoracic cage excursions; insufficient bronchial drainage; hypoventilation; abnormalities of acid-base balance. These complications frequently cause pneumonia which complicates the patients' recovery.

The authors examined the effect of vibration massage on the abnormalities in the respiratory function. The massage treatment was performed daily for 6-10 minutes, starting on the next day after the surgery. Electrical and manual vibration were performed daily for 6-10 minutes, starting on the next day after the surgery. Electrical and manual vibration were performed from lower to upper parts of the thoracic cage. The treatment was interrupted 1-2 times to let the patients to cough and clean the bronchial tree of sputum. Several respiratory and lab tests were performed to fully analyze the impact of massage treatment.

In 87% of patients, different abnormalities in the respiratory function were detected after the surgery. After treatment the authors observed the following positive changes: the decreasing of respiratory rate by 5-6 breaths per minute with the restoration of its normal depth; the tidal volume increased on 8%; the tidal capacity increased up to 11%; inspiratory reserve volume increased on 15-20%; capillary PO_2 increased on 4-6 mmHg. All these positive changes significantly speed up the patients' recovery and completely eliminated any pulmonary complications.

Beal, (1985) recommended **neuromuscular therapy** for the treatment of somatic dysfunctions caused by **chronic asthma**. The author recommended gentle introductory pressure on all detected areas of viscero-somatic reflexes followed by increased pressure after the superficial spasm and tension are reduced.

Ebner, (1985) used connective tissue massage for the treatment of patients with **dyspnea** (i.e., difficulty in breathing) caused by pulmonary disorders. The author reported that after treatment all patients start to breath more freely, deeply and regularly without visible difficulties. Similar effects were registered after segment-reflex massage (Glezer and Dalicho, 1955; Vasichkin, 1991) and periostal massage (Vogler and Krauss, 1975; Fokin, 1997).

Kuznetsov, (1979) and (1987) studied the effect of therapeutic and **asymmetric reflex massage** on the **acid-base balance** of patients with pulmonary disorders. In 1987 study all 64 patients had restrictive (i.e. tumor, bronchiectasis) or obstructive (i.e. chronic bronchitis, asthma, emphysema) pulmonary diseases. Thus, patients showed signs of hypoventilation and therefore had different degrees of respiratory acidosis, i.e. the decreasing body pH. Respiratory acidosis is a result of accumulation of excessive H^+ which is caused by lower blood oxygenation and insufficient H^+ elimination by the lungs.

61% of patients had compensatory respiratory acidosis. In such cases the insufficient pulmonary control of the acid-base balance was partly normalized by the increasing of urinary excretion H^+.

After the course of asymmetric segment-reflex massage, all patients showed improvement or complete restoration (in cases of moderate hypoventilation) of the acid-base balance. pH: 7.36 ± 0.003 before treatment (normal value = 7.40) and 7.40 ± 0.005 in 2 hours after the treatment. PCO_2: 39 ± 0.45 before treatment (normal value = 38) and 36 ± 0.63 alter. PO_2: $76\ 3 \pm 0.63$ before treatment (normal value = 80) and 80 ± 0.84 alter.

Based on the results of many years of studies, Dr. Kuznetsov concluded that massage is able to: enforce the elimination excessive H^+ through the lungs, increase blood oxygenation, and unload the kidneys. The last effect is especially important because increased urinary excretion of H^+ is the only one compensatory mechanism which supports the normal body pH in the patients with chronic pulmonary disorders. Unfortunately this mechanism is less effective compared to the balance of pH provided by the healthy lungs. Thus, massage is able to support the kidneys' function and therefore helps to normalize the acid-base balance.

The author also made the following practical recommendation: in cases of acute pulmonary disorder or relapse of chronic pathology, any type of massage treatment should start only on the 8-10th day. At this point the clinical symptoms have usually been calmed down by the medications and patients are able to handle the massage treatment well. The author additionally pointed out that therapeutic or segment-reflex massage are obligatory components of every treatment of pulmonary disorders.

Beeken, et al. (1998) examined the therapeutic impact of **neuromuscular massage** on 5 patients with chronic obstructive lung diseases (i.e. chronic bronchitis, emphysema, etc.). The authors measured 8 basic parameters of cardiac and pulmonary system functions during the 24 weekly treatments. Four patients showed significant improvement with increases in thoracic gas volume, peak flow and forced vital capacity. Besides this, saturation of the arterial blood and time of breath hold also significantly improved. Authors concluded that neuromuscular therapy improves pulmonary function, increases respiratory muscles strength and quality of life of patients with obstructive lung disorders.

Field, et al. (1998) examined effect of massage therapy on children with **asthma**. Patients in the clinical group (16 children) had regular massage treatment before bedtime for 30 days, delivered by their previously trained parents. The massage therapy included stroking and kneading techniques. Patients in the control group (16 children) had progressive muscle relaxation therapy under the same conditions.

Younger children (4-8 years old) from the clinical group showed the greatest improvements: the level of anxiety decreased dramatically; significant decrease of cortisol level was detected (from 1.2 to 0.8); forced vital capacity increased up to 24%; forced expiratory volume increased up to 27%; forced expiratory flow (FEF) increased up to 57%; peak expiratory flow rate increased up to 30%. The older children (9-14 years old) of the clinical group also exhibited signs of anxiety decrease, but among the pulmonary tests only FEF showed significant improvement of up to 57%.

The authors pointed out the importance of this particular parameter for the function of lungs affected by the asthma. FEF reflects the conditions of the air flow through the small airways which are mostly blocked by asthma. Thus, the authors concluded that daily massage normalizes the tone of airways, decreases their irritability and significantly improves parents' and children' quality of life by the better control over the asthma.

Zelenkin, et al. (1998) used low frequency vibration massage on patients with acute **maxillary sinusitis** alone and in its combination with **ethmoiditis**. Vibratory massage was performed daily over the area of projection of maxillary and ethmoidal sinuses. Clinical and immunological evaluation of results showed the positive dynamic in all patients with complete elimination of inflammation in the cells of the ethmoidal labyrinth detected by X-ray. The authors emphasized the effectiveness of treatment, its low cost and simplicity (i.e., it can be done by patients even at home).

Doering, et al. (1999) examined the effect of manual vibration massage over the thorax on 8 patients in intensive care unit after coronary artery bypass surgery (2 subjects), heart (3 subjects), and lung (3 subjects) transplantation. The authors found that percutaneous O_2 saturation was increased from 92% to 93.6%; central venous pressure was decreased by 11%; pulmonary vessels' resistance was reduced by 18.3%; the pulmonary resistance decreased from 10.5 H_2O/1/s to 9.2 H_2O/1/s.

After analyzing these data, the authors concluded that vibratory massage over the thorax improves respiratory function and lung perfusion by significantly decreasing ventilation/perfusion mismatch which plays negative role in the patients' recovery. The authors recommended manual vibration with the frequency of oscillation between 8 and 11 per second.

Fattah and Hamdy (2011) studied the effect of massage therapy on the pulmonary function of 60 children with **bronchial asthma**. The massage was given by previously trained parents every night before sleep for 5 weeks. At the end of the study, the clinical group's Forced Expiratory Flow in First Second was 2.3 ± 0.8 L *versus* 1.9 ± 0.9 L in the control group; the ratio of Forced Expiratory Flow in First Second/Forced Vital Capacity was 92.3 ± 21.5 in the clinical group versus 69.5 ± 17 in the control group ($p<0.01$). Thus the authors concluded that massage therapy improved the key pulmonary functions of the children, with bronchial asthma.

G. DIGESTIVE SYSTEM

The digestive system includes the esophago-gastrointestinal tract and hepato-pancreatic system. The principal functions of the digestive system are digestion and absorption of nutrients. The liver also provides the detoxification, phagocytosis, storage of vitamins A; B_{12}; D; E; K and minerals Fe and Cu.

Light massage strokes on the abdomen are used in all cultures and countries to relieve abdominal pain and discomfort. The first scientific approach was done by Prof. Botkin in 1888. He used massage as an important component of the treatment of patients with gastric and hepatic pathologies. He was the first author who recommended local massage in the epigastric area in the direction of gastric musculature instead of general abdominal massage in cases of gastric disorders.

In 1900 Dr. Kellogg the inventor of cornflakes, recommended abdominal massage with a leather-coated cannon ball to restore bowel movements in cases of constipation (Richards, 1998).

Kalistov, (1930) studied the motor activity of the gastro-intestinal tract during and after massage treatment. The author reported an increase in intestinal peristalsis as well as in the time it took food to pass through the gastro-intestinal tract.

Mattem, (1934) successfully used massage techniques on the upper splanchic region and **liver pump technique** as a part of non-surgical treatment of patients with gastro-duodenal ulcers.

Pogorelova, (1948) conducted a long clinical study on the patients with gastric ulcers. The control group of patients went through the traditional treatment of ulcers and patients in the clinical group additionally got massage treatment. The comparison of X-ray pictures from both groups showed that granulations filled the base of ulcer quicker and final ulcer epithelization occurred earlier in the clinical group compare to the control one.

Rumin, (1950) studied the effect of vibration massage on the gastric secretory activity of patients with **atrophic gastritis**. One of the main pathological symptoms of atrophic gastritis is the decreasing of gastric secretion. After permanent and interruptive vibration in the epigastric area the author registered stimulation of the gastric secretion with an increase its basal and maximal values.

In 1955 Glezer and Dalicho tested the gastric peristalsis using X-rays and acidity of gastric secretion in patients with gastritis and peptic ulcers after a course of **segment-reflex massage**. The authors reported a significant reduction of peristalsis and the normalization of gastric secretion acidity at the end of the treatment. Kunichev, (1985); Predel, (1987); and Vasichkin, (1991) also recommended segment-reflex massage treatment for patients with gastro-intestinal disorders.

Dubrovsky, (1973) studied the effect of abdominal massage on the **biliary secretion** in healthy volunteers. In the clinical group the amount of excreted bile exceeded the control group by 100-200 ml. Later, Matveeva, et al. (1997) used thermal vibromassage on the right epigastric area in cases of **biliary dyskinesia**. The authors registered the restoration of biliary system motility with the drainage of normal amount the bile into intestine. The stable remission persists for 6-8 months.

Kametani, et al. (1979) experimentally proved that **gastric motility** can be stimulated or inhibited by the cutaneous stimulation of different areas of the skin. The experiment was conducted on 20 anesthetized rats. Gastric motility was inhibited after abdominal skin stimulation and was stimulated after hind paw stimulation. After complete spinal cord transection at the cervical level, the facilitated impact of paw stimulation on the gastric motility was abolished, but the inhibitory effect of abdominal skin stimulation was preserved since this is a spinal reflex. The same results were obtained earlier by Sato, A. et al. (1975) after the activation of nociceptive receptors in the abdominal skin of 14 anesthetized rats.

In another study from the same laboratory at the Tokyo Institute of Gerontology Koizumi, et al. (1980) examined the effect of strong mechanical stimuli on **intestinal motility**. With the same experimental protocol, authors detected a so called " inhibitory cutaneo-intestinal reflex" after stroking and pinching of the abdominal area and "facilitatory cutaneo-intestinal reflex" after mechanical stimulation of the upper chest, neck, and forepaws.

The authors considered both reflexes a result of increasing (in the case of inhibitory reflex) or decreasing (in the case of facilitatory reflex) efferent activity of the sympathetic part of the autonomic nervous system. The activation of the skin nociceptors by strong compression in the abdominal area for 20 seconds also showed significant inhibition of peristaltic waves and basal pressure in the duodenum. However, the same stimulation on the neck and chest did not evoke any changes in duodenal motility (Sato and Terui, 1976). Results of these studies should be considered when an appropriate regime of massage treatment is designed for patients with gastro-intestinal disorders.

Ebner, (1985) examined the effect of **connective tissue massage** on patients with gastric disorders. After a course of massage treatment in the area of gastric connective tissue zones, all patients reported decreases in pain, belching and other uncomfortable sensations.

Bashnyak, (1989; 1993) established a new concept of **abdominal massage**. The author conducted numerous clinical studies on 829 patients to determine the effect of massage on different pathologies of the gastro-intestinal system. The author used gastrointestinal endoscopy, rectosigmoidoscopy and ultrasonography before and after the massage treatment.

The gastrointestinal endoscopy showed the following visible changes after the course of abdominal massage in the patients with **chronic gastritis**: stomach walls returned to their normal color because the venous stasis was reduced or completely eliminated; regular motor activity of the stomach and duodenum was restored; there was not any bile reflux from duodenum into the stomach. Similar positive changes (restoration of venous drainage and peristalsis) were detected by the rectosigmoidoscopy in the rectum and sigmoid colon of the patients with **Crohn's disease** and **irritable bowel syndrome**.

Fesmire, (1988) and Odeh, et al. (1990) reported that rectal digital massage was able to immediately terminate **intractable hiccups**. Because of its high effectiveness, all authors recommended the digital rectal massage as a first choice of treatment of intractable hiccups before the prescription of any pharmacological agents.

Field, (1995) examined the effect of massage therapy on 13 children with diabetes. The massage treatment was given by the previously trained parents. Regular massage sessions over the course of a month gave the parents and children a more positive attitude, reduced their stress and at the end of massage treatment helped to decreased the children's blood glucose level from 159mg/dL to 118 mg/dL.

Fokin, (1997) considers general body massage with very light strokes on the abdominal area as an important method of restoration of normal gastro-intestinal peristalsis after abdominal surgery.

Matveeva et al., (1997) used thermal vibromassage in the treatment of children with **biliary dyskinesia**. The authors registered a normalization to the biliary system's mobility while remission which lasted 6 to 8 months.

Aksenova and Romanova, (1998) conducted a clinical study on 80 patients with **chronic gastric ulcers** during the period of recurrence. In all cases the gastric ulcer was complicated by other chronic pathologies of digestive system: chronic hepatitis, cholecystitis or pancreatitis. The authors examined the effect of segment-reflex massage in combination with the stretching of skeletal muscles from the myotomes supported by same spinal nerves as the stomach.

All patients were separated into two groups. The patients from the first group had the traditional modern schema of drug therapy: antibiotics, antacids and H-2 receptor antagonists. The patients from the second group received the segment-reflex massage treatment in combination with stretching of affected skeletal muscles, corresponding diet and sucralfate. A 15-30 sessions course of segment-reflex massage with 30-50 minute treatments every day or every other day was applied. Because all patients had recurrences of acute clinical symptoms the abdominal reflex zones were not involved in the treatment.

The results of the treatment were examined by gastroendoscopy and ultrasound. The healing of gastric ulcers was registered in 85% of patients from the first group and in 83% of patients from the second group. Based on obtained results the authors concluded that segment-reflex massage treatment with muscle stretching in the reflex zone areas should be used as an alternative to drug therapy or in combination with it. In the last case, the segment-reflex massage treatment allows significant reduction of the drug dosages with maintenance of the same therapeutic potential.

Richards, (1998) examined the effect of abdominal massage on 10 patients with chronic **constipation** as a complication of cerebral palsy, Huntington's chorea, multiple sclerosis, irritable bowel syndrome, lung cancer, etc. In all cases the regular bowel movements were restored or improved after course of abdominal massage.

To be effective the treatment should be done daily, best of all at the morning, for at least 10 minutes. The complete course takes usually about 1 month. The author also pointed out the high effectiveness of self-massage by using the tennis ball. The patient rolls the ball over the abdomen following the pathway of large intestine, i.e. from right iliac area up to the right costal margin then across the abdomen to the left costal margin and down to the left iliac area.

Ernst, (1999) also pointed out significant benefits of abdominal massage therapy for the treatment of chronic constipation. The author reviewed several controlled clinical trials. Despite the long history of abdominal massage for the treatment of constipation the clinical interest in this method faded for several decades. It is only recently that this interest is restored. The author concludes that abdominal massage is a promising method of natural treatment for patients who suffer from chronic constipation.

Lämås et al, (2009) conducted a randomized controlled study to examine the effect of abdominal massage on 60 patients with chronic constipation. The control group showed a significant improvement in constipation syndrome (p=.013), abdominal pain syndrome (p=.019), and also had a significant increase of bowel movements compared to the control group (p=.016).

H. URINARY SYSTEM

The kidneys are responsible for the removal of waste products from the body; maintenance of the electrolyte balance; regulation of blood pressure; participation in the body's metabolism and acid-base balance. Massage can be a helpful treatment for patients who suffer from some disorders of the urinary system.

Sister Elizabeth (1966) used paravertebral effleurage strokes from the parietal area of the head to the sacrum at a speed of about 60 strokes per minute for at least 3 minutes to promote **urinary retention** in poststroke patients.

Griffith and Hansell, (1925); Zotov, (1981); Kunichev, (1985); Dubrovsky and Dubrovsky, (1995) reported increased diuresis after intensive full body massage with simultaneous stimulation of nitrogen, urea, P and NaCl excretion.

Kurz, et al. (1978) studied the effect of **lymph drainage massage** on urinary excretion of neurohormones and minerals in 29 patients with chronic lymphedema. The authors founded that excretion of epinephrine increased up to 50%; norepinephrine up to 19%; histamine up to 129%. At the same time the urinary excretion of 17-OH was down by 31%; serotonin by 22% and 5-HIAA by 21%.

Bashnyak, (1993) used **abdominal massage** for treatment of patients with **nephroptosis** (i.e., floating kidney). The author conducted intravenous urography before and after the treatment. After the course of specially designed abdominal massage and visceral manipulations, urograms showed significant improvement in the kidney position and in several cases its complete relocation to the normal anatomical site.

Dubrovsky, (1995) also recommended a combination of segment-reflex massage, abdominal massage and special exercises as a part of the nonsurgical treatment of patients with **nephroptosis**. The author also used back massage with special attention to the lower thoracic and lumbo-sacral areas along with a combination of sauna and increased water consumption as a preventive therapy of development of nephrolithiasis (i.e. urinary calculi).

Witort, (1999) offered a simple treatment of the urinary **stress incontinence syndrome**. The patients should tap the urine bladder reflex zone in the middle of palm with the ring finger of the same hand during every urination. With regular 5-7 day application of this simple procedure the patients are able to strengthen the external urethral sphincter and prevent the urinary stress incontinence.

Raviv et al., (2009) examined the effect of cranio-sacral therapy on the intensity of lower urinary tract symptoms (urinary incontinency) in 28 patients with **multiple sclerosis**. The authors found that patients in the clinical group showed significant improvements in post voiding residual volume, lower urinary tract symptoms, and quality of life compared to the control group ($0.001>p>0.0001$).

I. GENITAL SYSTEM

1. FEMALE GENITAL SYSTEM

The first work on using massage in cases of gynecological disorders was published in Sweden by T. Brandt (1868). He can be considered as a father of **gynecological massage** which is still practiced today in many countries by gynecologists or specially trained massage practitioners. Brandt used the combination of massage influence from the intravaginally placed fingers of one hand and the other hand located on the anterior abdominal wall. Thus, the operator massaged the uterus and ovaries between both hands. This treatment was used in cases of infertility, chronic ovaritis and atony of the uterus.

Later, in the 1930-1940s Kramarenko (1953) improved Brandt's method. The author used a combination of internal (gynecological) massage as it was used by Brandt and external therapeutic massage in the lumbo-sacral and abdominal areas. The author recommended this type of treatment for patients with complications of chronic salpingitis (adhesions in the areas of ovary and fallopian tubes), dysmenorrhea, premenstrual syndrome and uterine retroversion.

The value of this treatment was proved by decades of its clinical application as reported by Kunichev, (1985); Shterngertz and Belaya, (1992). For the same clinical purposes Glezer and Dalicho, (1955) used segment-reflex massage and Ebner, (1985) connective tissue massage.

Makarova, et al. (1998) examined the effect of therapeutic and segment-reflex massage on the skeletal muscles and blood coagulation of 74 women with chronic **salpingo-oophoritis** (i.e., chronic inflammation of fallopian tubes and ovaries). All the women complained about lower abdominal and back pain, fatigue, sleep disturbance, headaches, and fertility problems (57%). During palpation numerous cutaneous trigger points, abnormalities of connective tissue structures as well as hypertonuses and trigger points in the skeletal muscles were detected. The rectus abdominis, iliopsoas, piriformis and gluteus maximus muscles were mostly affected. More than half of the patients (51%) had abnormal position of uterus and restriction of its mobility.

The authors used classical therapeutic massage only on the abdomen (first group); classical therapeutic massage only on lumbo-sacral area (second group); segment-reflex massage in the Glezer/Dalicho reflex zones first on the abdomen and after that on the lumbo-sacral area (third group); and segment-reflex massage in the Glezer/Dalicho reflex zones in the opposite sequence: lumbo-sacral area and abdomen (forth group). In all groups the massage treatment started on 7th day of the menstrual cycle and included 10-12 daily sessions. Results were estimated clinically, by electromyography and by lab tests.

After the massage treatment stopped all patients in the third and forth groups complained about lower back and abdominal pain and discomfort. The physiological position of the uterus was restored in 20% of the patients in the first group, 30% of the patients in the second group, 63% of the patients in the third group and 56% of the patients in the forth group.

The electromyography test showed increased electrical activity in the affected muscles. However, the restoration of electrical properties in the third and forth group was more profound and stable. The difference between the patients of the third and forth groups were also significant. In the third group (abdomen -- lumbo-sacral area) the electrical potentials were increased on average by 48 mkV while in the forth group (lumbo-sacral area -- abdomen) the bioelectric activity increased an average of 120 mkV. Thus, the authors recommended the segment-reflex massage treatment of the patients with chronic, salpingo-oophoritis on the Glezed/Dalicho zones in the sequence: lumbo-sacral area -- abdomen.

Kuznetsov, et al. (1998) also studied the effect of therapeutic massage on 30 patients with chronic salpingo-oophoritis. The massage was conducted every day for 10 sessions (first group). On the second group of patients the authors also used the method of deep therapeutic massage for 5 sessions with 2-3 day breaks. The pain and uncomfortable sensations in the abdomen and lower back disappeared in 40% of patients from first group and in 72% in the second group. The uterus was restored to its physiological position in 33.3 % of first group and 80% of second group. 16.3% of patients from the first group were restored their reproductive function. The same result occurred in 33.3% of patients in the second group.

Valiani et al., (2010) examined the effect of massage therapy on the intensity of menstrual pain in 23 patients with **endometriosis**. The treatment consisted of 20-minute massage sessions in the painful areas on the anterior and lateral surfaces of the abdomen and the lumbo-sacral area. In the clinical group the authors registered an immediate pain relief after massage (34.8%) but interestingly enough the analgesia continued and reached its peak at six weeks after the intervention (65.2%). The statistically significant difference was ($p < 0.001$).

2. MALE GENITAL SYSTEM

Massage for the treatment of male sexual dysfunctions was used back in ancient time and is still in actual use today as well. Sexual massage is used by sex therapists and psychologists with the help of specially trained female massage practitioners. With appropriate psychological and drug support it is an effective type of therapy.

Another important type of massage application for male genital disorders is **prostatic massage** through the anterior wall of the rectum. This type of massage treatment is still an important part of modern treatment of prostatitis in many countries. However, as it pointed out by Nickel, et al. (1999) prostatic massage disappeared from the American medical scene approximately 30 years ago. Until recently it was only anecdotal experiences but the author concluded that prostatic massage slowly coming back and more and more North American urologists have interested in its clinical possibilities.

There are two approaches to the prostatic massage: diagnostic and therapeutic. The **diagnostic prostatic massage** is used to confirm diagnosis and detect inflammatory or neoplasmic disorders in the prostate. **Therapeutic prostatic massage** is used as a medical treatment procedure of chronic prostatitis in combination with other therapeutic modalities. Both approaches have the same massage protocol but different goals. The prostatic massage is usually conducted by the physician, the physician assistant or a specially trained massage practitioner.

a. Diagnostic Prostatic Massage

Bologna, et al. (1988) used prostatic massage to confirm diagnosis of **prostatic carcinoma** by harvesting abnormal cells from prostatic fluid. The authors concluded that prostatic massage is a much safer and effective procedure than the commonly used rectal needle biopsy especially for the early diagnosis of the neoplasm.

Sahin, et al. (1992) studied the effect of prostatic massage on the serum levels of acid prostatic phosphatase (PAP) and prostatic specific antigen (PSA) in patients with prostatic **benign hypertrophy** and metastatic **prostate carcinoma**. Six patients with urinary lithiasis served as control group. PAP and PSA are serum markers which allow doctors to estimate the development, results of treatment and prognosis for patients with prostate carcinoma. The authors found that both markers were significantly increased in the group of patients with benign hypertrophy and in the control group and returned to normal values in 48 hours. Thus, serum levels of both markers in cases of suspected carcinoma have to be evaluated only after 48 hours after prostatic massage. In such a case the real diagnostic picture can be detected.

Dolivo, and Askienazy, (1993) examined the value of prostatic massage for detection of *Chlamydia Trachomatis* in the male urethra. This microorganism is one of the major causes of chronic prostatitis and male infertility and frequently still stays undetected during the ordinary procedure of urethral swabbing.

The authors examined 105 men by urethral swabbing with following collection of urine and by collecting prostatic fluid after the massage. The *Chlamydia Trachomatis* was detected in 22 samples. In 9 patients the infection was detected by both methods of material collection but in 13 patients the result was positive only after the collection of prostatic fluid after the prostatic massage. The swabbing did not show any signs of Chlamydial infection in these same patients. The authors concluded that prostatic massage is highly effective diagnostic method for chronic, hidden forms of Chlamydial infection.

Hennenfent and Feliciano, (1998) also used the prostatic massage as a diagnostic tool to detect the changes in the white blood cell counts in the prostatic fluid of 35 men with genitourinary disorders.

Fahmy, et al. (1999) suggested another useful application of prostatic massage. To perform the artificial fertilization in case of **anejaculation**, the authors obtained the necessary spermatozoa after the vigorous prostatic massage. Spermatozoa were immediately used for intercytoplasmic injection in oocyst or cryopreserved for the future. The authors concluded that prostatic massage is a very helpful method of obtaining spermatozoa in cases of primary anejaculation.

b. Therapeutic Prostatic Massage

The therapeutic prostatic massage used as an important therapeutic component of treatment of **chronic prostatitis**. Its goals are: mechanical stimulation of receptors in the prostate; activation of arterial circulation and venous-lymphatic drainage in the prostate and surrounding tissues; and stimulation of prostate secretion. All these effects significantly reduce the chronic inflammation if prostatic massage is conducted 2-3 times per week for a total number of 10-15 sessions (Vasichkin, 1991). The course of massage can be repeated after 2-3 weeks break.

The prostatic massage is best conducted with the patient lying on the right side with his knees bent up to the chest. The necessary condition is full urine bladder which keeps the prostate from displacement during the massage treatment. The massage procedure usually takes only 1-2 minutes. The operator works from the peripheral parts of the prostate to its center to support prostatic fluid drainage (Dubrovsky, and Dubrovsky, 1995).

J. MASSAGE THERAPY DURING PREGNANCY

Pregnant women receive a great benefits from massage therapy. More and more women have begun to use massage during pregnancy to eliminate its negative symptoms.

Hedstrom and Newton, (1986) compared the application of touch during labor in different cultures and eras. The authors concluded that touch in the form of massage during labor is one of the most popular remedies for the pain and relief of muscle tension during contractions. At the same time in the USA, touch during the labor is used mostly as hand-holding between women and her partner. The authors also enumerated main massage techniques for pain relief during labor:

1. Effleurage.
2. Firm pressure on the lower back.
3. Firm and energetic frictions on the lower back.
4. Stroking of arms and legs.

As I already mentioned above Kaaja and Tiula, (1989) used lymph drainage massage for the treatment of the **nephrotic syndrome** during pregnancy. The authors considered 2-4 weekly massage sessions with a duration of 1-1.5 hours enough to control edemas caused by the nephrotic syndrome.

Stillerman, (1992) described the main benefits of maternity massage: decreasing the accumulation of everyday mental and emotional stress and anxiety; reducing the muscle tension of the upper and lower back muscles; increasing the tone of the overstretched abdominal and gluteal muscles; support of lymph drainage; increasing the general blood circulation and red cell count; stabilizing the hormonal levels.

Cox, (1994) considered the balancing effect on the hormonal state of the pregnant women as an important benefit of massage therapy. The normalization of the increased levels of thyroid and adrenal hormones eliminates or reduces a lot of discomforts of the pregnancy: irritability; "hot flashes"; tachycardia; tachypnea; and peripheral edemas.

Shipman, et al. (1997) examined the effect of antenatal (i.e. before delivery) **perineal massage** on 861 pregnant women who had delivery in the Watford General Hospital, England. Each woman in the clinical group performed perineal massage 3-4 times per week for 4 minutes, starting 6 weeks before estimated date of delivery.

The authors registered decreases of second and third degrees perineal tears to 69% in clinical group compared to 75% in control group. Besides this a decrease in the rate of instrumental deliveries was also detected: 34% in clinical group compared to 40% in the control group. The mothers over the age of 30 received mast benefits from the perineal massage because of the natural decreasing of soft tissues' elasticity.

The authors concluded that this simple procedure prevents complications during and after labor; significantly improves women's health and recuperation; and reduces the cost of the treatment. The same results were obtained earlier by Avery, and Van Arsdale, (1987) alter a study on a smaller number of women (55 subjects).

In 1999 Labercque, et al. also examined the effectiveness of perineal massage as a preventive measure to reduce complications during labor on 493 women compared to control group of 1034 women who did not use perineal massage during the pregnancy. The study was conducted in 5 hospitals of the Quebec province of Canada. In the clinical group there were registered 9.2% more vaginal births with intact perineum compared to the control group.

The general recommendations for perineal massage are: 5-10 minutes every day or every other day. Perineal massage can be performed by the woman or her partner using appropriate amount of lubricant over the perineum and lower vaginal wall. The woman should place her 3rd finger on perineum and thumb inside the vagina, slightly compress tissue and stroke from side to side. These strokes should alternate with gentle compression and vibration over perineum.

Geranmayeh et al., (2012) studied the effect on perineal massage during the second stage of labor on the integrity of perineum and rate of episiotomy. The authors found that even such a late application of perineal massage significantly reduced perineal trauma ($P = 0.004$) and rate of episiotomy ($P < 0.001$).

Field, (1998) examined the effect of massage (clinical group) on pregnant women versus relaxation therapy (control group). After the treatment all women from the clinical group experienced lower anxiety and depression; had lower stress hormone levels (i.e. norepinephrine and cortisol); had fewer sleep problems and less pain in the lower back and legs; and lower prematurity rate. The positive influence of massage was also detected during labor: the massaged women needed less medication; their labor period was shorter; they had a lower rate of postpartum depression and stayed in the hospital fewer days. The author explained the phenomenon of labor facilitation by the possible stimulation of oxytocin production caused by pregnancy massage.

Findley and Chamberlain, (1999) reported that 90% of surveyed women considered massage during the labor as a major tool of pain relief. The authors pointed out the importance of paravertebral massage strokes from the level T10 to sacral area. According to the "gate control" theory of the pain, firm massage on these areas will block pain impulses produced during the contractions.

Mortazavi et al., (2012) examined the effect of massage as an alternative tool to control the intensity of pain during labor and the level of anxiety in 120 women. The clinical group received strong and rhythmic 30-minute massages during the three stages of labor. After a massage at each stage, pain and anxiety level were measured. The authors found that women in the massage group were in a lower pain and anxiety state at each stage in comparison with the control group ($p < 0.05$).

Massage has very important benefits for breast-feeding mothers. Sister Angela Murdaugh and Miller, (1997) summarized their recommendations on how to correctly use massage for increasing lactation. The authors described 3 major components of breast massage: opening of the lacteal ducts; alternate massage; manual expression.

1. Opening of the Lacteal Ducts

This part of breast massage should start during the first days of milk production before the actual breast feeding. It can be conducted by the woman or massage practitioner by applying squeezing massage strokes directed from the upper portion of the breast to the nipple.

2. Alternate Massage

Alternate massage is performed by women during feeding (see Fig. 1). This procedure includes emptying of alveoli first from the upper medial part of the breast (area #1) then from the upper lateral part (area #2) and finally from lower sector of the breast (area #3).

3. Manual Expression

Manual expression is also performed by the mother before the feeding to soften the nipple and after the feeding to completely empty the breast of the milk which baby did not use. If a woman correctly performs all three parts of breast massage she can stimulate lactation for a longer period of time and save herself from congestion of the milk in the breast and inflammatory complications.

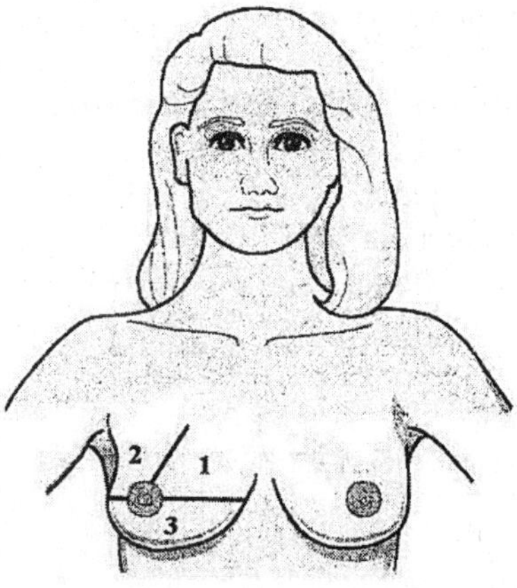

Fig. 1. Correct sequence of alternate massage on the right breast

Ahn et al., (2011) found that when breast massage is started as soon as possible, it greatly reduces the intensity of breast pain ($p < .001$), increases the number of times newborns suckled after the first and second massage ($p < .001$), and decreases the concentration of sodium in breast milk ($p = .034$).

K. MASSAGE IN PEDIATRICS

Massage plays a significant role in pediatrics. It is an extremely important method of supporting and stimulating the health and development of pre term and full-term infants.

Prof. Maksimovich-Ambodik back in the 1800s was the first scientist who persistently recommended massage for stimulating development of pre term infants. Thanks to his authority massage therapy is still a valuable part of modern pediatric throughout all republics of the former Soviet Union and other East European countries.

The massage for full-term and premature infants can be done by the professional massage practitioner and/or by the parents. As correctly pointed by Stillerman, (1992): "Babies need touch to survive" and "... massage enhances all characteristics of bonding between infant and parents".

Belaya, (1974) offered following explanation of the benefits of massage therapy for premature and full-term infants. The infant, in contrast with an adult, has a larger skin surface compared to its body mass. Thus, massage forms the greater afferent nervous input to the central nervous system which accelerates the child's verbal, mental and emotional development. The author pointed out the common psychological phenomenon: the child always produces the first verbal reactions during the light touch and effleurage of the abdomen and legs.

White-Traut and Goldman, (1988) examined effect of 10 minutes of massage and 5 minutes of rocking on 33 healthy premature infants. The authors pointed out the importance of the right selection of infant and procedure for the massage treatment. The following conditions should met:

1. Massage has to start before feeding. In this case infant is more alert and active during the feeding and able to consume and digest more food. This is an extremely important matter which speeds up the infant's development.
2. If an infant exhibits any negative reactions during massage of some particular areas these areas should be avoid. If the infant still exhibits negative reactions for more than one minute, massage should be discontinued.

3. An infant can exhibit delayed autonomic responses to massage (e. g. vomiting). Thus, the infant should be watched after a session is completed.

Vasichkin, (1991) pointed out the importance of **infant massage** for speeding of child's physiological and mental capability. As it is known, the infant has increased tonus of muscle-flexors on the upper and lower extremities compared to muscle-extensors. Later, after 3 months, balance between flexors and extensors is established. This is a first critical step to future walking. The massage therapist should relax the group of flexors and stimulate muscle-extensors during the treatment. Children who received regular massage during the first 3-4 months obtain balance between these muscle groups earlier. It allows them to sit, walk and even talk sooner.

A lot of interesting results on the matter of massage in pediatric practice were reported by T.M. Field from Touch Research Institute at the Miami School of Medicine. At this point she is the leader of scientific exploration of massage benefits in USA. In 1996 Field, et al. examined the effect of massage therapy on the 40 healthy infants. Children in the clinical group got 15 minutes of massage therapy by their previously trained mothers for 12 days over six weeks. In the control group only rocking was performed. Children in the clinical group cried less, slept better, gained more weight, showed signs of better emotional and sociable development. Lab tests showed lower salivary cortisol levels, decreased urinary excretion of norepinephrine and epinephrine, and increased levels of serotonin. Thus, the author pointed out that massage had significant benefits on the health and development of healthy infants by reducing their stress level.

In an earlier report authors Kuhn, et al. (1991) showed that urine epinephrine and norepinephrine levels are increased in premature infants after massage therapy. This is a clear indication of the stimulation of the sympathetic nervous system which increases infant's maturation.

In 1998 Dr. Field conducted another important clinical study on the effect of massage therapy on premature infants. Each infant from the clinical group got 15 minutes of massage 3 times per day for 10 days while each subject was still in an incubator in the neonatal intensive care unit. In the control group, premature infants got regular treatment. The subjects from the clinical group gained 47% more weight compared to the children from the control group. They also stayed in the hospital for 6 fewer days with cost savings of $10 000 per patient. The author detected increased norepinephrine and epinephrine levels in the patients from the clinical group. This allows Field to conclude that stimulation of these hormones production by massage therapy caused detected effects. The author followed both groups during the first year of their life. Children from the clinical group still had weight prevalence and they showed significant improvement in the mental and motor development compared to patients from the control group.

Thomsen and Koltai, (1989) examined the effect of massage in combination with passive stretching on **strernomastoid tumor of infancy**. This perinatal disorder is fibrosis of sternomastoid muscle which is visible as firm, painless spindle-like mass usually located in the distal 1/3 of affected muscle. It occurs frequently, about 4 cases per 1000 births. Some cases of sternomastoid tumor spontaneously regress; however without the proper medical attention torticollis can develop with head tilt to the affected side, neck torsion and facial deviation.

After the establishing diagnosis of sternomastoid tumor the authors applied two daily massages of the distal end of the affected muscle with following passive stretching by bending and turning head to the opposite side. In all 7 cases fibrotic masses in the sternomastoid muscles disappeared within 6 weeks after start of the therapy. Thus, the authors considered massage and passive stretching as a valuable conservative treatment of this disorder which should be performed as early as possible before any decisions about surgical intervention are made.

Larsen, (1990) considered massage as an ultimate help for **infants' colic**. The author recommended training the parents on this matter. Belly massage should start with very gentle clockwise circular strokes around navel. As circles become larger, massage strokes should become more firm. For the next part the parent should massage along the course of the colon starting at 8 o'clock, passing 12 and finishing at 5 o'clock. At the end the parent can lift one or both legs to the belly and/or make a circular movements. The author recommended to start the massage 15-30 minutes after the meal. Massage relaxes the smooth muscles of intestine by the activation of cutaneo-visceral reflex with a subsequent decrease of flatus and increase of feces passage. Whole body massage should start only after the belly massage is done with appropriate amount of oil.

Dietz, et al. (1990) discussed the effect of mobilization and massage on 5 patients with **reflex sympathetic dystrophy**. This type of pathology affects mostly adults but the authors described 5 cases which where diagnosed in children. The main clinical symptoms are: severe pain, vasomotor instability with trophic changes of soft tissues, osteoporosis and contractures in joints. The typical treatment includes complete immobilization in a cast, analgesic and anti-inflammatory medications, and surgery (i.e., sympathectomy) recommended in cases of conservative therapy failure. The authors used the combination of weight bearing, light exercise and massage 3 times per day.

To formulate a massage therapy protocol authors used the "gate control" theory of the pain with idea of inhibition pain analyzing system through the stimulation of large afferent fibers (see below in the Chapter III. In four cases the patients had complete recovery and stayed asymptomatic during a follow-up period of 14.5 months. In one case, a 14-year old girl had several relapses but they were successfully controlled by the discussed therapy and she still had only mild pain and discomfort during the following 9 months.

Guzzetta et al., (2011) reported important findings of a clinical study conducted on brain development in pre-term infants who where treated with massage therapy. The massage started 10 days after birth and continued for two weeks. Using electroencephalography the authors detected an increase in brain maturation in the group where massage was used. The authors concluded that massage affects the maturation of the brain's electrical activity in a way which is similar to that observed in utero-term infants.

L. MASSAGE IN DERMATOLOGICAL PRACTICE

Massage can be used only as an important therapeutic component of treatment of noninfectious dermatological disorders. The benefits of massage in the treatment of dermatological disorders are more significant when the nervous system is involved into pathogenesis of disease, for example, psoriasis, neurodermatitis, etc.

The first successful medical application of massage in dermatological practice was made by the French physician L. Brocq (1907). He offered a special type of massage treatment he called massage-mobilization on patients with **scleroderma**. Later this treatment became known as a **Brocq's method**. The author recommended pressing one or both palms tight against the skin in the affected areas and stretching tissues in different directions between both hands. The hand(s) has to move with the skin. At the end the operator has to try to create the fold of skin in the areas of cutaneous fibrosis.

Kramarenko, (1953) highly recommended therapeutic massage for the treatment of **eczema**. The author observed positive results in some cases when even drug therapy did not help the patients. He offered following a protocol of treatment on the example on the eczema of the hand: the whole upper extremity, excluding hand; massage along the pathways of major nerves; the area of eczema (slow effleurage, gentle kneading and light percussion by fingertips); the whole upper extremity, excluding the hand; the energetic friction, deep kneading and compression on the cervical and upper thoracic back; vibration on the paravertebral areas.

One of the most frequent clinical symptoms which accompanies a lot of dermatological disorders is **pruritis** or itching. Generalized pruritis can be also one of the symptoms of more serious inner organ pathologies: hepatitis, hyperthyroidism, lymphoma, etc. Pruritis is a very unpleasant sensation which produces the desire to scratch. Persistent scratching to relieve the itching sensation causes different secondary dermatological lesions or cutaneous infections. Thus, the control of itch especially generalized pruritis is a very significant problem.

Mezlack and Schester, (1965) conducted an important experimental study on this matter. The authors examined the effect of vibration massage on the **itching sensation** on 50 healthy individuals. To produce the itch authors applied cowage to the flexor surface of the wrist joint. After subjects reported a desire to scratch, vibration massage was applied to the stimulated area (wrist joint), to the flexor surface of the forearm, and to the opposite wrist joint. In all groups the intensity of itch was reduced. However the complete block of the itching was obtained only if vibration massage was applied to the itch stimulated area and to the opposite wrist.

The authors offered the following explanation of the itch reducing effect of vibration. The vibration stimuli have the dual, opposite effect on the itch (i.e., stimulation-inhibition). The C fibers which are activated by the vibration facilitate the conductance of the itch sensation to the CNS. At the same time the vibration activates A fibers which stimulate substantia gelatinosa in the spinal cord with the following inhibition of conductance of sensory impulses (i.e. itch) to the CNS. However, the number of low threshold A fibers activated by the vibration is much larger than the number of activated C fibers. Thus, the overall effect of vibration on the itch sensation is inhibitory. Because the substantia gelatinosa accepts impulses from the both sides of body, the vibration massage on the opposite non-stimulated wrist will also inhibit the itching sensation on the stimulated wrist.

Patino et al. (1999) registered significant decrease of pruritis by massage therapy in the areas of hypertrophic scars after severe burns.

Kunichev, (1985); Vasichkin, (1991); and Dubrovsky, and Dubrovsky, (1995) recommended segment-reflex massage for the patients who suffer from **psoriasis**. All authors agreed that massage treatment should be applied only during periods of stable remission to prevent relapses. The actual areas of psoriatic lesions do not undergo the massage treatment. The correct application of segment-reflex massage significantly decreases the frequency of psoriatic relapses.

Antoniyev and Belova, (1985) examined the effect of a combined treatment consisting of therapeutic massage, segment-reflex massage, self-massage by the patients and physical therapy on 123 patients with chronic **eczema, neurodermatitis** and **psoriasis**. The results of treatment were estimated after 12-13 months. During the period of treatment the frequency of relapses compared to the previous year decreased for the patients with chronic eczema in 4.1 times; for the patients with the neurodermatitis in 3.7 times; and for patients with psoriasis in 5.2 times. In 65.7% of the patients the pruritis was completely eliminated. The authors defined the primary goals of massage therapy on the patients with chronic noninfectious dermatologic disorders as: the stimulation of blood circulation and lymph drainage in the affected areas of the skin, the regulation of central nervous system to suppress the pruritis, and decreasing the frequency of relapses.

Vasichkin, (1991) recommended Nikolsky's method of psoriasis treatment. The main difference of this technique is the use of massage directly on the psoriatic lesion. In small areas the operator places the tip of the thumb on the one side of the lesion and the rest of fingers on the opposite side. The fingertips have to be placed tight against the skin exactly on the borders of normal and pathologically changed areas of the skin. With spread fingers, the operator stretches the area of psoriatic lesion and brings the fingers close together with a rhythm of about 50-60 changes per minute for 3-5 minutes. If the lesion is large a two hand variant of this treatment recommended. It is best if this type of treatment is performed in a direction perpendicular to the lines of cleavage.

Putt, et al. (1994) reported a case study treatment of 16-year old patient with **alopecia areata**. Alopecia areata is sudden hair loss which is caused by an autoimmune conflict. During the course of disease the patient's body forms antibodies against its own hair follicles with the following hair loss. Stress is considered one of the possible mechanisms that triggers autoimmune reactions. From this point of view the authors conducted 7 months of treatment which included 2 behavioral techniques (relaxation and a reward program) and 10 minutes daily scalp massages. The patient had this disorder from the age of 12 and had previously received all possible methods of modem treatment without any significant improvement.

At the beginning of the discussed treatment the patient had two completely bald areas on his head: 78 x 55 mm on the left side and 94 x 61 mm on the right side. At the end of the treatment the bald area on the left side was 58 x 45 mm and on the right side was 87 x 63 mm. One year after the beginning of treatment the patient did not have any bald areas and his normal hair production was restored. Because only one case was examined the authors did not draw any conclusions from the obtained result. However they pointed out the importance of further studies on these simple but highly successful (for this patient) methods of treatment.

Dubrovsky and Dubrovsky, (1995) used the following schema of treatment of severe pruritis: back massage along the paravertebral areas (deep friction, kneading and vibration); permanent vibration strokes on the every areas where the patient feels the pruritis; ice cube massage in the areas of the most severe itching sensation.

Field, (1995) examined effects of massage therapy on children with **psoriasis** and **allergic dermatitis**. The author registered reduced stress levels and positive impacts on the immune system. However author concluded that more studies need to be done in regard to this matter.

Schachner, et al. (1998) recommended massage to reduce the symptoms of chronic **atopic dermatitis** in children. The study was conducted on 20 children: a control group (10 subjects) was treated by standard medical care (i.e. emollients and topical corticosteroids) and clinical group (10 subjects) was additionally treated by 20 minute daily massages by the trained parents for 1 month.

The results were estimated by the dermatologists who were blind to the child's group assignment. The following clinical parameters were estimated focally and globally: redness, lichentification, scaling, excoritaion and pruritis. Clinical and statistical evaluation of the obtained results showed that all tested parameters significantly improved in the clinical group. In the control group only scaling improved after one month of treatment. Because of a strong correlation between atopic dermatitis and stress accumulation, the authors explained the therapeutic impact of massage therapy by the decreasing anxiety level and stimulation parasympathetic part of the autonomic nervous system with the resulting peripheral vasodilation. The result of this study are very important because approximately 22.5% of the general population have different forms of allergic reactions: dermatitis, asthma, atopic rhinitis, etc. (Diepgen and Fartasch, 1992).

Roh et al (2007) studied the effect of rehabilitative massage on **scars** and depression level of burn victims. The authors found that burn survivors who were treated with massage exhibited lesser pruritus, improved skin status, and lesser depression. The remaining scar showed improvement in skin pigmentation, pliability, vascularity, and height (compared to the surrounding skin) as measured on the Vancouver Scar Scale. Similar results were obtained earlier by Patiño et al., (1999).

M. OTHER EFFECTS OF MASSAGE THERAPY

Pedini and Zaietta, (1975) examined the effect of massage on splitting triglycerids in the adipose tissue. The authors found increased level of glycerol in the blood after massage treatment. This is clear evidence of the stimulation of lipolysis in adipose tissue. To chronically enhances lipolysis the massage has to be repetitive. The authors considered the increasing release of catecholamines by tissue nerve endings in the massaged area as a major contributor to observed effect.

Pendini and Zaietta discovered this mechanism by administrating beta-blocking drugs which inhibit cathecholamines secretion. If drugs were administrated before massage session there was not any signs of massage-induced lipolysis in same subjects.

Hemdl, et al. (1984); Becker and Prysi, (1990) recommended **postoperative breast massage** after breast augmentation surgery. This procedure, which consists of daily breast compressions, prevents the development of capsular contracture. This treatment should start approximately 4 weeks after the surgery.

Hsu-Cy, et al. (1995) studied the effect of local massage on adverse reactions and immunogenicity of diphteria-tetanus-pertussis (DTP) vaccine on 327 infants. In the clinical group, local massage of the **vaccination** site was performed. In the control group only the usual protocol of vaccination was administrated. Children in the clinical group showed more adverse reactions compare to the control group: more local pain and higher fever. However these reactions were still mild. At the same time children in the clinical group showed significantly better immunogenicity compared to the control group. The antibody production in both groups was tested at 2, 6, 7, 18, and 19 months of age. Children in the clinical group developed much higher levels of antibodies against filamenous hemagglutinin, petrussis toxin and petrussis agglutinogen compared to the control group. Thus, the authors concluded that local massage at the site of vaccination immediately after the injection significantly stimulated antibody production and child's immunity.

Sullivan, et al. (1997) reported another interesting case study. As a result of accident a 25-year old patient had **tetraplegia** (i.e. paralysis of all 4 extremities) after a complete lesion of the spinal cord on the level C4. One of the additional problem for this patient was increased tension in the laryngeal muscles. This tension was a compensatory reaction to the partial failure of the respiratory muscles to support normal respiration. As a result of this tension the patients had a strained strangled voice along with the normal structure of their vocal folds.

The authors studied the effect of 20 massage sessions on the fundamental frequency of the patient's voice. The patient had a 15 minute massage session 5-times per week on the laryngeal region, face, neck and shoulder muscles. The mean fundamental frequency before massage was 337.75 Hz and after treatment 293.30 Hz or 13% decrease. At the same time the patient reported feelings a 37.8% reduction in perceived regional laryngeal tension after the massage sessions. The authors detected this parameter with the help of a modified visual analogue scale. The authors did not register long-terrn effects, however they concluded that regular massage treatment reduces laryngeal tension, improves the pathologically changed vocal parameters and facilitates the other methods of treatment.

Several studies reported significant increases in the serum concentration of **insulin** after massaging site of its subcutaneous injection for 15-30 minutes. Berger, et al. (1982) examined the effect of temperature, massage, exercises, and changing site of injection on the absorption of insulin from subcutaneous tissues and its biological effect. Only massage and a hot bath dramatically increased serum concentration of insulin during 1.5 hours after the injection.

Dillon, (1983) reported a rise in the free insulin level of 10.14 ± 9.91 microU/ml with a subsequent serum glucose level drop of 8.3% lower than in control study (without massage).

Linde, (1986) registered serum insulin increases in 9 healthy volunteers from 13.8 ± 1.8 mU/L before massage to 56.4 + 8.7 mU/L after massage of the injected site, versus 15.3 ± 3.0 and 19.7 ± 2.2 mU/L during the control study. All the authors highly recommended this simple procedure to increase the effectiveness of insulin therapy for the diabetic patients.

Ueda, et al. (1993) reported the results of the clinical study in which authors examined the effect of gentle epigastric massage on regression of sensory **epidural analgesia** on 16 patients after obstetric and gynecological surgeries. As is known complete sensory restoration after spinal epidural anesthesia sometimes takes several hours. 30 minute epigastric massage significantly ($P < 0.001$) speeded up the regression of analgesia and restored the normal sensory innervation faster.

Trubetskoy, et al. (1998) opened new perspectives of clinical application of massage. The authors examined the effect of massage on the release of subcutaneously injected **liposome encapsulated drugs** to the blood circulation.

Liposomes are highly purified, synthetic membrane spheres made from phospholipids with a size of approximately 1/50 diameter of the human hair. Spherical shape and microsize allow liposomes to easily pass membranes and enter the cells. Different drugs or nutrients can be encapsulated inside liposomes to facilitate their delivery to the targeted tissue or organ. Liposomes with bioactive molecules inside (i.e. drugs) are usually injected intravenously. In such cases the bioactive molecules are released from liposomes gradually and a steady level of drug into blood circulation is supported for a longer time. However, intervenous injection of liposome-encapsulated drug does not provide its sufficient depot in the body. In other words the liposome-encapsulated drugs have to be injected again but less frequently compared to non-liposome forms of the same drug.

Another way of liposome delivery is subcutaneous injection. In this case the depot of liposomes is created in the place of injection but the process of liposome delivery to the blood is extremely slow. Different modalities which were introduced to increase the liposome-encapsulated drugs' release from the subcutaneous tissues into lymph and later into blood circulation included: ultrasound, temperature, electric-, magnetic-, and electromagnetic fiends. However, the release of liposomes from the subcutaneous depot still not sufficient.

The main barrier for this phenomenon is interendothelial gaps between the cells of lymphatic vessel walls. These gaps regulate any transport between the lumen of lymphatic vessel and interstitium (i.e. intercellular spaces). The interstitium-lymphatic transfer depends on the hydrostatic pressure and the size of transporting particles, for example liposomes. Small particles are easily absorbed by the lymphatic system while larger particles stay in the interstitium longer.

From these theoretical speculations the authors decided to examine the rate of release of liposome-encapsulated drug from the subcutaneous tissues after increasing the hydrostatic pressure in the interstitium by massage. The experiment was conducted on 17 rabbits. 200 ml of liposome-encapsulated hormone angiotensin II were injected subcutaneously into a front paw. The size of liposomes was larger than the normal size of interendothelial gaps. It allowed the authors to create permanent deposit of liposomes into subcutaneous tissues. For the experiment the authors used hormone angiotensine II which is a potent vasoconstrictor. Angiotensin II increases the arterial blood pressure and this parameter was recorded before and after a 5 minute massage of the injected side.

The authors detected up to a 40% increase in liposome concentration in the general blood circulation after massage treatment with subsequent increases in arterial blood pressure. These data were also supported by the results of gamma-scintigraphy. The results of this study have an incredibly important future for controlled drug release.

The authors discussed two practical outcomes of this study. One time subcutaneous injection of pain killing drugs encapsulated into liposomes creates its long lasting deposit in tissues. By massaging the place of injection the patient or nurse is able to release a new portion of the drug into circulation as soon as patient needs it. Thus, the patient actually controls the analgesic action of the drug. Diabetic patients on insulin treatment are another group which has significant benefits from this type of controlled release. Instead of regular insulin injections the patients can have one long-lasting subcutaneous shoot of liposome-encapsulated insulin and able to control its release from the depot by the massaging the site of injection.

Hemandez-Reif, et al. (1999) reported a reduction of intensity of **smoking craving** by self-massage. The study was conducted on 20 adult smokers. In an experimental group subjects were conducted self-massage of the hand and car during the craving for 1 month. The self-massaged group exhibited less anxiety, better mood, less intensive withdrawal symptoms and fewer cigarettes per day by the last week of the study. The author concluded that massage therapy can be an important method of adjunct treatment for adults who attempt smoking cessation.

II. PRESSURE AND MECHANISMS OF THE THERAPEUTIC EFFECT OF MASSAGE THERAPY

Massage therapy has a limited arsenal of therapeutic modalities. The massage practitioner can count only on different forms of pressure (including vibration), stretching and the activation of temperature receptors. Between these three modalities pressure is the main therapeutic tool with stretching and temperature receptors' activation playing a supportive role in the treatment. Thus, discussion of mechanisms of the therapeutic effect of massage treatment will refer us mostly to the mechanisms of pressure's therapeutic impact.

Pressure is a physical force which is used by massage practitioner to achieve therapeutic results. Thus, the operator converts the kinetic energy of massage strokes into various physiological phenomenons on tissue and cellular levels (e.g. changes of interstitial pressure) as well as into a chain of electrochemical reactions in the massaged area and whole organism.

The final success of therapeutic or medical massage treatment directly depends on the correct application of pressure. It includes the right combination of proper techniques; the form of application (i.e. permanent or intermittent); speed of application; intensity of application (i.e. light-moderate-deep pressure); and the area of application.

Only after careful evaluation of all these parameters and formulation of the right treatment protocol can a massage practitioner expect stable results from the therapy. If the chosen schema does not work adjustments to the protocol have to be made. Sometimes these adjustments can completely change the initial schema of treatment. One has to remember one important rule: If therapy is unsuccessful, of course in cases when massage is indicated, it means that the practitioner developed the wrong treatment protocol.

A. MECHANISMS OF THERAPEUTIC IMPACT OF MASSAGE THERAPY

The massage treatment has two mechanisms of therapeutic impact: reflex (indirect) effect and local (direct) effect. This classification is very approximate because for example the local mechanism is a component of reflex mechanism. However it makes representation of material easier.

1. INDIRECT, REFLEX MECHANISM OF MASSAGE THERAPY

Reflex therapeutic impact of massage therapy has a complex mechanism. I don't want to take the reader's time with a long discussion on this matter because information about the reflex mechanism of massage treatment already revealed in detail in the *Medical Massage* textbook. However, I want to emphasize one important point. The basic concept of this mechanism is the formation of reflex zones. In the cases of visceral (i.e., inner organ) disorders the reflex zones are formed only after 3 months of medical history of these pathologies. In the cases of somatic pathologies this period is shorter but still takes at least 2-3 weeks. Thus, in the every new cases of somatic disorders the local therapeutic effect of massage treatment is the leading mechanism. Thus, in this book we will concentrate the reader's attention on the local mechanism of massage therapy.

2. DIRECT, LOCAL MECHANISM OF MASSAGE THERAPY

Everyone who practices medical aspects of massage experiences cases when 2-3 sessions eliminate the patient's somatic problem with complete restoration of all affected functions. I don't mean just pain relief, I am talking about actual stimulation of the healing process with obtaining stable therapeutic results - for example in cases epycondylitis, tendinitis, muscular and ligamental injuries and so on. What mechanisms are responsible for such a "miraculous" effect?

If we analyze the information from previous chapter we can enumerate local effects which are proved to play role in therapeutic impact of massage treatment: pain relief; peripheral arterial vasodilation; increase of venous and lymph drainage; stimulation of local metabolism. However, practically all authors agreed that these positive changes have transitory character and slowly faded within 2-3 hours after the end of a session. Thus, to obtain stable therapeutic result the massage practitioner has to perform a course of treatment. If we accept this point of view as ultimately correct we cannot fit cases with rapid stimulation of the healing process into this concept or we should not take them in consideration. However they do exist and demand their explanation. Let us look at the cellular mechanisms which are responsible for the therapeutic effect of massage therapy.

a. Effect of Mechanical Stimuli on Cellular Metabolism. Role of Cytoskeleton

The therapeutic potential of different types of manual therapy started to slowly attract the attention of scientists in the various fields of medicine. If Russian scientists draw their conclusions mostly from the clinical experiments and observations, American scientists draw their conclusions from the experimental models as well. Technical devices with high resolution capacity allowed scientists to obtain important information which revealed mechanisms of physiological and therapeutic impacts of pressure on the cellular and subcellular level. To fully appreciate importance of this information I think it will be helpful to take a short trip into cellular biology and biochemistry.

Every cell composed from cellular membrane and cytoskeleton, cytoplasm with organelles, and nucleus with nucleous (see Fig. 2). The structure and functions of all cellular components are well known and it is not the subject of our discussion. However findings about the cytoskeleton and its relation to external mechanical stimuli applied to the cell are breakthroughs in the understanding of the therapeutic effect of the mechanostimulation of the living cells.

The cytoskeleton is a complex system of fibrillar structures located in the cytoplasm. It can be compared to the human skeleton which provides a frame for our body and its dynamic support. The cytoskeleton gives the cell its form. For example, fibroblast, which is a major repair cell of the body has shape because the fibrils of the cytoskeleton are arranged in a particular way.There are 3 types of fibrils in the cytoplasm which form cytoskeleton: mictotubules, actin filaments and intermediate filaments.

Microtubules

Microtubules have a diameter of approximately 25 nm and build up from protein **tubulin**. During mitosis microtubules form the spindle which pulls double set of chromosomes apart to form two new cells formed from one maternal.

Actin filaments

Actine filament have a diameter of approximately 10 nm and consists of proteins **actin**, myosin and energy source APT. They are a major contractile apparatus of the cell.

Intermediate filaments

Intermidiate filaments have a diameter of 7 nm and form a net throughout all the cytoplasm with especially high density around the nucleus. This net is not flat but a 3-dimensional structure through the entire thickness of cytoplasm. It links cellular organelles, the nucleus and cytoplasmic membrane together to form the cell.

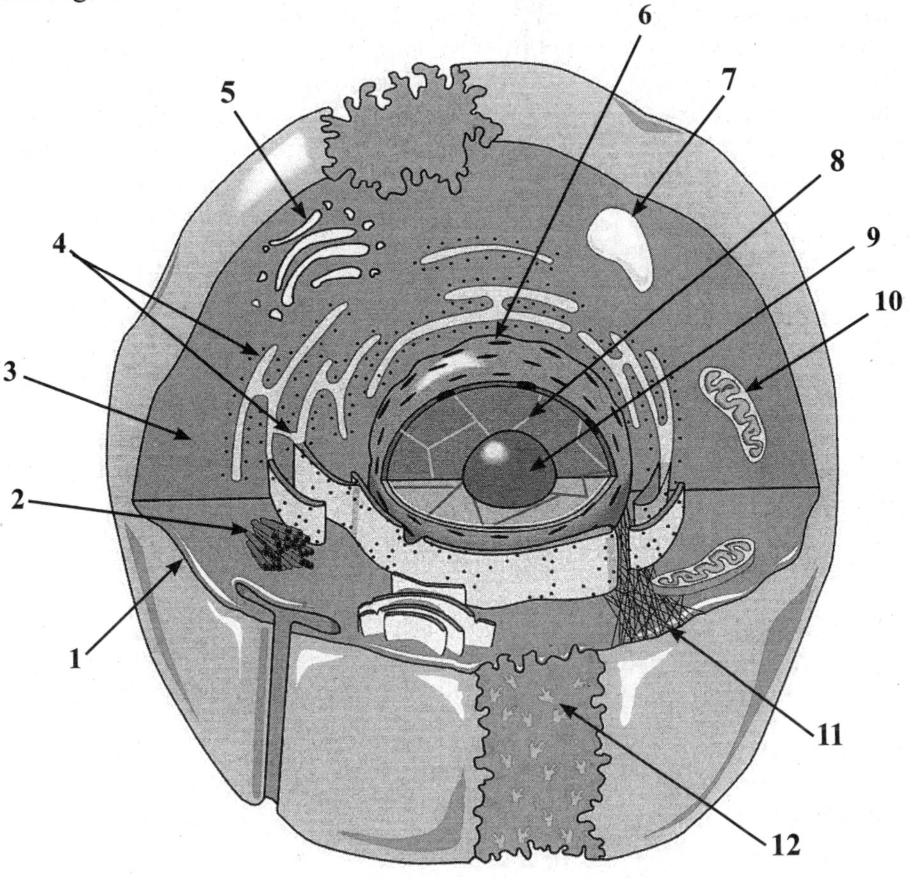

Fig. 2. Structure of the cell

1 - cytoplasmic membrane

2 - centriole

3 - cytoplasma

4 - rough endoplasmic reticulum with ribosomes

5 - Golgi apparatus

6 - nuclear membrane with pores

7 - lysosome

8 - nucleus

9 - nucleous

10 - mitochondria

11 - part of exposed cytoskeleton

12 - cytoplasmic pore

Jain, et al. (1990) in an experimental study on human fibroblasts showed that microfibrils of cytoskeleton have a special arrangement, which is responsible for an increase in intercellular stress in the direction of applied pressure and an decrease of intercellular stress when applied pressure is directed perpendicularly to the main orientation of fibrils in the cytoskeleton.

Opposite to the human skeleton, the cytoskeleton is an extremely dynamic structure. It is in a state of constant changes. The cell is able to completely dissolve and resynthesize the cytoskeleton in several minutes. Fig. 3 shows an electron microscopic picture of the cytoskeleton of a fibroblast.

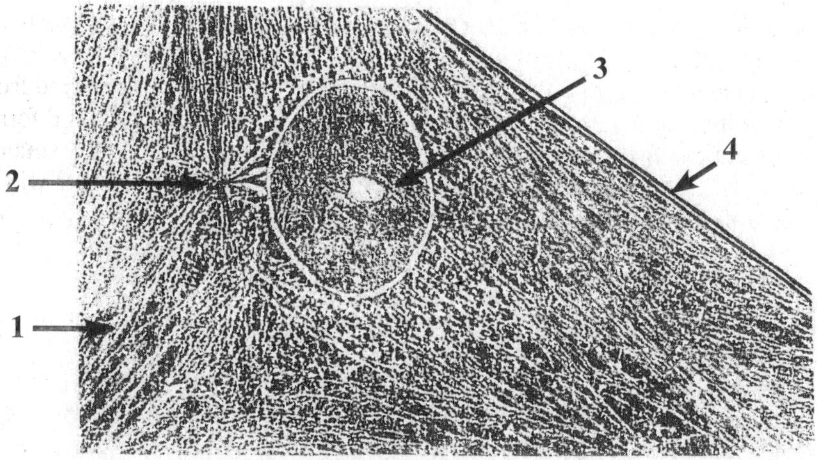

Fig. 3. Electronic microphotograph of cytoskeleton in the perinuclear area of human fibroblast.
1 - cytoskeleton
2 - fibrils of cytoskeleton form the dense structure in the perinuclear area
3 - nucleus with nucleoskeleton
4 - cytoplasmic membrane

From the time of its discovery at the beginning of the 20th century, the cytoskeleton was always viewed as a purely mechanical structure that provides the shape of the cell and participates in cell motility and migration (e.g., leukocytes, natural killer cells, etc.). The cytoskeleton was also viewed as one of the key mechanical components of cell division. However, modem experimental equipment allowed scientists to set up and conduct more detailed studies of the structure and functions of the cytoskeleton. Thanks to these studies, we now know the following functions of the cytoskeleton:

1. Providing the cellular morphology; i.e., shape of the cell.
2. Distribution of the cellular organelles.
3. Intercellular movements of cytoplasm and organelles.
4. Participation in cellular division.
5. Motility of the cell.
6. Control over the cytoplasmic membrane.
7. Connection of the cytoplasmic membrane to the nucleoskeleton and stabilization of the nucleus.
8. The regulation of protein production.
9. Control over genes' expression.

Functions #1-5 were always associated with the cytoskeleton. However, for our discussion, functions #6-9 are extremely important, and their discovery is one of the greatest achievements of modern cellular biology. Of course, we are interested in theoretical conclusions that can be projected on massage therapy and clarify its healing mechanisms. Let's see how the cytoskeleton and, consequently, cellular functions are affected by the external mechanical stimuli.

Control over cytoplasmic membrane

A cytoplasmic membrane surrounds the cells and actively interacts with the environment; i.e., extracellular matrix. It has a thickness of 7.5 nm, or 1/4000 of an inch, and is made up of double layers of phospholipids with integrated proteins. Fig. 4 shows the structure of the cytoplasmic membrane.

The integrated proteins work as gates that connect the external environment and inner part of the cell. Any macromolecules that the cell needs for its metabolism pass into the cell through these gates. They also allow the new synthesized proteins or waste to be secreted from the cell. **Cytoplasmic proteins** occupy approximately 50% of the membrane's mass and form the net of receptors over the entire outer surface of the cytoplasmic membrane. Thus, any outside molecule has to first interact with these receptors to be recognized. Only after this occurs will the gate open up and let macromolecule in.

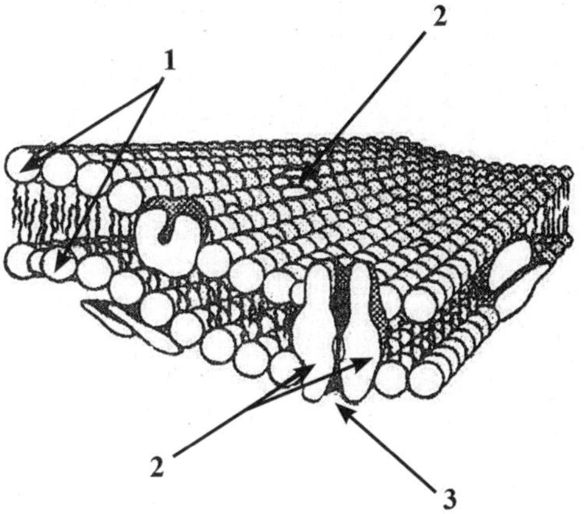

Fig. 4. Structure of cytoplasmic membrane

1 - double layer of phospholipids
2 - protein receptor (gate)
3 - inner part of the gate
4 - outer part of the gate (i.e., enter)

Any mechanical stimuli (e. g., changes in the interstitial pressure) affect the receptors on the cytoplasmic membrane. After exposure to the original stimuli, receptors are able to convert mechanical energy into chemical stimuli that can be conducted inside of the cell. Jain, et al., (1990) concluded that mechanical signals can be converted into chemical signals in the form of **cyclic-AMP**. Komuro, et al. (1991) also pointed out the activation and participation in this process of one of the key enzymes of cellular metabolism, **protein kinasa C**. Not all receptors in the cytoplasmic membrane act as mechanoreceptors. More likely, that one particular family of proteins, called **integrins**, reacts to the mechanical stimulation (Wang, et al., 1993).

The fibrils of the cytoskeleton are deeply anchored in the membrane including the protein receptors. The cytoskeleton has major regulatory control over the function, arrangement and even number of protein receptors incorporated into the membrane. Thus, by regulation of cytoplasmic proteins, the cytoskeleton changes the metabolism of the whole cell by controlling the number and intensity of impulses conducted from the extracellular matrix into the cell (Jain, et al., 1990).

Gataullin and Zaripov, (1988) examined the effect of **colchicin** on the mechanoreceptive ability of single Pacinian corpuscles that were isolated from the mesentery of a cat.

The conchicin is known to be selectively disrupt the intracellular microtubules of the cytoskeleton without any additional damage to the living cell. After the exposure of the Pacinian corpuscles to the colchicine the complete depression of this mechanoreceptor ability to generate action potentials was detected.

The results of this study leave no doubt about the controlling function of the cytoskeleton over the cytoplasmic membrane. The authors tested the single mechanoreceptor cell that normally produces the action potentials after the direct deformation of its cytoplasmic membrane by vibration stimuli. The colchicine disrupted the fibrils of cytoskeleton and, consequently, the Pacinian corpuscle lost its ability to generate action potentials because of interruption of conductance from the cytoplasmic membrane's receptors into the cell.

Connection of the cytoplasmic membrane to the nucleoskeleton

The nucleus stores the vital information of all living objects - DNA. The nucleus is surrounded by its own nuclear membrane, which has pores that open into the cytoplasm and endoplasmic reticulum (see Fig. 2). Through these pores, the permanent interchange of different molecules between the cytoplasm and the nucleus is occurs. The nucleus also has its own **nucleoskeleton** (see Fig. 3). Some authors consider the cytoskeleton and nucleoskeleton as the same continuous structure because of their striking similarity (McKeon et al., 1986). However, even if this hypothesis is wrong, the cytoskeleton still has very high density all around the nucleus (see Fig. 3), and is also able to control the activity of the pores in the nuclear membrane.

One of the most important functions of the cytoskeleton is its ability to conduct information from the cytoplasmic membrane receptors directly to the nucleus, with the following changes in cell growth and proliferation, protein synthesis and genes expression. Every mechanical stimulus which is applied to the living cell affects the mechanoreceptors first. Their activation immediately causes the reorientation of fibrils in cytoskeleton with subsequent nucleus distortion (Maniotis et al., 1977).

Wang et al. (1993) see cytoplasmic receptors, cytoskeleton fibrils and the nucleus as one "hard-wired" structure, where mechanical stimulation of the receptor's site immediately produces deep morphological and biomechanical changes in the whole cell, including the nucleus.

Regulation of protein production and genes expression

After we clarified the relationship between the external mechanical stimuli, receptors, cytoplasmic membrane, cytoskeleton and nucleus, we have to look at how this chain of events affects the cell functions; i.e., proliferation, protein synthesis and genes expression. Let's look on this process on the example of the human fibroblast with the help of Fig. 5.

The external mechanical stimuli activate the receptors in the cytoplasmic membrane of the fibroblast. These mechanical stimuli are converted into chemical signals and cause the reorientation of the cytoskeleton in the direction of the applied force. The cytoskeleton's reorientation causes nucleus distortion, and it responds with increased **DNA synthesis** and **replication** (Curtis and Seehar, 1978; Somjen et al., 1980; Brunett, 1984); increasing the synthesis of messenger-RNA (m-RNA); i.e., **transcription** of information from the replicated DNA (Kumoro et al., 1991).

The newly synthesized chain of m-RNA, which carries identical information about the structure of the original DNA, leaves the nucleus through the pores in the nuclear membrane directly into rough endoplasmic reticulum. Here m-RNA associates with ribosomes and the process of **translation** i.e., protein synthesis starts.

This process is also supported by transport-RNA (t-RNA), which pulls the required amino acids from the cytoplasm to the m-RNA-ribosomal complex and attaches them one by one to the new-synthesized molecule of **procollagen**. This transport of amino acids by t-RNA is also under control of the cytoskeleton (Bereiter-Hahn et al., 1987).

Procollagen which is formed inside of the fibroblast is a direct precursor of **collagen**. Procollagen needs to be secreted from the fibroblast into extracellular matrix, where its conversion into a newly formed molecule of collagen occurs. Thus, mechanical stimuli activate the fibroblasts and stimulate procollagen synthesis which leads to the increasing of collagen and extracellular matrix production at the injured site.

Collagen is the most abundant protein of any life organism and it comprises approximately 1/3 of all proteins in the body (Geneser, 1986). The role of collagen is critical for every living organism because it forms the actual frame of all tissues and inner organs.

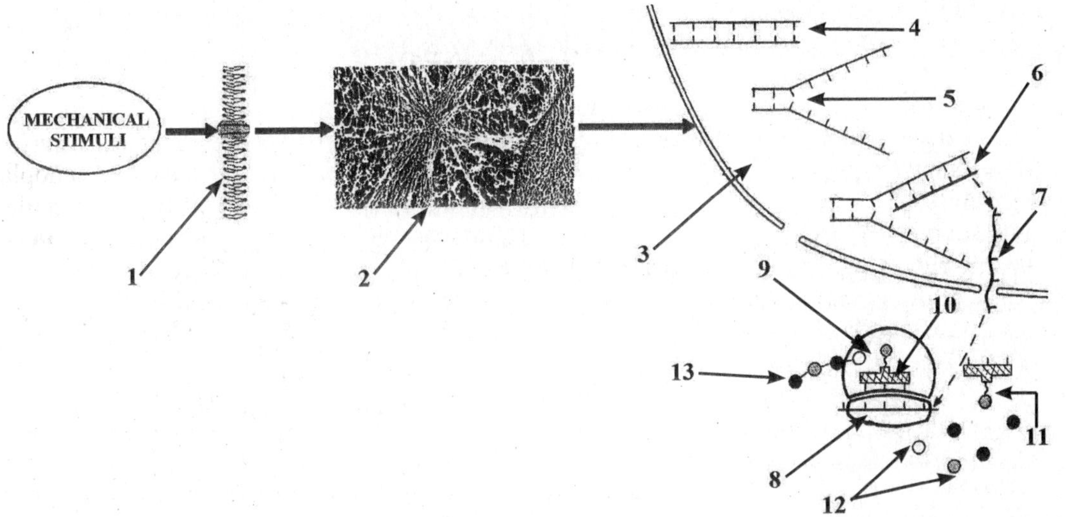

Fig. 5. Chain of events in the fibroblast triggered by the direct application of mechanical stimuli

1 - activation of mechanoreceptors in the cytoplasmic membrane and conversion of mechanical stimuli into chemical signals
2 - conduction of chemical signals by cytoskeleton to the nucleus with its following distortion
3 - nucleus
4 - "passive" double-chained molecule of DNA
5 - activation of DNA molecule by nucleus distortion and following DNA replication, i.e., splitting
6 - transcription of DNA, i.e., reading of DNA sequence and synthesis of messenger RNA(mRNA)
7 - m-RNA leaving nucleus through the pore in the nuclear membrane
8 - m-RNA attached to the ribosome of rough endoplasmic reticulum as a matrix for the future protein synthesis; i.e., translation
9 - ribosome
10 - transport-RNA (t-RNA) brought amino acid to the m-RNA-ribosomal complex
11 - another t-RNA transporting the next amino acid to the new synthesized protein molecule
12 - free amino acids in the cytoplasm
13 - new synthesized molecule of procollagen ready to leave the fibroblast into extracellular space

What practical outcomes of all these events on the cellular level, and how they explain the therapeutic impact of massage therapy?

Leung et al., (1976) reported that smooth muscle cells increased production of **collagen** after the application of mechanical stimuli. However, their proliferation was not detected.

Curtis and Seehar, (1978) showed that mechanical stress stimulates the **DNA synthesis** and division of fibroblasts from chick embryos. The authors detected the increase in the mitotic index in the experimental study up to 5.1 $\pm$ 1.5, versus the same parameter in a control study, 2.3 $\pm$ 0.7. Thus, mechanical signals are able to augment the cells' proliferation (especially fibroblasts), which is very important for the stimulation of the healing process at the site of an injury.

Shirinsky et al., (1989) showed that the mechanical deformation of human **endothelial cells** *in vitro* produces their rapid growth and elongation (within 3 hours), with the formation of a multi-layered structure. Within 48 hours, endothelial cells became uniformly oriented along the axis of the future vessel. Thus, mechanical energy is able to stimulate the new capillaries' formation.

Jain et al., (1990) showed that direct mechanical pressure on human fibroblasts causes **cellular growth** to increase 1.7 times, increasing protein synthesis up to 48%, and increasing intercellular C-AMP 3.7 times in 24 hours after the mechanical stimulation. The fibroblast activation and collagen production are major components of healing that affects every tissue in the human body.

Wirtz and Dobbs, (1990) reported that after a single application of mechanical stimuli to the alveolar type II cells they were able to increase Ca^{+2} exocytosis and **surfactant secretion** during the next 15-30 minutes. The surfactant is a special fluid that covers the inner surface of alveoli and prevents their collapse during expiration. Thus, the authors showed that the functions of the inner organs' cells also can be affected by mechanical stimulation.

Komuro et al., (1991) found in an experimental study on rats' neonatal cardiocytes that mechanical stress stimulates the cardiac cells' hypertrophy and specific **genes' expression**. The authors showed that total RNA content in the experimental group increased up to 45%, versus no increase in the control group during 24 hours. The genes' expression is one of the most intimate processes of nature. The ability of mechanical stimuli to affect the genes' expression brings a new understanding of the mechanisms that are responsible for many visceral disorders.

Chen and Grinnel, (1995) found that stretching the skeletal muscle of a frog in the physiological range (up to 2 mm) more than doubled the spontaneous and evoked release of the neurotransmitter **acethylcholine** from its motor nerve terminal, with an accompanying increasing of frequency of end-plate potentials. The mechanism of this effect is the activation of integrins in the cytoplasmic membrane, and additional mobilization of Ca^{+2} from internal and external sources. These data allow us to conclude that light stretching of the skeletal muscles at the end of massage treatment will stimulate the muscle tone and muscle performance.

Davidson et al., (1997) examined the effect of soft tissue mobilization (intense cross-friction) on experimental tendinitis caused by the injection of collagenase into the Achilles tendon of 20 rats. The results obtained from experimental and control groups were examined with light microscopy, electron microscopy, immunoelectron microscopy and by gait analysis. The authors found that the mean increase of the fibroblast count in an experimental group was to 15 ± 11, versus 3 ± 3 in the control group. All fibroblasts in the experimental group exhibited a highly developed rough endoplasmic reticulum, which is clear evidence of the stimulation of collage production. Thus, the mechanical stimuli, cross-friction in this case, attract the neighboring fibroblasts to the site of treatment, with a following stimulation of **collagen production** and healing of affected tendons.

Gehlsen et al., (1999) also examined the effect of soft tissue mobilization with different amounts of applied pressure on the **fibroblasts count**. The authors used the same experimental model of tendinitis in the Achilles tendon. They found that the application of strong pressure stimulated the healing process in the tendon much faster (fibroblast count = 375) compared to the treatment with light (fibroblast count = 190) or moderate (fibroblast count = 250) pressure. For the first time in modem literature, the authors also established a clear connection between mechanical stimuli, their therapeutic effect on somatic pathology in the form of soft tissue mobilization, and their effect on cellular functions.

To really understand the significance of all this information the reader should realize that some of reported effects were obtained from cells that were placed in the experimental conditions outside of the body (i.e., *in vitro*). Thus, stimulation of cellular activity was a result of purely mechanical stimulation of these cells without the participation of any other systems traditionally responsible for the coordination of cellular activity: nervous, humoral or immune.

At the end of this review, I would like to quote the conclusion from an article by Maniotis, Chen and Ingber (1997) published in *Proc. of the National Academy of Sciences of the USA*:

> "... direct mechanical linkages throughout living cells raise the possibility that regulatory information, **in the form of mechanical stress or vibration** (em-

phasized by R. T .), may be rapidly transferred from these cell surface receptors to distinct structures in the cell and nucleus, including ion channels, nuclear pores, nucleoli, chromosomes, and perhaps even individual genes, independent of ongoing chemical signaling mechanisms."

b. Effect of Pressure on the Orientation of Collagen Fibrills Phenomenon of Piezoelectricity

As we discussed in the previous section, the mechanical stimuli applied to the place of injury is able to increase collagen production by the stimulation of fibroblasts' functions and by attracting new cells from neighboring areas. However, increased collagen production alone is not enough to heal the injured site. The correct orientation of collagen fibers is an equally important element. Without the proper orientation of collagen fibers, an increase in collagen production is useless. Are mechanical stimuli somehow able to affect this process as well? We should answer this question positively. Numerous scientific reports support this conclusion. However, we should start this discussion with a quick review of the piezoelectrical phenomenon because of its direct connection to this matter.

Piezoelectricity is the ability of inorganic and organic substances to generate electrical potentials in response to pure mechanical deformation without any external electrical or magnetic field. The effect of piezoelectricity was discovered in inorganic crystals by the Curie brothers in 1880 (Williams, 1974). It was also found that the application of an external electrical field to these crystals causes their mechanical deformation as well. For several decades the piezoelectricity was considered as a feature of asymmetric inorganic crystals only. However, in 1957 two Japanese scientists, Dr. E. Fukada and Dr. L. Yasuda, detected the existence of the piezoelectric effect in the human bone. This effect was detected as electrical potentials registered in the bone during the application of mechanical stimuli which cause bone deformation.

Let's discuss this matter with the help of Fig. 6. At the moment of application of pressure, the negative potentials can be registered on the compressed side of the bone because of displaced electrons inside of the specimen. The electrical activity returns to "0" as soon as there is not a further increase in pressure, but already achieved pressure is still maintained. However, at the moment pressure is released and bone returns to its previous shape, the smaller positive potential is registered as well. This positive charge is detected on the stretched side of the bone specimen and indicates the return of electrons to their places. Thus, mechanical deformation of bone (e.g., during regular walking) produces the constant bi-polar electrical potentials.

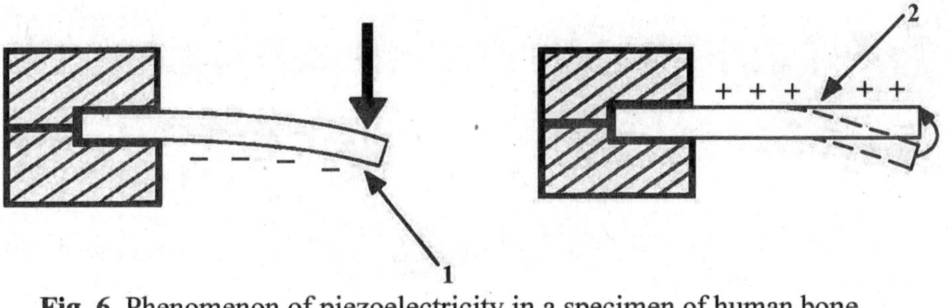

Fig. 6. Phenomenon of piezoelectricity in a specimen of human bone
1 - specimen of bone under the external mechanical pressure
2 - same specimen of bone with restored shape after the pressure released
"—" - negative charge on the compressed side of specimen
"+" - positive charge on the stretched side of specimen at the moment of releasing pressure

The first attempts to explain the piezoelectric properties of bone reasonably concluded that the inorganic part of the bone is responsible for this phenomenon. This assumption seemed correct because the inorganic part of the bone is arranged in crystals as well. These crystals are called **apatite**. However, in the beginning of the 1960s two American scientists, Dr. R.O. Becker and Dr. C.A.L. Basset, conducted a series of brilliant electro-physiological experiments which proved that the collagen in bone is mostly responsible for the phenomenon of piezoelectricity.

The collagen molecules produced the negative potential during the bone's deformation, compared to the apatite crystals which exhibited the positive charge. Now we know that negative potentials are responsible for tissues' growth. Positive potentials have the opposite effect because they inhibit healing process in the tissue. This discovery had enormous impact on medicine, especially on orthopedy. Today, the acceleration of fracture healing and callus formation in nonunion fractures by external and internal electrical devices is a common medical procedure.

After Becker and Basset published their results, scientists in different countries started to examine the piezoelectric properties of other biological materials. The results were astonishing. It was found that keratin (Fukada, 1982), elastine of the skin (Shamos and Lavine, 1967; Basset, 1971) and ligaments (Fukada and Hara, 1969), collagen in the tendon (Anderson and Eriksson, 1968), actine and myosin in the skeletal muscles (Fukada and Ueda, 1970), hyaluronic acid (Barrett, 1975) and even DNA molecules (Fukada, 1982) and some individual amino acids (Vasilesku, et al., 1970; Furukawa and Fukada, 1976) exhibited piezoelectric properties as well. Gross et al. (1983) considered the possibility of the piezoelectricity playing a role in the conduction of nervous impulses along the nerve. All of this allowed Shamos and Lavine, (1967) to conclude that "piezoelectricity is a property of most, if not all, tissues in the plant and animal kingdoms."

In 1977, Prof. B. Lipinski, in *Medical Hypotheses*, formulated the theory which links the therapeutic effects of soft tissue manipulations, acupuncture, Hatha Yoga and the action of negatively charged air ions with piezoelectrical properties of the biological tissues. According to the author's hypothesis, proteins, nucleic acids and mucopolysaccharides, which compose all tissues of the human body, exhibit piezoelectric properties. Thus, they are capable of transducing a mechanical energy into an electric energy. The author assumed that stimulation of specific areas on the surface of the body produces the electrical current. This piezoelectrically induced current activates the healing processes in the stimulated area, and/or is able to flow "towards the internal organs along the semiconductive channels of biological macromolecules." Thus, this mechanically induced electrical energy has great regulatory effect on the cellular and molecular levels.

What is the meaning of these findings for massage therapy? They are crucially important for understanding the therapeutic mechanism of massage. The collagen in the bone is absolutely identical to the collagen in any other tissue. Thus, piezoelectrical properties of collagen are similar throughout the body. Collagen is the most abundant protein in the human body, and its piezoelectric properties have been sufficiently examined. Let's look at the local electrophysiological response of collagen molecules to the external application of mechanical stimuli in the form of massage strokes.

A molecule of collagen is a strong **dipole**; i.e., it has two oppositely charged ends. The head has a positive charge and the tail has a negative charge. However, the overall charge of a collagen molecule is positive. Collagen molecules unite together to form anatomical structures (tendon, fascia, aponeurosis, bone, etc.) and consequently, these structures exhibit the **fixed electrical charge**. Massage therapy delivers mechanical stimuli to the soft tissues, and two major electrophysiological effects will be triggered there: piezoelectric phenomenon and streaming potentials.

Piezoelectric phenomenon

External mechanical stimuli deform the collagen molecules, causing the piezoelectric effect and changes in the fixed charge of collagen molecules. This process can be seen as increasing the negative fixed charge of collagen molecules or decreasing their positive fixed charge. Both descriptions are equally correct. Thus, the mechanical deformation of collagen during the massage treatment is responsible for an increase in the negative charge in the soft tissues. These negative potentials have strong proliferative (i.e. restorative) impact on the tissues in the massaged area.

As Shamos and Lavine showed in 1967, human skin from the forearm exhibited piezoelectric properties under direct mechanical stimulation. Collagen was mostly responsible for this phenomenon; however, the piezoelectric properties of elastine and keratin also played a role. The authors also pointed out that the largest magnitude of piezoelectric effect was registered when mechanical stimuli were applied at an angle of 45 degrees to the main orientation of collagen fibrils.

This is an important practical outcome, which can be used by practitioners to optimize the therapeutic results of massage treatment. The main orientation of collagen fibers can be easily detected in the skin according to the lines of cleavage (see below Fig. 60) and in other soft tissues according to their anatomical structure.

Streaming potentials

As I mentioned above, the molecule of collagen exhibits a fixed electrical charge. The extracellular collagen is surrounded by extracellular fluid, which is extremely movable and carries a large number of different molecules, anions, cations and dipoles with different electrical charges (e.g., Na ; Cl ; K ; amino acids, etc.) When they pass by the molecule of collagen with its fixed electric charge, the difference of electric potentials creates an electric field (see Fig. 7 'a'). These electric potentials are called **streaming potentials** (Basset, 1971; Lee, et al. 1979; Guzelsu, 1982). The magnitude of these potentials is mostly dependent on the local pH (Gross and Williams, 1982).

The streaming potentials were originally detected inside the blood vessels, when charged particles passed with the flow of blood near the endothelial cells which form vascular walls and also have a fixed charge. However, later the streaming potentials were also detected in the soft tissues; e.g., in the fascia and tendon (Anderson and Eriksson, 1968; Basset, 1971). Gross, et al. (1983) considered the transmembrane streaming potentials, that are a result of fluctuations in the hydrostatic pressure, as one of the possible mechanisms of conductance of impulses along the nerve.

Massage strokes deliver interruptive mechanical stimulation to the soft tissues and cause a fluctuation of interstitial pressure in the extracellular space. Thus massage increases the interstitial pressure and stimulates the flow of interstitial fluid, which carries the charged particles around the structures with fixed electrical charges - collagen, cellular membranes, etc. Because now charged particles move quicker with the increased flow of intersitial liquid, a stronger electrical field develops between these structures and particles (see Fig. 7 'b'). Thus, an additional amount of stimulating electrical energy is produced in the massaged area.

Both of these events (i.e. piezoelctric phenomenon and streaming potentials) in equal degree, are responsible for the collagen deposit at the injured site and, more important, the proper orientation of collagen fibrils. Basset, (1971) concluded that "tension exerts a major influence on the alignment of collagen bundles in tendons, fascia, ligaments, and arteries."

Myers et al., (1984) in an experimental study on human cartilage showed that changes in the extracellular fluid movement and structure of collagen fibers are mostly produced when mechanical stimulation is applied in the form of direct compression. When mechanical stimuli were applied to produce a pure shear deformation, no changes of these parameters were detected. This matches exactly with the clinical observations of the therapeutic impact of different massage techniques. The healing potential of effleurage and light friction on the tissues' regeneration is significantly lower compared to strong friction, vibration and kneading techniques.

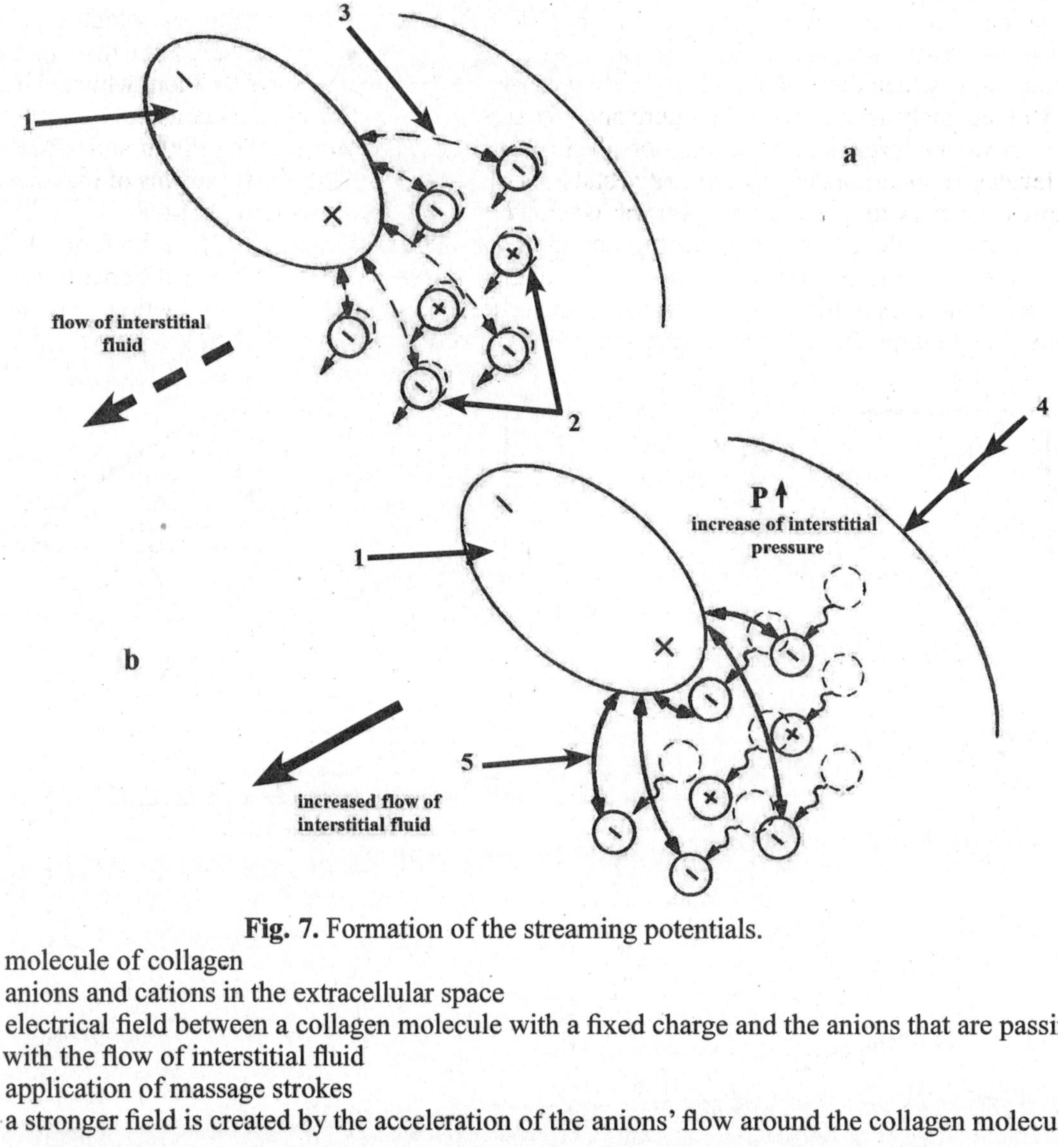

Fig. 7. Formation of the streaming potentials.

1 - molecule of collagen
2 - anions and cations in the extracellular space
3 - electrical field between a collagen molecule with a fixed charge and the anions that are passing it with the flow of interstitial fluid
4 - application of massage strokes
5 - a stronger field is created by the acceleration of the anions' flow around the collagen molecule

As we can see, mechanical stimulation produces the changes in the electrical environment of the extracellular matrix. These changes immediately affect the cellular membrane and receptor-proteins, with the stimulation of cellular activity follows, as discussed in the previous section. Thus, mechanical stimulation introduces some kind of electrical commands into the extracellular matrix, which affects the extracellular events and intracellular activity as well.

3. GENERAL RECONSTRUCTION OF EVENTS RESPONSIBLE FOR THE LOCAL THERAPEUTIC EFFECT OF MASSAGE

From all the information we discussed above, a cellular theory to explain the local stimulation of the healing process by massage is slowly emerging. I don't want to mislead the reader with a well established theory. It does not exist at this point. These are only preliminary results and speculations, but all authors in the discussion part of their articles made conclusions which support and complete each other as missing parts of the same puzzle. In significant degree, the theoretical considerations which the reader will find below reflect the author's personal opinion, which is based on a detailed analysis of modern literature and 17 years of personal clinical experience.

If we analyze the new information about the effect of pressure on the cellular and subcellular levels and incorporate it into already established views on the local mechanisms of massage therapy, we can try to generally reconstruct the chain of events with the help of Fig. 8.

For example, the massage practitioner applies strong mechanical stimuli in the form of deep friction and compression in the place of somatic pathology. In such a case, the practitioner triggers five major processes in the massaged tissues: pain relief, peripheral arterial vasodilation, stimulation of venous and lymph drainage, microtraumatization of soft tissues and cellular stimulation.

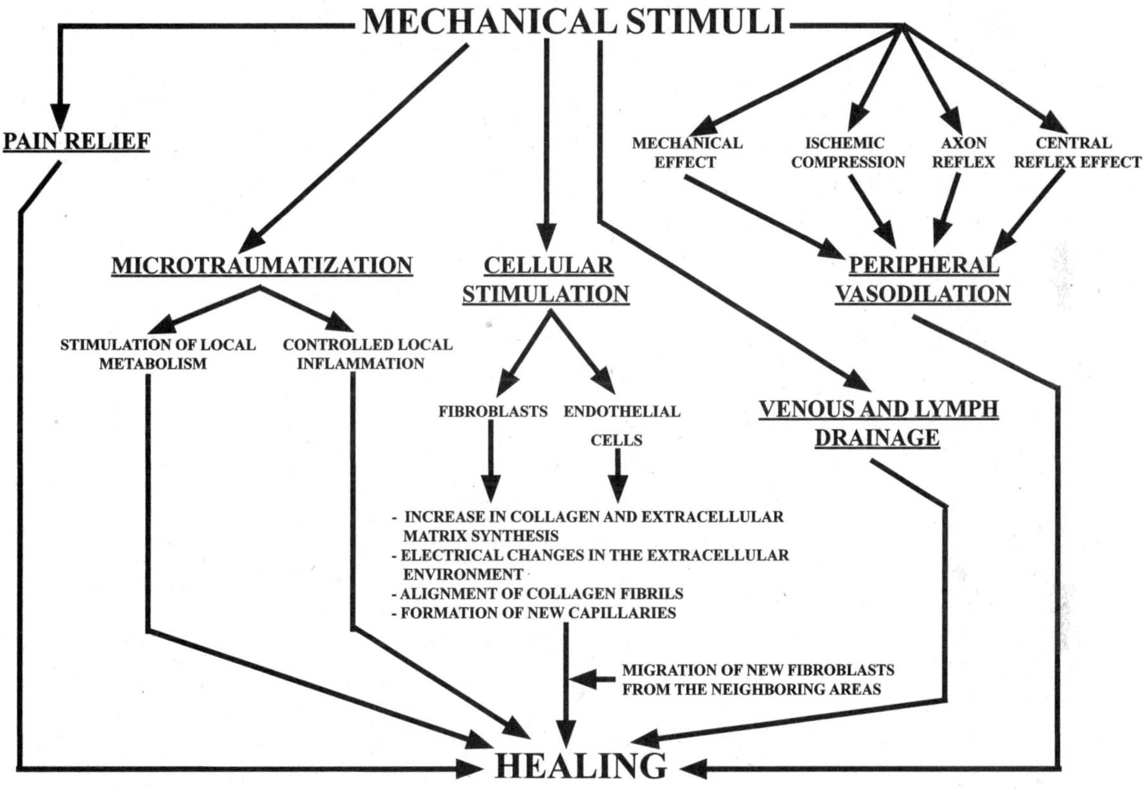

Fig. 8. General reconstruction of the local therapeutic effect of massage therapy

a. Pain Relief

We will discuss this important subject in detail in chapter III.

b. Peripheral Arterial Vasodilation

Peripheral vasodilation has two components: vasodilation of already functioning capillaries and the opening of reserve capillaries. Four different mechanisms are in charge of peripheral vasodilation:

Mechanical effect of massage strokes
As a result of the mechanical effect of massage strokes, more blood is pushed through the massaged area. Besides this, the massage strokes support the venous and lymphatic drainage.
Axon reflex
For information about the axon reflex, see page 16.
Ischemic compression
The ischemic compression causes the reflex vasodilation. For this purpose, soft tissue compression should be applied several times, then a quick release of pressure should follow. During soft tissue's compression, pressure should be maintained for at least 30 seconds. See chapter V for more details about ischemic compression.
Reflex vasodilation
Vasodilation in the area of reflex zones is caused by reflex mechanism, which involves the central nervous system. This mechanism is employed in cases of chronic somatic or visceral disorders. The reflex vasodilation also can be a result of the release of vasoactive substances from the massaged tissues into the general blood circulation.

c. Stimulation of Venous and Lymph Drainage

Trauma or chronic inflammation are always accompanied by a decrease of venous and lymph drainage. It forms a vicious cycle since insufficient drainage delays the healing process. Massage therapy, especially in form of Lymph Drainage Massage, speeds up the healing process by stimulating venous and lymphatic drainage which helps to remove waste products and restore normal circulation.

d. Microtraumatization of Soft Tissues by Intensive Massage Strokes

Energetic friction, vibration and strong compression cause microtraumas of soft tissues and capillaries that lead to **microhemorrhages** (i.e., microbleedings) and controlled inflammation. When microhemorrhages occur, the blood that leaks into the tissues acts as a natural biological stimulator. In such a case, the blood protein and the remains of cellular elements should be oxygenated and removed from the tissues, but to do this the local metabolism has to be stimulated. Thus, this activation of local metabolism at the site of an injury stimulates the healing of somatic disorders or post-traumatic rehabilitation.

More changes occur from evoking local **controlled inflammation**. This process starts after the end of massage treatment and continues for 24-48 hours. The physiological reaction of the body to any kind of trauma is local inflammation. Thus, after the massage, the first reaction to the tissues' damage is the emergence of neutrophils from circulation into these tissues, with the accompanying attraction of macrophages (Smith et al., 1994). Their major function is to clean up tissue debris at the place of trauma.

These cells engulf the remains of damaged cells and release enzymes which, additionally, produce **cytolysis** (i.e., cell distraction) in the tissues that have little chance of survival after the trauma. Thus, at the beginning of inflammation the actual trauma becomes even worse. However, this is the signal for fibroblasts from neighboring regions to migrate into the area of controlled inflammation to restore the normal structure of soft tissues.

e. CELLULAR STIMULATION

As we discussed above, the mechanical stimuli activate the fibroblasts that are normally present in soft tissues, and they start to produce new collagen and components of extracellular matrix to repair the injured site. Additionally, newly migrated fibroblasts increase the amount of extracellular matrix and collagen production. Repetitive application of mechanical stimuli during the following sessions further stimulates the activity, proliferation and collagen production by all fibroblasts in the massaged area.

The formation of a new capillary network as a result of mechanical stimulation of the endothelial cells is another equally important healing factor in the place of initial abnormality.

Newly synthesized procollagen molecules leave fibroblasts and form collagen deposits at the site of injury. Mechanical stimuli applied to the same area produce the chain of electrophysiological events which speed up the process of collagen deposit as well as the correct orientation of collagen fibrils. This process restores the normal anatomical structure in place of injury or somatic pathology.

All these events don't happen during one day. This is why the massage practitioner and the patient can expect stable results of treatment only when massage therapy is performed as a course of treatment. Only in such cases do massage employing a correctly developed protocol deliver the combination of different healing factors on the organic, cellular and subcellular levels and produce the maximal therapeutic effect.

B. ADVERSE EFFECTS OF PRESSURE

Excessive pressure can be a very destructive power. Uncontrolled strong mechanical stimulation without necessary adjustments to the patient's needs can cause serious medical complications of massage treatment. To emphasize the importance of this matter, I want to briefly represent some cases of adverse effects of strong pressure that were published in medical journals in 1990es.

Tachi et al., (1990) described the case of a 57 year old woman who had autoimmune thyroiditis or Hashimoto's disease. After she went through a vigorous and painful massage on her neck and shoulders for the relief of muscular tension, she developed a case of severe destructive thyrotoxicosis.

Herkovitz, (1992) reported the case of massage-induced injury of the recurrent motor brunch of the median nerve after the inappropriate compression of soft tissues proximally to the transverse carpal ligament. The patient suffered paralysis of thenar musculature, and had to undergo a long and expensive treatment of the median nerve injury.

Danchik et al., (1993) reported the case of myositis ossificans traumatica after inappropriate massage treatment in a 20 year old professional hockey player. The patient was hit in the lateral thigh during a game. At the time of the injury, the athlete was inappropriately treated with heat and deep massage, and subsequently developed a large hematoma and a severe case of myositis ossificans. Myositis ossificans, or ossification, is a condition in which damaged muscle tissues are replaced by a calcific mass.

Lin, (1993) reported the case of dissection of the extracranial part of the internal carotid artery, which caused the formation of a mural hematoma, after the deep tissue massage on the neck. The pathology was detected by MRI. This is an example of a life-threatening complication.

Mumm, (1993) reported the case of an unusual complication of massage therapy. A 64 year old woman suffered from a severe vesicular zoster over all eight cervical dermatomes, with the predominant spreading of viral infection along the ulnar nerve, after a brutal massage on the left cervical and suprascapular areas. The patient previously had a varicella virus infection at age 11. The authors concluded that damage of the peripheral nerves during the massage activated the latent zoster virus and triggered the new wave of infection.

Medvedev, (1994) reported the case of an acute unilateral neurosensory hearing loss caused by deep tissue massage on the upper portion of the trapezius muscle at the place of its insertion into the occipital bone. The possible cause is the compression and damage of the lesser occipital nerve against the occipital bone.

Yeo et al., (1994) reported the case of a massive hematoma resulting from digital massage of an anticoagulated patient. The massage therapist used excessive pressure despite the patient's warnings. As a result of this type of "treatment", the patient had a large hematoma of soft tissues, and it took a long period of time for complete recovery.

Kerr, (1997) reported the case of a 51 year old woman who had long history of ureteral stenosis, caliculi, and had a double J stent permanently placed in her ureter. During deep massage treatment with uncontrolled pressure, she suddenly felt severe pain in her flank. In the emergency room, the displacement of the ureteral stent was detected. The pain was gone as soon as the stent was restored in its position.

Mikhail, (1997) reported the case of a renal artery embolization caused by deep tissue massage on the back of a patient with a partial aortic occlusion. As a result, the function of the patient's kidney was severely affected.

Geise, (1998) reported the case of posterior interosseus syndrome after deep tissue massage on the forearm. The posterior interosseus nerve is a branch of the radial nerve which innervates extensor digitorum, extensor digiti minimi and extensor carpi ulnaris muscles. For a long period of time, the patient had pain and weakness in the hand and fingers during the extension.

As you can see, inappropriate application of excessive pressure can cause severe medical problems. These articles were published in different countries by medical doctors who dealt with patients suffering from the complications of massage treatment. Unfortunately, these cases are not exceptional. Complications following inappropriate pressure application can cause a serious medical problem.

All of these articles have one striking similarity. During the massage treatment all patients reported to the operator about the excessive amount of applied pressure. However, in all of these cases the massage practitioners did not pay attention to the patient's complaints, and even encouraged them by relating the future 'benefits of this 'treatment.' The proper application of pressure can be described by one simple rule: It must be applied at the right time, on the right place, with the right intensity while patient controls it.

III. PATHOPHYSIOLOGY OF PAIN. THE PAIN-ANALYZING SYSTEM AND ITS CORRECT ACTIVATION BY MASSAGE THERAPY

The relationship between pain and massage therapy is a very important subject, one that is frequently misunderstood or overlooked. As soon as the massage practitioner stimulates the pain receptors he or she activates a unique system of the human body. The elements of this system are carefully balanced. To use this system for therapeutic purposes, the massage practitioner has to know exactly what he expects from the treatment and how to use massage manipulations for the patient's benefit.

Pressure is the principal method by which the massage therapist can activate the pain system. Thus, the application of the right amount of pressure is a tool which can be used for the patients' benefit as well as against the patient's health when it is applied inappropriately. First, let's briefly review the pathophysiology of pain.

A. PATHOPHYSIOLOGY OF PAIN

Generally, pain can be characterized as a person's subjective response to trauma or illness. But the conception of pain is much more complex than this general description. This concept has profound philosophical, social and economic meanings and definitely played an important role in the development of our civilization. Pain has always haunted humans and despite modem achievements, its control is still an important medical and social problem. It is impossible to discuss all the aspects of pain in one chapter, this is why we will look at the pain concept from the massage therapy point of view.

Pain receptors (i.e., nociceptors) are the free nerve endings which are located practically in every tissue of the body. Pain receptors are activated by a variety of noxious stimuli of different nature: mechanical, thermal or chemical. As with any peripheral receptors, free nerve endings have their own firing levels, or thresholds. If, for example, the massage therapist touches the patient's skin, the touch receptors are stimulated, send afferent (i.e., ascending) discharge to the central nervous system, and the perception of touch is formed. In this case, the free nerve endings are not activated. If the amount of pressure increases and exceeds the firing level of free nerve endings, they are now activated and send their own afferent discharge to the central nervous system and the patient feels pain. Thus, the sensory receptors in the skin which are responsible for touch, pressure, temperature, and vibration sensations are never activated by noxious stimuli. Only free nerve endings or pain receptors are activated by noxious stimuli. About 20% of nociceptors serve as mechanical nociceptors; i.e., they react to excessive pressure, pinching, etc. (Iggo, 1974).

The firing level of free nerve endings is called the **threshold of pain**. The threshold of pain differs not only from person to person, but also it varies on different parts of the same individual's body. Fig. 9 shows differences in the threshold of pain on the surface of the human body according to Bojarsky, (1973). In that study, the threshold of pain was determined by the registration of the patient's responses to electrical current.

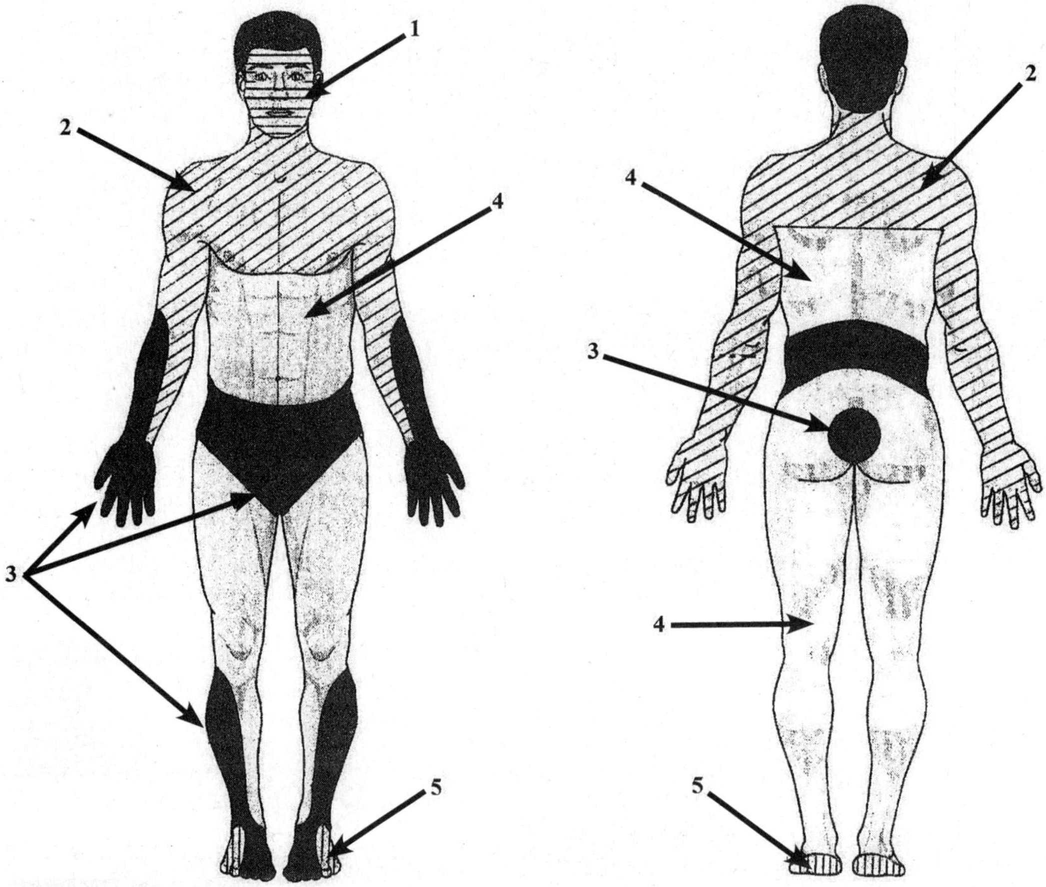

Fig. 9. Threshold of pain on the skin of the human body (Boyarsky, 1973)
1 - area of highest sensitivity (electric current 0.2-0.3 mA)
2 - area more sensitive than area #3 (electric current 0.4-0.5 mA)
3 - area of medium sensitivity (electric current 0.5-0.6 mA)
4 - area less sensitive than area #3 (electric current 0.6-0.7 mA)
5 - area of lowest sensitivity (electric current 0.7-0.8 mA)

The action potentials (i.e., nervous impulses) are generated in the free nerve endings and conducted to the central nervous system via two types of nervous fibers. Large, **unmyelinated C** fibers conduct the action potentials at **low speed** (about 0.5-2 m/s). Small, **myelinated A** fibers conduct the action potentials at **high speed** (about 12-30 m/s). Thus, we have two types of pain: slow and fast pain respectively. The fast pain is sharp and precisely localized. The slow pain is dull, aching and poorly localized. The predominance of fast or slow pain completely depends on the activity in the A or C nervous fibers.

In 1939, Zotterman reported the results of an important experimental study which is still classical today. The author conducted many experiments to study the electrophysiology of the cutaneous sensory nerves, using the saphenous nerve of a cat as an experimental model. He examined the effect of different types of cutaneous stimulation: strong stroking, gentle feathering, tickling, needle prick, electric shock, heat and vibration. The author also examined their reciprocal relations.

The effect of each type of cutaneous stimulation was tested by the electrode inserted into the saphenous nerve to register size, number and velocity of the afferent (i.e., ascending) action potentials, which were generated in the peripheral receptors after the different types of cutaneous stimulation.

Dr. Zotterman reported many important findings and I want to especially emphasize one of them. Comparing the results of skin stimulation by firm stroking and needle prick, the author concluded that both types of cutaneous sensation elicited the **same pattern** of action potentials which propagated to the central nervous system through the same afferent sensory fibers.

If one compares both strips in Fig. 10, it is easy to notice almost complete similarity of action potentials generated in the skin's peripheral receptors by the application of the firm stroke and needle prick. The large beta-potentials are followed by smaller sigma-potentials, which form the **afterdischarge**. The main difference between both strips is the prolonged registration of beta waves after firm stroking of the skin compare to the needle stimulation.

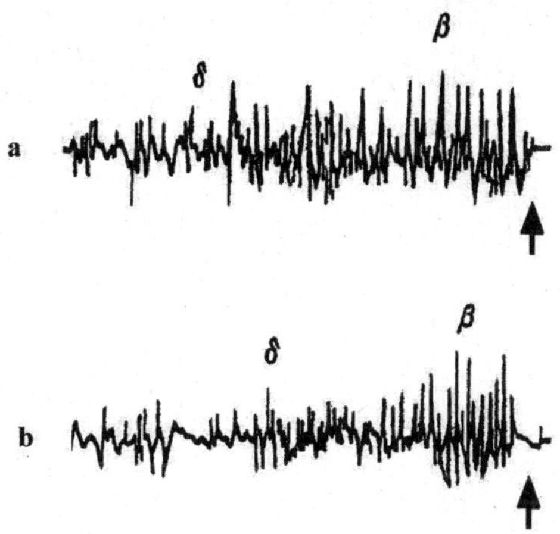

Fig. 10. The pattern of action potentials registered in the saphenous nerve of a cat after skin stimulation by firm stroke and needle prick. (To be read from right to left. Zotterman, 1939).
a - action potentials registered after firm stroking of the skin
b - action potentials registered after needle prick stimulation
arrows - application of stimuli
ß - beta waves: large potentials of very short duration
δ - sigma waves: small potentials which form the afterdischarge

By measuring the velocity of conductance of both types of action potentials, Dr. Zotterman also found that stimuli evoked by strong skin stroking reached the central nervous system with the same speed as a fast pain. From this data the general analgesic effect of massage therapy (also known as counterirritation) can be easily explained. In the case of chronic visceral or somatic pain, massage techniques mechanically deform the skin's mechanoreceptors and elicit action potentials which propagate to the central nervous system with greater speed than chronic pain stimuli which are mostly conducted through slow pain afferent fibers. Thus, the action potential produced by skin stroking reaches the brain **earlier** than chronic pain stimuli reach the spinal cord. In such cases, the activity of the hypothalamus is inhibited and the hypothalamo-cortical discharge ceases with the following inhibition of areas of cortex which previously were overstimulated by the permanent bombardment of chronic pain stimuli. Besides this, the brain also has time to elicit central control over the "gates" (see below) in the spinal cord to suppress the continuous flow of pain stimuli from the affected area of the body.

The free nerve endings are a **slowly adapting** type of peripheral receptors. This means that they will continue to fire for some time even after the withdrawal of the noxious stimuli. If we compare the free nerve endings of A and C nervous fibers we can see that the level of adaptation is much lower for the C fibers compared to the A fibers. Thus the pain receptors of the A fibers are the most slowly adapting peripheral receptors. Therefore, acute pain is the most excruciating feeling.

The information from the free nerve endings is coded as the sequence of action potentials. They propagate along the A and C nervous fibers which are part of the afferent (i.e., ascending) sensory pathways to the CNS. All sensory information about pain is delivered to the central nervous system through the dorsal horns of the spinal cord in the lateral spinothalamic tract which delivers information from the spinal cord to the brain.

B. "GATE -CONTROL" THEORY OF PAIN

The biggest breakthrough in understanding the pathophysiology of pain happened in 1965. Journal *Science* published the classic article of Prof. R. Mezlack and Prof. D. Wall: "Pain Mechanisms: A New Theory." This article introduced now widely accepted "gate-control" theory of pain.

1. MAIN COMPONENTS OF GATE-CONTROL SYSTEM

According to the "gate-control" theory of pain, the spinal cord has three systems which primarily modulate information from pain receptors before transferring it to the brain (see Fig. 11). These systems are the Substantia Gelatinosa, the T-Cells and the Central Control Trigger.

a. Substantia Gelatinosa

The substantia gelatinosa consists of small, tightly packed cells of grey matter which are located at the top of the **dorsal (posterior) horns** of spinal cord in the lamina I. The substantia gelatinosa can be viewed as a kind of somatic map which consists of a great number of tiny cellular compartments. Each of them is responsible for handling information from the sensory receptors of a particular, small area of the skin (Mezlack and Wall, 1989).

The existence of two types of regulatory cells in substantia gelatinosa is another of its important features. These cells exhibit the stimulating or inhibitory control over the activity of T-cells. Thus, the substantia gelatinosa is a major regulatory relay station which conveys and primarily modifies the afferent (i.e., ascending) sensory and noxious stimuli from all peripheral receptors located in various receptor fields of human body.

b. T-Cells

T-cells are also part of the grey matter of dorsal horn.. However, they are larger than the substantia gelatinosa cells, and they are located next to the substantia gelatinosa in the lamina V of dorsal horns. T-cells have a direct ascending and descending exchange of information with the brain. The activity of T cells is to a significant degree, regulated by the substantia gelatinosa.

c. Central Control Trigger

A human's strong emotions, moods and even memories also play significant roles in pain perception. From this point of view, Prof. Mezlack and Prof. Wall developed the concept of the Central Control Trigger. The authors considered the central control trigger to be a main factor of higher control over the "gates." Mezlack and Wall attributed the central control trigger to the **dorsal columns** of the spinal cord. Fibers originated there have direct access to the thalamus, and later to the cortex, and they conduct information to them with greater speed. This allows the brain to project the efferent (i.e., descending) control over the "gates." Thus, slowly increased pain (pressure in the case of massage) can be controlled in significant degree by the central nervous system. If the patient understands the importance of treatment, uses a slow pattern of breathing, employs muscle relaxation and the practitioner distracts the patient (bring up a topic interesting to the patient), the central control trigger can be activated and it will increase the amount of control over pain.

2. APPLICATION PRESSURE AND GATE-CONTROL SYSTEM

Pressure is one of the main therapeutic tools of massage therapy. Therefore, we will discuss the formation of pain perception (see Fig. 11 and 12) using the examples of correct and inappropriate pressure application on the pathologically changed area (e.g., trigger point).

a. Correct Application of Pressure

The special cells called substantia gelatinosa or 'gate-keepers' are located in the dorsal or posterior horns of the spinal cord, just after the dorsal root of each spinal nerve enters the spinal cord. Mild stimuli, in our case initial gentle pressure, activates the touch receptors. If the pressure continues to increase **slowly** and reaches the pain threshold the C nervous fibers are activated. As soon as stimuli reach the substantia gelatinosa via C fibers, its cells keep the "gates" between the substantia gelatinosa and next layer of cells called T cells in the closed or partly closed position (see Fig. 11). As a result, the number of nervous impulses which is generated in the T cells and conducted to the brain via spinothalamic tract decreases, and little or no pain is felt, even if applied pressure s deep and strong. The closing "gates" also blocks the afferent (i.e., ascending) flow of pain impulses from the area of the trigger point or any other affected area. It decreases chance of referred or radiating pain.

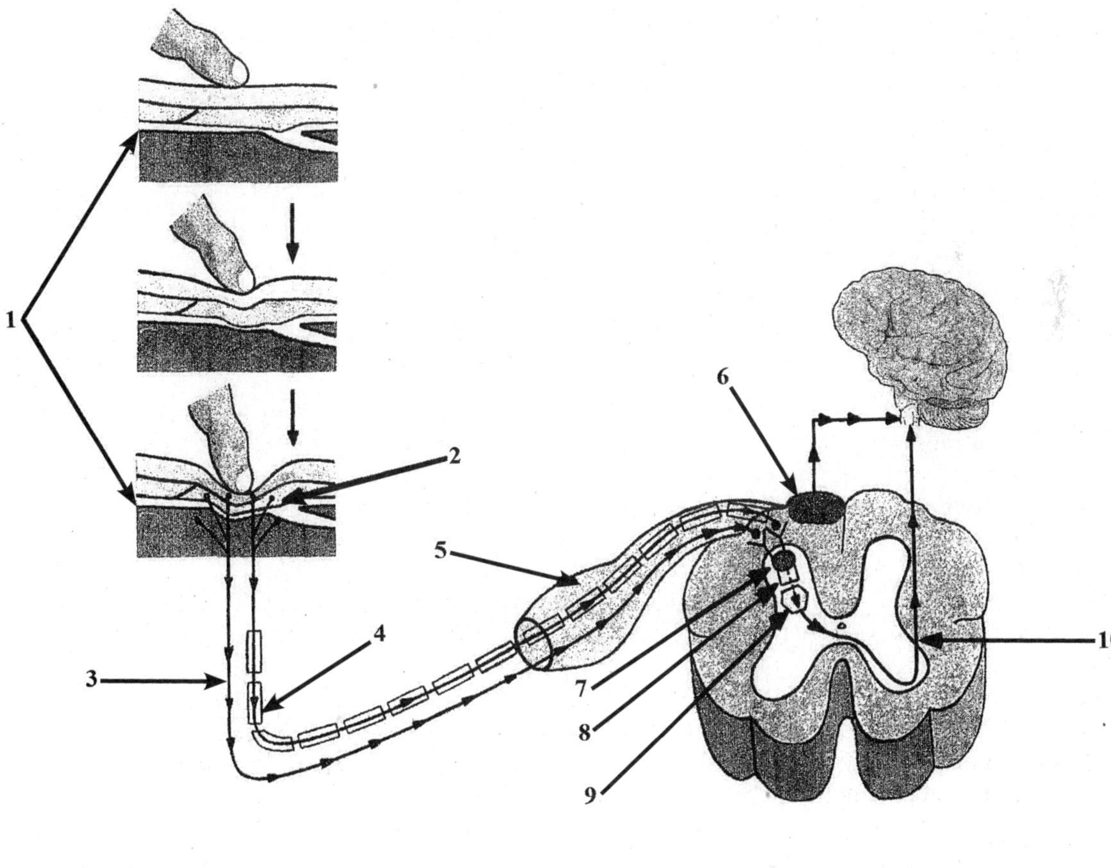

Fig. 11. "Gate-control " theory of pain. Physiological response to the correct application of pressure in areas with a low pain threshold.

1 - slowly increased pressure in combination with permanent vibration (about vibration see below)
2 - nociceptors (i.e., pain receptors)
3 - increase in action potentials' conductance via large, slow, unmyelinated C fibers
4 - inhibition of action potentials conductance via small, fast, myelinated A fibers.
5 - dorsal root
6 - dorsal column nuclei (activation of central control trigger system with fast afferent flow to the brain)
7 - substantia gelatinosa
8 - closed "gates"
9 - T -cells
10 - block of afferent flow of pain stimuli to the brain

Besides controlling the "gates" the substantia gelatinosa modulates the sensory input from A and C nervous fibers. Thus the substantia gelatinosa is able to suppress the activity of A nervous fibers and stimulate the activity of the C nervous fibers if pressure is applied correctly.

b. Inappropriate Application of Pressure

Strong noxious stimuli (e.g., strong pressure way beyond the personal pain threshold) activates mostly the A fibers (i.e. fast pain), which overcome the activity of C fibers (i.e., slow pain) as it is shown in Fig. 12. The noxious stimuli arrive at the substantia gelatinosa and its cells open the "gate" between the substantia gelatinosa and the T-cells as wide s possible. As a result, the T-cells are activated and start to generate nervous impulses, which are conducted to the brain via the lateral spinothalamic tract and pain perception is formed.

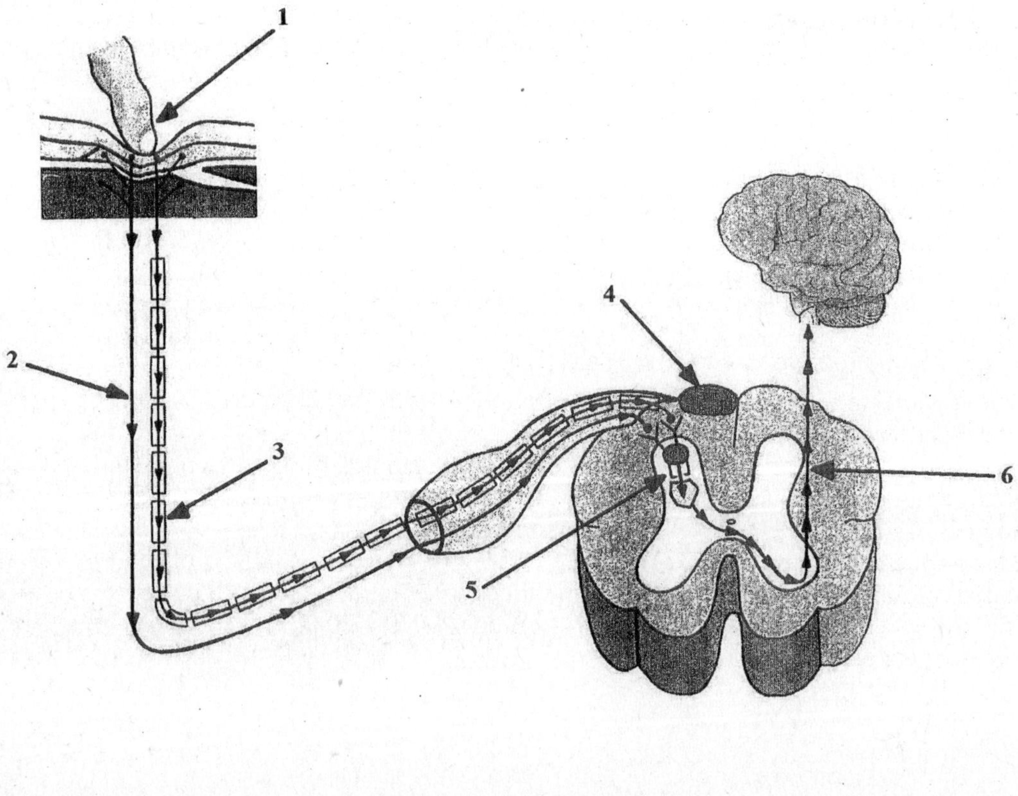

Fig. 12. "Gate-control" theory of pain. Physiological response to the application of excessive pressure in areas with a low pain threshold (e. g., trigger point).
1 - excessive pressure application
2 - inhibition of action potentials' conductance via large, slow, unmyelinated C fibers
3 - increase in action potentials' conductance via small, fast, myelinated A fibers
4 - dorsal columns nuclei (central control trigger system does not active)
5 - opened gates between the substantia gelatinosa and the T cells
6 - afferent (i.e., ascending) flow of pain stimuli from nociceptors to the pain analyzing centers in the thalamus and cortex

C. PAIN AND MASSAGE THERAPY

Now we should look at the relationship between pain and massage from the point of view of the "gate-control" theory. As mentioned previously, the threshold of pain varies from person to person. In many cases, the massage practitioner deals with clients who ask about deep tissue massage. With this category of clients, the practitioner does not have to worry about the amount of applied pressure. These clients have high thresholds of pain, and they feel comfortable about the excessive pressure during the treatment.

The matter of this discussion is the patients who have a low pain threshold or who suffer from hypertonic muscular pathology, cutaneous or periostal trigger points. In these areas, the patient's pain threshold is significantly or even critically low. For the patient's health benefit, the practitioner has to pay special attention to these areas. During the therapeutic massage treatment the operator can activate nociceptors and hit the threshold of pain. Besides this, some methods of medical massage treatment employ extra pressure in the form of ischemic compression. In both cases, the massage practitioner has to correctly apply pressure for the patient's benefit.

The therapist activates the pain analyzing system for therapeutic purposes. However, in many cases the patient is already exhausted from the long chronic pain suffering. Thus, additional pain during the massage treatment can make the situation worse. First of all, it is unpleasant, and no one likes pain in any form. These unpleasant sensations can increase or initiate negative mental and emotional reactions. Secondly, if the massage therapist does not control the pain during the treatment the patient will reflexively generate **protective muscular tension**, which makes the treatment more difficult and its final results questionable. Thus, control over the pain if this system is activated is an extremely important matter for a successful massage treatment.

In the case of therapeutic massage, the first contact of the operator's hand with the massaged area activates touch, pressure and temperature receptors. They form the afferent (i.e. ascending) sensory discharge that is analyzed by the brain. At the beginning of treatment these impulses are the most powerful stimulators of the hypothalamus, which can be viewed as a main relay station to convey information to the cortex. As was shown by Gellhorn (1958), the changing state of the hypothalamus can alter the state of excitability of the cerebral cortex, including its motor areas via hypothalamo-cortical nervous pathways.

Any kind of noxious stimuli stimulates the hypothalamus and, consequently, the cerebral cortex. With prolonged massage therapy, especially if the **inhibitory regime** is applied (see below), the flow of sensory impulses from the massaged area blocks the sympathetic part of the hypothalamus and, consequently, inhibits the hypothalamo-cortical discharge and activity of cerebral cortex. The inhibition of the motor areas of the cortex produces a reflex relaxation of the skeletal muscles. Thus, if the massage treatment **does not reach** the threshold of pain, the sympathetic part of the hypothalamus is suppressed.

Goats and Keir, (1991) discuss another possible mechanism of analgesic effect of massage therapy. The authors considered the earlier work of Watson (1982), who pointed out the mechanism of releasing **endogenous opiate** substances in the segment of the spinal cord at which spinal nerves from the affected area enter.

Discussing the therapeutic effects of connective tissue massage, Goats and Keir reasonably assumed that massage employs this analgesic mechanism as well. As discussed previously, massage blocks the noxious stimuli' conductance by closing the "gates." At the same time, the noxious receptors which were activated by the massage strokes "initiate reflex activity leading to the release of endogenous opiate substances in the spinal segment at which the pain bearing nerves enter."

The major proof of this assumption is the long-lasting analgesia produced by massage, compared to the simple activation of the "gate-closing" mechanism, seeing in an ice cube massage.

In sensitive areas, massage strokes can, and in many cases have to, reach the threshold of pain. The massage therapist can use four tools to help the patient actively control pain sensations: an inhibitory regime of massage, gradual increasing of pressure, permanent vibration, and central control trigger.

1. INHIBITORY REGIME OF MASSAGE TREATMENT

The therapist must always start treatment in pain-sensitive areas using massage in the inhibitory regime. It is also helpful to briefly apply this treatment after ischemic compression, or any other treatment that exceeds the patient's threshold of pain.

Any kind of inhibitory treatment has one goal: reducing pain and tension in the soft tissues and skeletal muscles. All strokes in the inhibitory regime are united by one common principle: the applied pressure has to be moderate, while the massage influence on the affected area has to be prolonged. Thus, there should not be any painful stimuli application during inhibitory treatment.

Another special feature of the inhibitory treatment is the type of applied techniques. To successfully perform inhibitory treatment, the massage therapist must use no more than 1-2 massage techniques, and must repeat them over and over. The therapist can use effleurage or slow kneading techniques. No percussion, interruptive vibration, strong kneading or compression is applied to the massaged area.

As it was experimentally proven by Goldberg, et al. (1992, 1994), massage in the inhibitory regime decreases activity in the pool of alpha-motoneurons in the lower motor centers of the spinal cord with accompanying muscle relaxation. Experimentally, it can be seen as a inhibition of the amplitude of H-reflex in the massaged muscles.

Let's discuss the physiological mechanism of the inhibitory treatment. If the operator starts to work on the affected area where peripheral receptors already have low threshold of activation, the afferent (ascending) flow of sensory impulses from the peripheral receptors in the massaged area is conducted to the spinal cord and excite the lower motor centers (Fig. 13 'a', #6) located in the posterior horns of the spinal cord. After reaching posterior horns the afferent sensory flow speeds up to the upper motor centers in the cortex (Fig. 13 'a', #9).

As a result, the efferent (descending) motor flow from the upper motor centers is conducted via the lateral corticospinal and rubrospinal tracts (Fig. 13 'a', #7) to the lower motor centers located in the anterior horns of the spinal cord The simultaneous stimulation of lower motor centers by afferent (ascending) impulses from peripheral receptors and efferent (descending) impulses from upper motor centers in the brain evokes the efferent (descending) flow of motor impulses, which are conducted back to the same massaged area and it will initially increase the protective reflex tension in the massaged soft tissues.

Protective muscle tension forms because the peripheral receptors consider the initial application of massage strokes as a potential threat (in the affected areas). In such a case, an alarm in the form of an ascending sensory flow generated by peripheral receptors in the massaged area rushes up along the afferent nervous pathways: from peripheral receptors, to the posterior horns of the spinal cord and finally to the lower motor centers in the anterior horns of the spinal cord (see Fig 13 'a').

However, this situation changes quickly. If the operator continues to work with the same techniques, on the same area, with the same pressure for couple minutes - the peripheral receptors soon will reach their adaptation level and the production of action potentials will decrease. The 'sensory computer' in the posterior horns of the spinal cord is also inhibited by the massive, continuous flow of the afferent harmless stimuli. Thus, the membranes of the peripheral receptors, as well as spinal neurons in the posterior horns of the spinal cord, become depolarized and are unable to generate or conduct a sufficient amount of afferent (ascending) nervous impulses to the lower and upper motor centers (see Fig. 13 'b'). As a result, the amount of efferent (descending) nervous impulses generated in the lower and upper motor centers decreases and reflex protective tension is slowly eliminated, and tension in the pathological areas is reduced in some degree (Turin, 1992).

The inhibitory regime of massage treatment is able to suppress pain in significant degree. Massive afferent flow of sensory impulses generated by massage strokes helps to keep the "gates" in the spinal cord in the closed or partly open position, blocking pain stimuli conduction to the upper levels of central nervous system. This effect of inhibitory treatment can be successfully used for pain reduction on patients following surgery, or for those with cancer, causalgia, etc.

Marin, et al. (1991) analyzed the effect of massage treatment on 116 patients following a thoracotomy. The massage therapy treatment started on the first day after surgery and continued for eight days. The analgesic effect of massage therapy was estimated using a visual analog scale. The degree of pain suppression reported by all patients after massage treatment was significant.

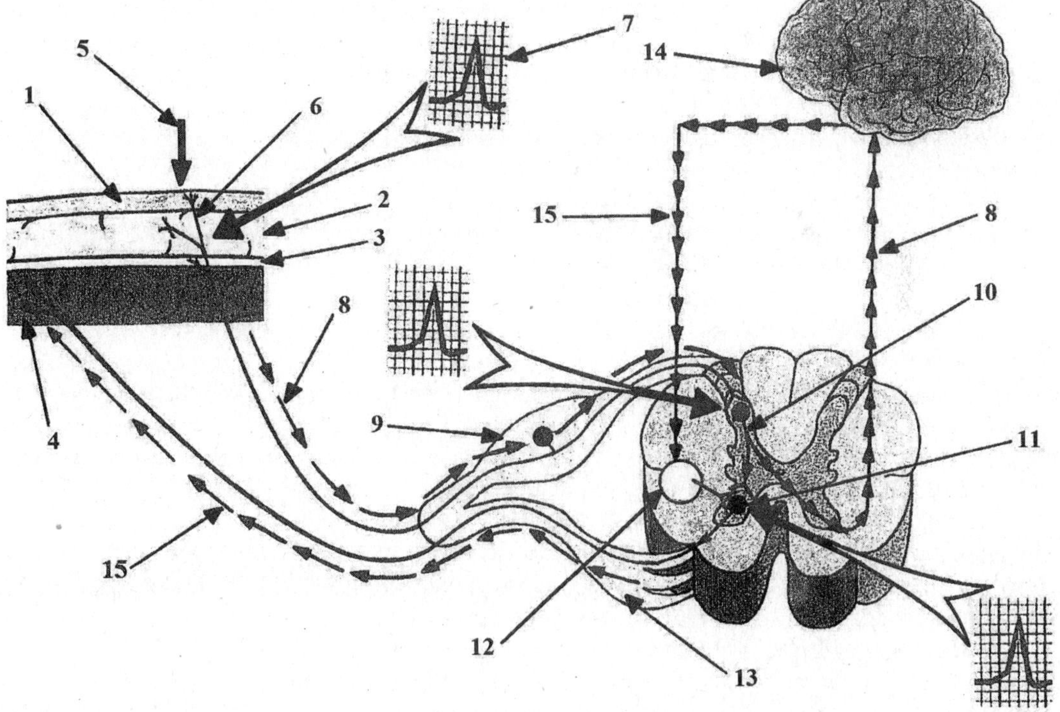

a - chain of neurophysiological events at the beginning of massage treatment

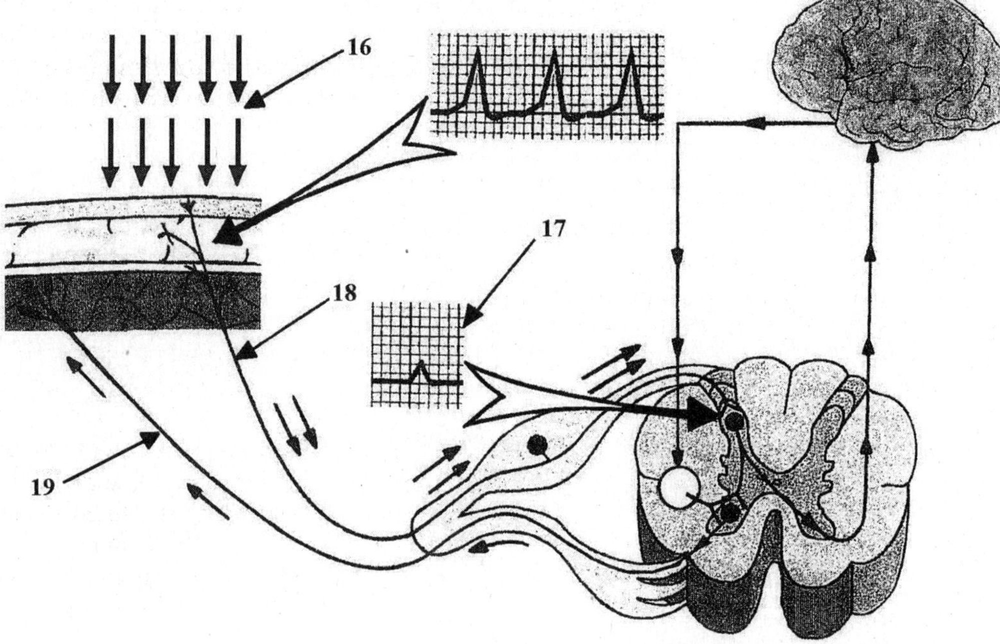

b - neurophysiological changes caused by massage in the inhibitory regime

Fig. 13. The mechanism of inhibitory massage treatment

1 - skin
2 - subcutaneous tissue
3 - fascia
4 - skeletal muscle
5 - initial massage stimulation
6 - peripheral sensory receptors
7 - generation of standard action potential
8 - flow of afferent (ascending) sensory impulses
9 - dorsal (posterior) root .
10 - intermediate neuron
11 - lower motor center
12 - lateral corticospinal and rubrospinal tracts
13 - ventral (anterior) root
14 - higher motor center
15 - flow of efferent (descending) motor impulses
16 - application of massage in the inhibitory regime
17 - depolarization of nervous centers with decease of action potential production
18 - weak flow of afferent (ascending) sensory impulses caused by the inhibitory massage
19 - weak flow of efferent (descending) motor impulses

2. GRADUAL INCREASING OF APPLIED PRESSURE

The massage therapist has to increase pressure slowly and gradually, and only after the preparation of the affected area using massage in the inhibitory treatment. In this case, only the C nervous fibers will be activated during the treatment (see Fig. 11 and 12). They send information to the substantia gelatinosa to keep the "gates" in the partly open position. The patient feels less pain, even if the amount of pressure is significant. Thus, by gradually increasing pressure, the operator stimulates C nervous fibers to create an imbalance between the inputs of slow and fast (i.e., A nervous fiber) pain systems. Only in this case will the therapeutic impact of massage treatment be physiological, and the results are stable.

3. PERMANENT VIBRATION

Another way to control pain in the sensitive areas is with permanent vibration. According to Zotterman (1939), Mezlack and Wall (1965 and 1985) permanent vibration stimuli reduce low-intensity pain and itch and stimulate high-intensity pain and itch at the first moment of their exposure on the tested area. However, the further application of permanent vibration stimuli activates both A and C nervous fibers, but the fast pain system reaches the adaptation level faster while the slow pain system is still firing. Thus, the overall effect of permanent vibration is strong pain inhibition (Mezlack and Schecter, 1965).

Wall and Crowly-Dillan, (1960) in a series of experiments showed that vibration inhibits all types of nociceptors and proprioceptors (i.e., touch, pressure, temperature). The authors also pointed out the central inhibition of proprioceptors, especially pain receptors. The authors considered two possible mechanisms of central inhibition of pain by the vibratory stimuli: presynaptic blocking with the following reduction of afferent impulses in size and number, and the increasing of the threshold of nervous cells activation. Thus, the massage practitioner should use pressure in combination with permanent vibration in all sensitive areas. It will set the gates in a more closed position and help to pain stimuli during the treatment.

4. ACTIVATION OF CENTRAL CONTROL TRIGGER

Another important mechanism of pain suppression during treatment is the central control trigger (see Fig. 12 and 13). The massage practitioner can activate this system by using two approaches. First of all, every step of the treatment has to be explained, or even shown to the patient using examples, **before** the session. The patient has to clearly understand what to expect after this particular session and also during the entire course of treatment. There should be no sudden changes or additions to the treatment without an explanation to the patient. Secondly, just before and during the activation of the pain analyzing system the practitioner should talk to the patient on the subject that he or she is interested in (e.g. patient's hobby). Arrange the conversation in such a way that the patient tells you a story while you are concentrating on the treatment process. Frequently remind the patient about complete muscular relaxation and slow pattern of breathing.

These four basic principles should be applied during every massage treatment when the practitioner reaches the patient's personal pain threshold. Massage therapy that follows these rules has an expressive analgesic effect in the case of severe chronic pain. For these purposes, therapeutic massage can help to control the general pain syndrome in the cases of fibromyalgia, diabetic or alcoholic neuropathy, causalgia, cancer, etc.

Weinrich, (1990) examined the effect of 10 minutes of massage therapy on 28 patients with different types of cancer. They found that immediate pain relief was detected with patients having the strongest pain. The patients with moderate or low pain did not report significant relief. At the same time, pain medications caused significant pain relief in only 2 hours after their administration.

Thus, the authors made the following practical recommendations: massage should be used for the immediate reduction of strong pain until the medications start to work; i.e., massage should be applied in combination with pain-controlling drugs.

D. OUTCOMES OF INAPPROPRIATE APPLICATION OF PRESSURE DURING THE MASSAGE TREATMENT

Now, let's take a look at what has happened with patients for which pressure has been applied inappropriately during massage treatment. If the amount of pressure is not adjusted to the patient's pain threshold three reflex protective mechanisms are activated: withdrawal reflex, fast pain analyzing system, and indirect activation of the muscle spindle receptors.

1. WITHDRAWAL REFLEX

The exact location of the trigger point, or hypertonus, can be found by the application of the so-called '**Jump Test.**' If strong pressure is applied in the correct direction of the entrance into the trigger point, the patient withdraws body or part of the body from the practitioner. This is a classic example of withdrawal reflex, which is used in this case for diagnostic purposes. In our everyday life, this reflex protects us from any strong noxious stimuli (hot stoves, pin prick, etc.).

The withdrawal reflex is a simple reflex which is activated on the level of the spinal cord (see Fig. 14). It uses the fast pain system to conduct the impulses to the spinal cord without involving higher sensory and motor centers in the brain. The same protective reflex can be elicited by the sudden application of strong pressure on a sensitive area or on unprepared muscles. The activation of the withdrawal reflex is wrong approach to any massage treatment. It can be used only for diagnostic purposes. Its permanent activation during the therapy triggers the protective muscle tension, supports the development of hypertonic muscular pathologies and, finally, ruins all efforts.

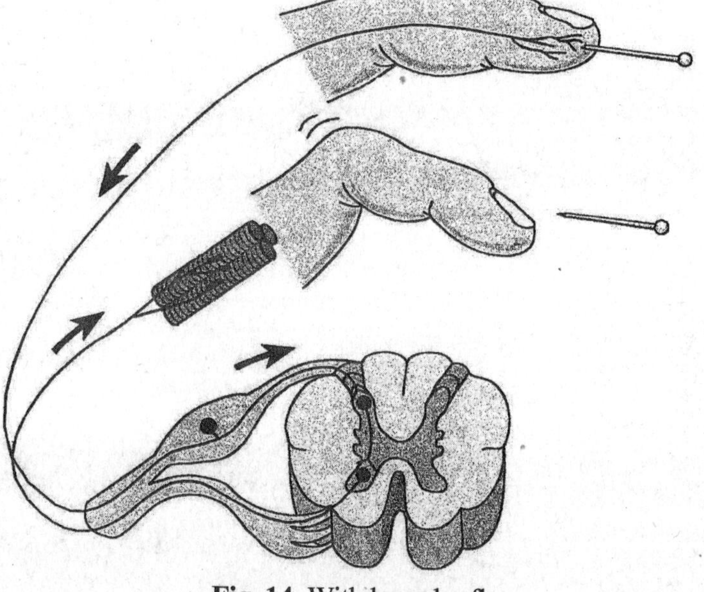

Fig. 14. Withdrawal reflex

2. FAST PAIN SYSTEM OR "A" NERVOUS FIBERS

If noxious stimuli (e.g., strong pressure) are applied to sensitive area incorrectly, the balance between slow and fast pain systems is shifted to the latter one. The substantia gelatinosa opens the "gates", and T cells generate the impulses which reach the brain and form the perception of pain (see Fig. 13). The next step is the activation of the motor cortex which triggers efferent, motor discharge to the area where noxious stimuli applied. This motor, descending flow forms the protective muscle tension and is responsible for building up tension in the already affected muscles.

3. INDIRECT ACTIVATION OF MUSCLE SPINDLE RECEPTORS

Indirect activation of the muscle spindle receptors, or evoking a stretch reflex, is a more complicated process. Let's discuss this subject with the help of a diagram (see Fig. 15).

As discussed previously sudden, sharp pain evokes a withdrawal reflex. Constant intensive pain stimuli activate nociceptors in the skin, connective tissue structures and skeletal muscles, and elicit afferent (ascending) sensory input to the spinal cord and the brain (see Fig. 15, #2). As a result, the spinal cord increases its gamma motor (efferent) discharge to the muscle spindle receptors of the skeletal muscles located in the same region (see Fig. 15, #7). This discharge causes the ends of the muscle spindles to contract and, subsequently, the central parts of the spindles are stretched. Following this, the sensory elements of the muscle spindles located in the center start to generate their own action potentials, which travel to the lower motor centers of the spinal cord through afferent sensory neurons (see Fig. 15, #10). Lower motor centers then send an alpha motor (efferent) discharge back to the skeletal muscles in the same area where the original pain stimuli were applied (see Fig. 15, #11). This motor discharge causes muscle contraction and increases local tension.

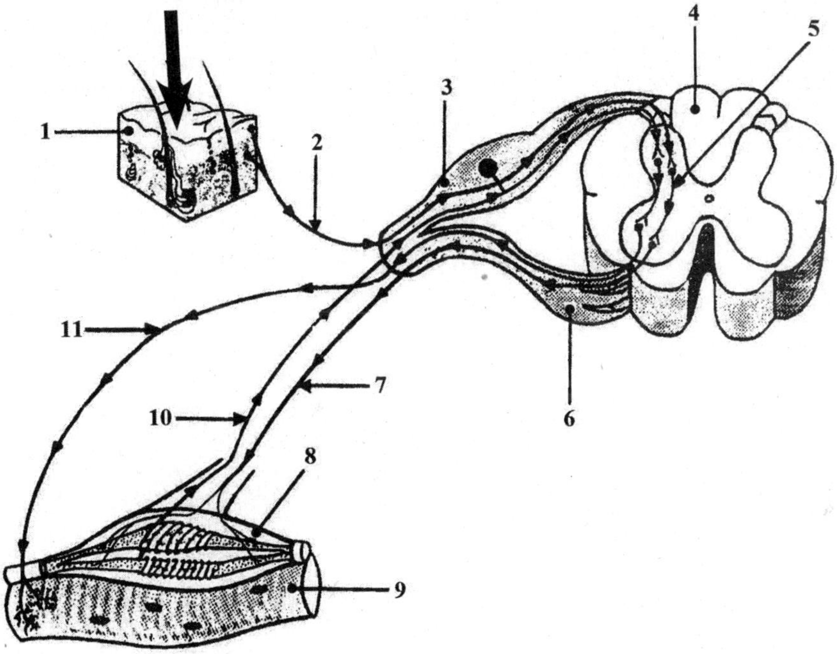

Fig. 15. Indirect activation of muscle spindle receptors (stretch reflex)

1 - excessive pressure in the tissue with a low pain threshold
2 - flow of sensory afferent impulses
3 - dorsal (posterior) root
4 - spinal cord
5 - intermediate neuron
6 - ventral (anterior) root
7 - gamma motor efferent neuron
8 - muscle spindle receptor
9 - skeletal muscle
10 - sensory afferent neuron
11 - alpha motor neuron to the skeletal muscle

Withdrawal reflex and, especially, the activation of the fast pain system are responsible for the formation of protective muscular tension. If the practitioner does not pay attention to protective muscular tension and tries to overcome it with stronger pressure, he or she can easily damage the soft tissues, especially the skeletal muscles.

The indirect activation of the muscle spindle receptors has an even more negative effect on the physiology of muscle contraction. It is actually responsible for the formation of new trigger points and hypertonuses, or makes their clinical picture worse. Thus, the application of excessive pressure worsens the clinical picture of hypertonic muscle pathology in the long run despite apparent pain relief directly after the session. This is a very important matter for anyone who practices medical massage, especially the methods of ischemic compression. We will talk about the correct application of ischemic compression later in chapter V.

E. RULES OF CORRECT APPLICATION OF STRONG PRESSURE

At the end of this chapter, I want to outline one more time the rules of the correct application of strong pressure during massage treatment:

1. Always explain the goals and methods of treatment to the patient. The patient has to cooperate with the massage practitioner during the treatment. Both of them should work in partnership to optimize the effect of the treatment.
2. Define the patient's personal pain threshold in the massaged area by slowly pressing the fingertip of the thumb or index finger into the soft tissue. Coordinate the amount of applied pressure with the patient's reactions.
3. Determine the exact location of all trigger points or any other types of painful areas (i.e. myogelosis). The massage practitioner has to be able to detect the trigger points in all tissues (i.e. skin, skeletal muscles, periosteum) and 'entrance' into each trigger point.
4. Always start with effleurage strokes of gentle and medium pressure to reduce the patient's anxiety about the first touch in sensitive or painful areas.
5. To prepare the massaged area, use effleurage and slow kneading in the inhibitory regime. At the same time, these strokes will activate C nervous fibers (i.e., the slow pain analyzing system). It will help to control pain stimuli during the subsequent application of deep tissue strokes or compression.
6. Try to avoid creating protective muscular tension. Apply pressure slowly and increase it gradually. Always remind the patient of the necessity complete muscle relaxation. If you feel that the patient generates protective muscular tension, **do not** overcome it with stronger pressure. Make the patient relax first.
7. Apply pressure in combination with permanent vibration on the sensitive areas to control pain analyzing system.
8. Activate the patient's central control trigger system during the massage treatment.
9. After deep tissue treatment or compression, always use fast effleurage and gentle vibration over the whole massaged area. You can find a description of compression techniques in chapter V.
10. Apply pressure at the right time, on the right place and with the right intensity.
11. To see the protocol of ischemic compression in video mode please visit our main educational website: **www.scienceofmassage.com**, click on the *Journal of Massage Science* icon where you will find a 4-part article on "Science of Trigger Point Therapy" in the Jan/Feb-Sept/Oct 2009 issues of the Journal.

IV. THE HAND AS A THERAPEUTIC TOOL. THE CONTACT AREAS FOR MASSAGE TREATMENT

During the long period of evolution, only humans developed the hand as a unique instrument for effectively exploring and interacting with the environment. With its truly unique characteristics the hand is the main therapeutic and diagnostic tool for anyone who practices any type of manual treatment. In this chapter we will look at the anatomy and biomechanics of the hand from the massage therapy point of view. First, let's review some anatomo-biomechanical characteristics of the human hand, and discuss their role in the massage therapist's professional performance.

A. ANATOMO-BIOMECHANICAL CHARACTERISTICS OF THE HAND FROM THE MASSAGE THERAPY POINT OF VIEW

Many textbooks represent the anatomy of the hand in detail. In this section we will discuss the anatomo-biomechanical characteristics of the human hand only from the position of the hand as a therapeutic tool. If we examine the human hand's shape and anatomy from this point of view, we can see that different parts of the hand can deliver different types and intensities of therapeutic impact. The bony, prominent parts and the fingertips are great instruments for the stimulation or compression of soft tissues. The padded areas of hand can be successfully used for soft, sedative strokes. Different types of hand prehensions also create optimal conditions for the various massage techniques.

The hand is the main diagnostic tool for everyone who practices massage, especially medical massage. The experienced therapist closes his or her eyes during the palpatory examination to fully analyze the tactile information conducted from the hand's receptors to the brain. Thus, the therapeutic and diagnostic ability of the hand originates from its unique blend of anatomo-physiological characteristics.

1. SKELETON OF THE HAND

The bones of the hand provide the frame for the soft tissues and are used as levers for movements in the joints. The human hand is formed by the following bones (see Fig. 16):

a. Capal Bones

Eight carpal bones are arranged in two rows. The proximal row includes the scaphoid, lunate, triquetral and pisiform. The distal row includes the trapezium, trapezoid, capitate and hamate. Both rows form the midcarpal joint, with little gliding movements between two rows.

b. Metacarpal Bones

The metacarpal bones are the five longest bones in the hand and support its frame. Proximally they form the carpometacarpal joint with the distal row of carpal bones, and distally they form the metacarpophalangeal joints with the proximal phalanges.

Carpometacarpal joints

The 2nd to 5th carpometacarpal joints have some insignificant movements in flexion-extension; adduction-abduction and circumduction. The 1st carpometacarpal joint is more mobile and it has several degrees of freedom: flexion-extension, adduction-abduction, circumduction and opposition-reposition. The opposition is a combination of flexion and medial rotation, while repositon is a combination of extension, abduction and lateral rotation. These seemingly simple movements in the 1st carpometacarpal joint are an absolutely unique feature of human hand. They definitely played an important role in human evolution.

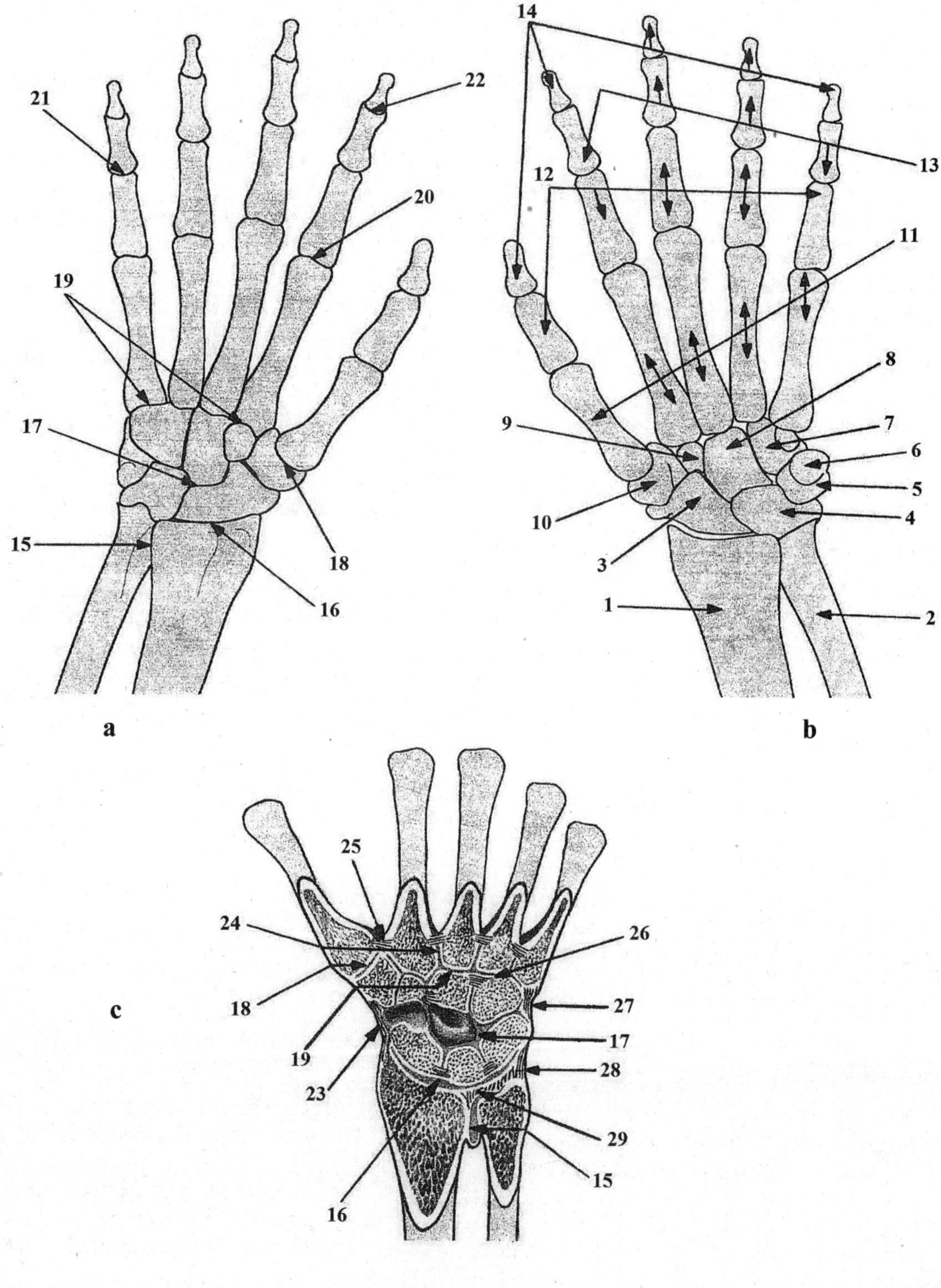

Fig. 16. Skeleton of the hand

1 - radius
2 - ulna
3 - scaphoid
4 - lunate
5 - triquetrum
6 - pisiform
7 - hamate
8 - capitate
9 - trapezoid
10 - trapezium
11 - metacarpals
12 - proximal phalanges
13 - middle phalanges
14 - distal phalanges
15 - distal radioulnar joint
16 - radiocarpal joint
17 - midcarpal joint
18 - 1st carpometacarpal joint
19 - carpometacarpal joints
20 - metacarpophalangeal joints
21 - proximal interphalangeal joint
22 - distal interphalangeal joint
23 - radial collateral ligament
24 - intermetacarpal joint
25 - metacarpal interosseus ligament
26 - intercarpal ligament
27 - carpometacarpal ligament
28 - ulnar collateral ligament
29 - articular disk

a - palmar hand
b - dorsal hand
c - palmar hand with the frontal cut of the carpometacarpal area (Kovanov and Travin, 1983).

Metacarpophalangeal joint

Metacarpophalangeal joints are visible as knuckles with the 3rd one most prominent. Metacar pophalangeal joints have two degrees of freedom: flexion-extension, adduction-abduction and their combination - circumduction. The metacarpal bones, especially their heads, form the transverse arc, with the head of the 3rd metacarpal bone as a higher point in the arc. This is especially noticeable when one makes a fist. The vertical axis of the hand continues from the forearm along the capitate bone, 3rd metacarpal bone and 3rd finger.

c. Phalangeal Bones

The 2nd to 5th fingers have proximal, middle and distal phalanges, while the thumb has only proximal and distal phalanges. Thus, there are nine interphalangeal joints in the human hand. They have only one degree of freedom: flexion-extension.

d. Wrist Joint

The wrist joint is one of the key components of professional massage therapy. It has to provide stability and flexibility to the hand simultaneously. Effective palmar, digital or palmar-digital prehension is available only with a strong, stable joint. The wrist joint is also one of the most common sites of professional hand injuries.

As is represented in Fig. 25 the wrist joint has three degrees of freedom: flexion-extention, adduction-abduction and circumduction. All movements in the wrist joint are executed around axises that cross each other on the level of the head of the capitate bone (Palastanga et al., 1989).

Thus, to reduce tension in the hands build by massage work, one has to gently mobilize the area around the capitate bone (see Fig. 34).

The wrist is formed by three joints. The **radiocarpal joint** (or wrist joint) is formed proximally by the radius and articular disk, and distally by the scaphoid, lunate and triquetrum bones. The articular disk separates this joint's cavity from the **distal radioulnar joint**, and disk forms the articular surface for the triquetral bone, while serving as a shock absorber between the hand, ulna and elbow joint. This is why the hand is vulnerable to injuries if the practitioner applies pressure while keeping the hand in ulnar deviation because the triquetrum bone squeezes the articular disk instead of the lunate bone which would makes more equal contact with the articular disk and radius. The **ulnacarpal joint** is formed by the ulna and triquetrum bone.

e. Skeleton of the Hand From the Massage Therapy Point of View

Now let's look at the hand's skeleton from the massage therapy's point of view.

1. The different bony prominent parts of the hand should be used as contact areas for massage treatment (see Fig. 43). Optimally, they should be employed for friction or compression techniques.

2. During the any deep tissue work, try to keep the applied pressure (e.g., during compression) as close as possible to the axis, which is formed by the wrist joint and radius or by the 1st through 3rd fingers, wrist joint and radius (see Fig. 17).
When the hand is placed in the preferable position, the main pressure is transferred proximally in the following sequence: hand - wrist joint - radius and interossei membrane - ulna - elbow joint (see Fig. 17 'a'). If the main pressure is applied along the axis of the ulna, it directly reaches the elbow joint without the unloading function of the radius and interosseus membrane. On Fig. 17'b' pressure spread along the interosseus membrane is shown as four short arrows. In this case, the elbow joint becomes more vulnerable to early degenerative changes (i.e., osteoarthritis) and various somatic disorders in the area of elbow (e.g., periostitis, epycondylitis, etc.).

3. The 1st carpometacarpal and wrist joints are the most vulnerable to professional injury. The practitioner has to be extremely careful in cases when strong pressure is applied. This is especially important when extra pressure is combined with massage strokes (e.g., during strong kneading). In this case, the wrist joint has less stability and is more susceptible to the injury. Some wrist injuries (e.g., de Quervain's disease) can severely affect the practitioner's professional performance and even career.

4. When the massage practitioner spreads his or her fingers widely and simultaneously compresses the soft tissues he or she puts a lot of pressure on the periosteum which covers the shaft of the metacarpal bones and proximal phalanges. It makes them susceptible to injuries, and to the development of a very painful complication called **periostitis**. Thus, try to keep the fingers as close together as possible during the application of massage techniques. If the treatment demands wide spread fingers, do not stay in this position for a long period of time and use your body weight as a tool. Alternate these strokes with other techniques or use two hands application.

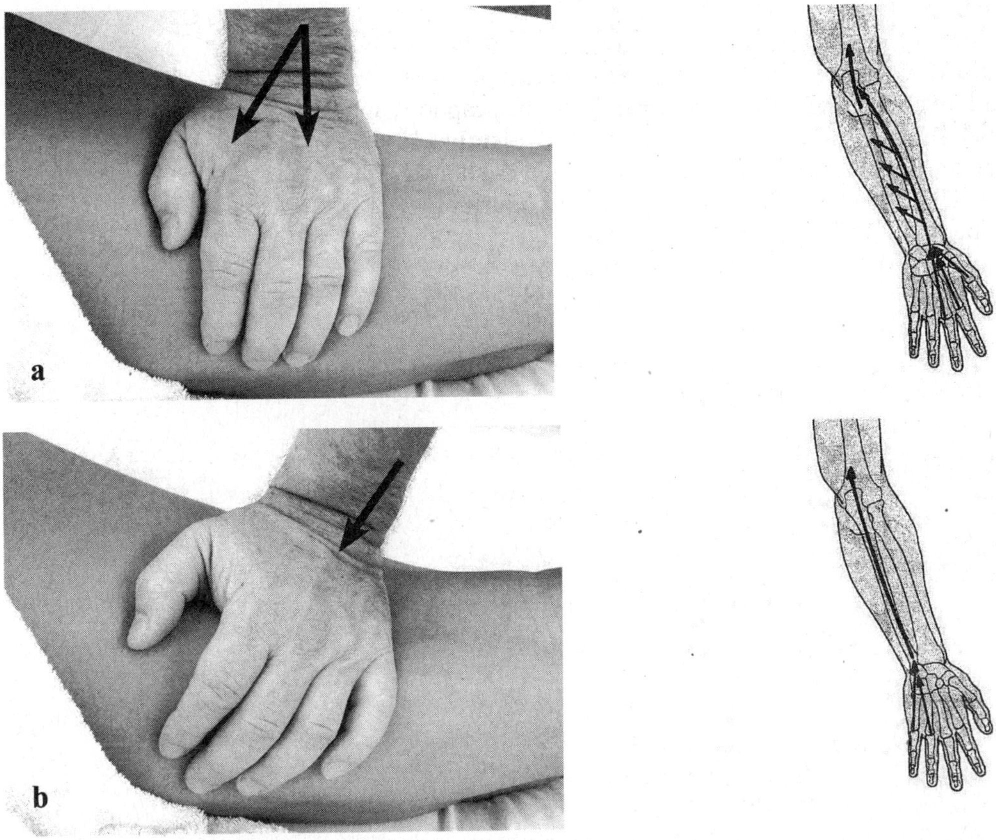

Fig. 17. The preferable and nonpreferable distribution of pressure during massage treatment
a - preferable hand position **b** - nonpreferable hand position

2. LIGAMENTAL SUPPORT OF THE HAND

The human hand is formed by a lot of different size of bones and joints. The best combination of hand's rigidity and flexibility is provided by sophisticated ligamental support, which is shown in Fig. 18. The complex system of ligaments deserves a separate discussion. This information can be found in any anatomy textbook. However, some important facts should at least be briefly mentioned from the position of massage therapy. From this point of view, we will discuss several important ligaments:

a. Radial Collateral Ligament

The radial collateral ligament reinforces the lateral side of the wrist joint (see Fig. 16 and 18). This ligament starts from the styloid process of the radius and inserts into the scaphoid bone. The radial collateral ligament can be damaged by hyperadduction in the wrist joint (i.e., excessive ulnar deviation). If the ligaments in the wrist are not strengthened by exercise, and the amount of massage work is not increased gradually, another scenario can occur. The permanent traumatization of the ligaments and the capsule of the joint will produce chronic inflammation in these tissues and in the periosteum of the styloid process of radius; i.e., causes Radial Styloiditis which can severely affect the therapist's professional ability.

b. Ulnar Collateral Ligament

The ulnar collateral ligament reinforces the medial side of the wrist joint and distal radioulnar joint as well (see Fig. 16 and 18). This ligament starts from the styloid process of the ulna and inserts into the triquetrum bone. Everything discussed previously with regard to radial collateral ligament applies to the ulnar collateral ligament with one difference: This ligament is vulnerable to injury when the hand in the position of hyperabduction (i.e., excessive radial deviation).

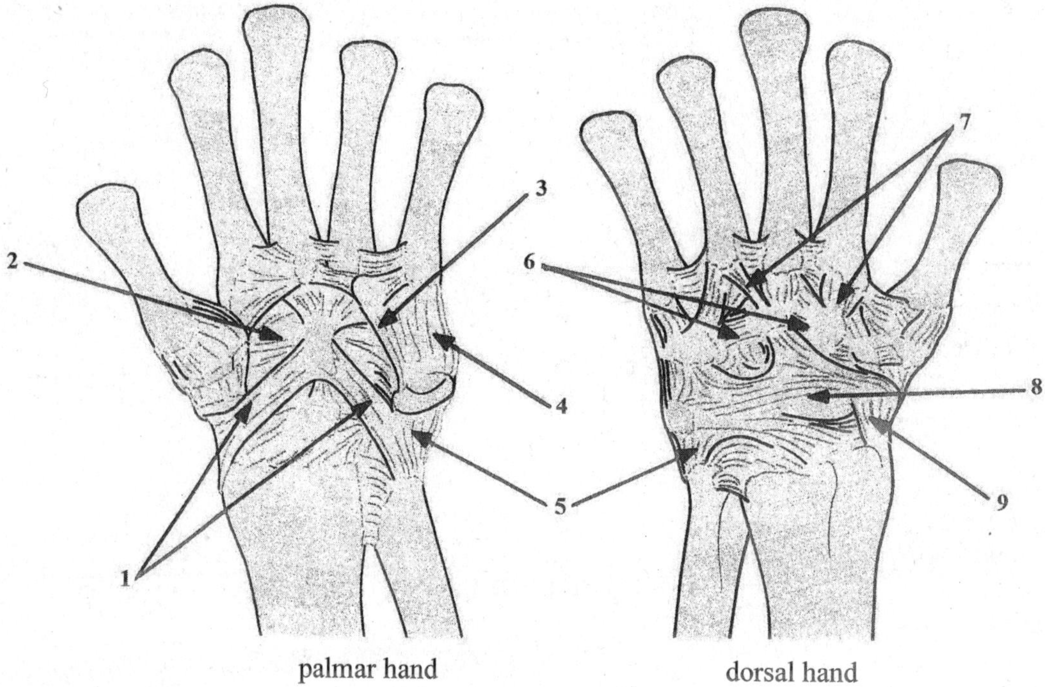

Fig. 18. Ligaments of the hand

1 - palmar radiocarpal lig.
2 - radial carpal lig
3 - pisohamatum lig
4 - pisometacarpal lig
5 - ulnar collateral lig.
6 - intercarpal lig.
7 - carpometacarpal lig.
8 - dorsal radiocarpal lig.
9 - radial collateral lig.

c. Flexor Retinaculum

The flexor retinaculum is a ligament which runs in a perpendicular direction to the vertical axis of the palmar hand. It consists of two layers: superficial - volar carpal ligament and deep - transverse carpal ligament (see Fig. 19 'a'). The transverse carpal ligament is the roof of the carpal tunnel. This ligament also consists of two bands. The **proximal band** runs between the scaphoid and pisiform bones and the **distal band** runs between the trapezium and hamate bones. The carpal bones form the bottom of the carpal tunnel. The carpal tunnel contains nine tendons (four tendons of flexor digitorum superficialis, four tendons of flexor digitorum profundus, and one tendon of flexor pollicis longus muscles) and the median nerve (see Fig. 19 'b'). The entry into the carpal tunnel can be projected on the distal volar skin crease of the wrist.

This tunnel has a conical shape with the following average dimensions: length - 0.5 inches; width at the entrance - 1 inch; width at the exit - 0.5 inches. Compression of the median nerve between the transverse carpal ligament and tendons causes Carpal Tunnel Syndrome.

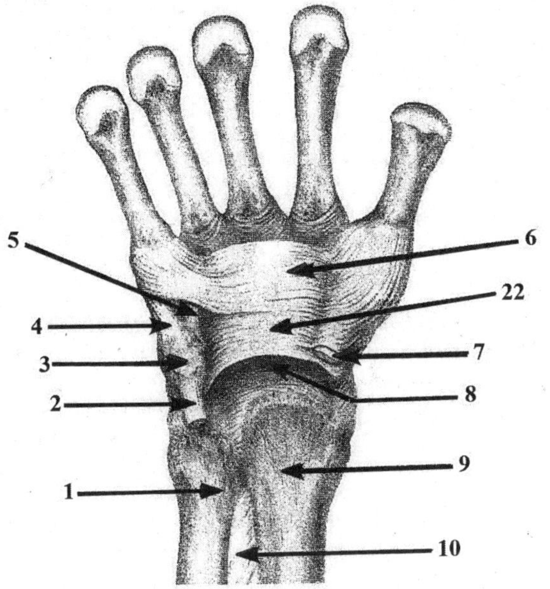

a

b

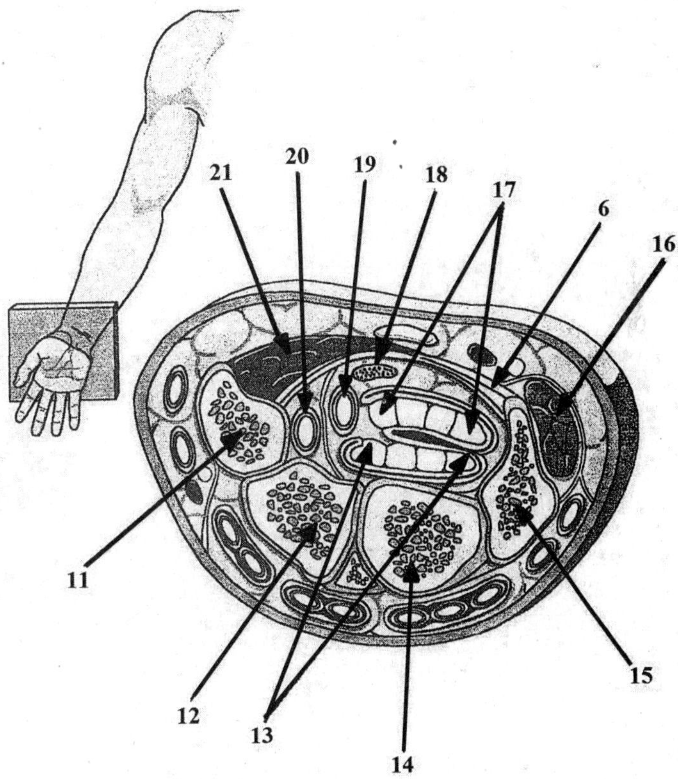

Fig. 19. Anatomy of the carpal tunnel

Fig. 19. Anatomy of the carpal tunnel

1 - ulna
2 - tendon of extensor carpi ulnaris m.
3 - pisiform
4 - pisometacarpal lig.
5 - pisohamatum lig.
6 - distal band of transverse carpal lig.
7 - tendon of flexor carpi radialis muscle
8 - carpal tunnel
9 - radius
10 - interosseus membrane
11 - trapezium
12 - trapezoid
13 - tt. flexor digitorum profundus muscle
14 - capitate
15 - hamate
16 - m. abductor digiti minimi
17 - t. flexor digitorum superficialis muscle
18 - median nerve
19 - t. flexor pollicis longus muscle
20 - t. flexor carpi radialis muscle
21 - m. abductor pollicis brevis
22 - proximal band of transverse carpal lig.

3. MUSCLES OF THE FOREARM AND HAND

The movements of the hand and fingers are supported by the 39 forearm and hand muscles (see Fig. 20 and 21). Among them there is not even one muscle which participates in a singular movement; i.e., absolute flexor or absolute adductor. All have combined actions. For example, the extensor carpi radialis longus muscle participates in the radial deviation (i.e. abduction) and extension in the wrist joint (see Fig. 43). Thus, each forearm and hand muscle supports different movements.

a. Biomechanical Classification of Forearm Muscles

Depending on the type of movement, each muscle can be a prime mover, synergist, antagonist, fixator or neutralizer of the movement.

1. The muscle **prime mover** is directly responsible for the desired movement. If several prime movers are involved in the movement they are called **agonists**.

2. Muscle **synergists** help the prime movers to execute the same movement. However, they only play a supportive role.

3. Muscle **antagonists** relax during the movement.

4. Muscle **stabilizators** are under isometric contraction and provide stability in the place of origin or insertion of the prime movers and agonists.

5. Muscle **neutralizers** eliminate some unnecessary contraction of other muscles during the movement.

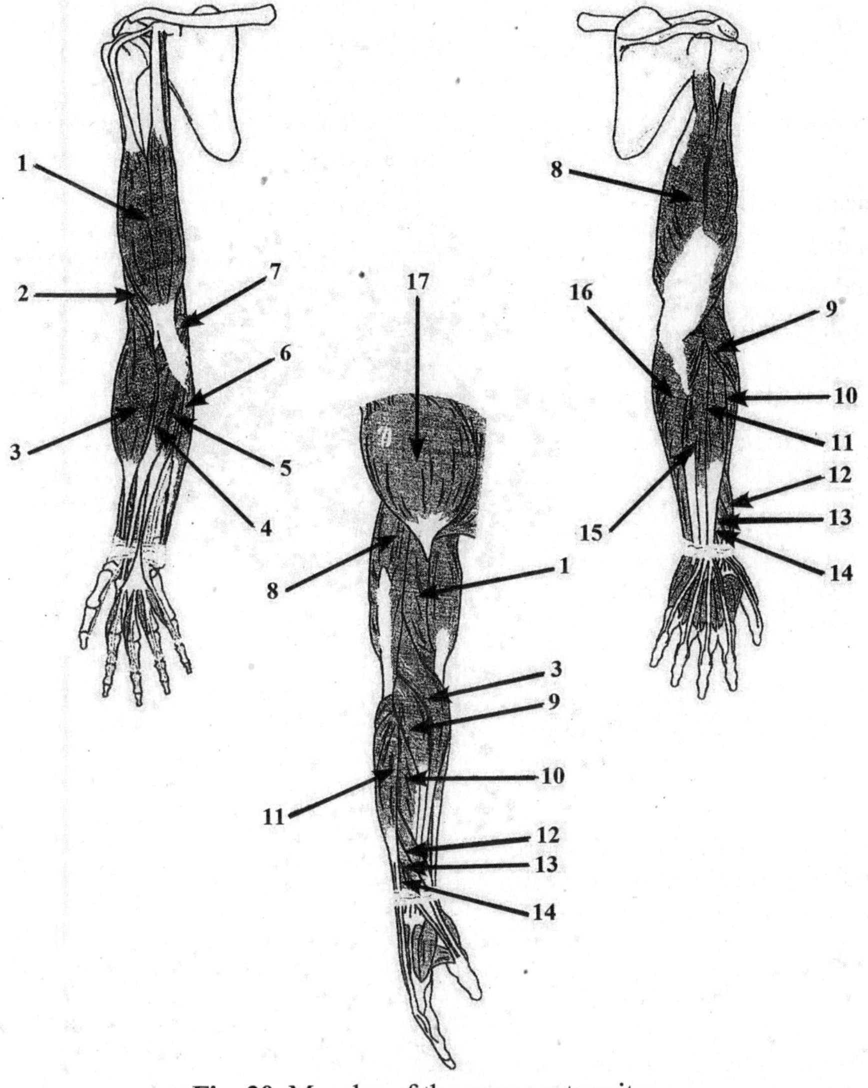

Fig. 20. Muscles of the upper extremity

1 - biceps brachii m.
2 - brachialis m.
3 - brachioradialis m.
4 - flexor carpi radialis m.
5 - flexor digitorum superficialis m.
6 - flexor carpi ulnaris m.
7 - pronator teres m.
8 - triceps brachii m.
9 - extensor carpi radialis longus m.
10 - extensor carpi radialis m.
11 - extensor digitorum communis m.
12 - abductor pollicis longus m.
13 - extensor pollicis brevis m.
14 - extensor pollicis longus m.
15 - extensor digiti minimi m.
16 - extensor carpi ulnaris m.
17 - deltoid m.

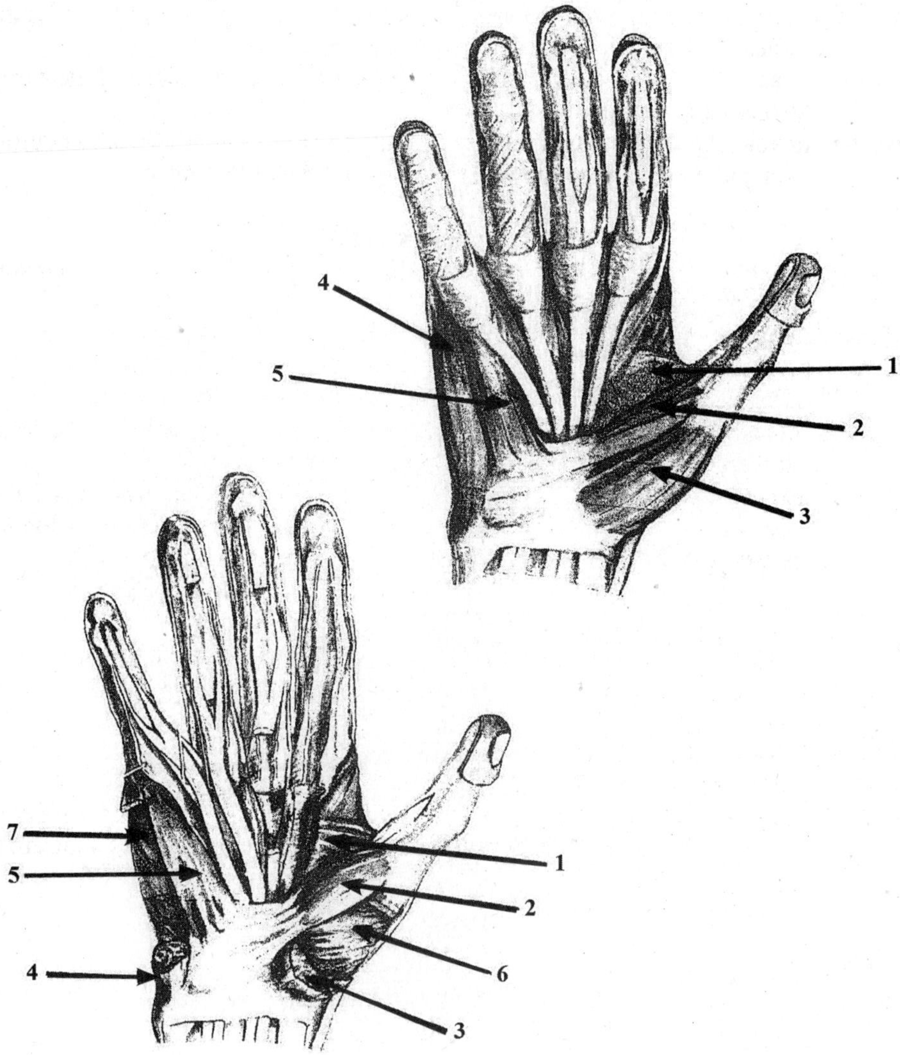

Fig. 21. Muscles of the hand (Kiss, Szentagothai, 1960)

1 - adductor pollicis m.
2 - flexor pollicis brevis m.
3 - abductor pollicis brevis m.
4 - abductor digiti minimi m.
5 - flexor digiti minimi m,
6 - opponens pollicis m.
7 - opponens digiti minimi m.

Let's look at the movements in the wrist joint from the point of view of reciprocal coordination between different muscle groups (Matev and Bankov, 1981):

Hand Flexion

Prime movers: flexor carpi radialis, flexor carpi ulnaris muscles
Synergists: palmaris longus, flexor digitorum superficialis and profundus, flexor pollicis longus muscles

Antagonists: extensor carpi ulnaris, extensor carpi radialis longus, extensor carpi radialis brevis, extensor digitorum, extensor pollicis longus muscles
Stabilizators: triceps brachii muscle stabilize the hand flexors at the place of their origin during strong hand flexion
Neutralizers: flexor carpi radialis and flexor carpi ulnaris muscles reciprocally neutralize abduction and adduction in the wrist joint during hand flexion

Hand Extension

Prime movers: extensor carpi radialis longus, extensor carpi radialis brevis, extensor carpi ulnaris muscles
Synergists: extensor digitorum, extensor indicis, extensor pollicis longus muscles
Antagonists: flexor carpi radialis, flexor carpi ulnaris, palmaris longus, flexor digitorum superficialis and profundus, flexor pollicis longus muscles
Stabilizators: biceps brachii, brachialis, and triceps brachii muscles stabilize the origin of prime movers during the forceful extension of the wrist joint
Neutralizers: extensor carpi ulnaris neutralizes the possibility of abduction or radial deviation in the wrist joint during hand extension. The extensor carpi radialis longus and brevis muscles neutralize the adduction or ulnar deviation of the wrist joint

Abduction or Radial Deviation

Prime movers: extensor carpi radialis longus, extensor carpi radialis brevis muscles
Synergists: flexor carpi radialis, extensor pollicis longus, extensor pollicis brevis, abductor pol licis longus muscles
Antagonists: extensor carpi ulnaris, flexor carpi ulnaris muscles
Stabilizators: biceps brachii muscle
Neutralizers: flexor carpi radialis muscle neutralizes hand extension during abduction in the wrist joint; extensor carpi radialis longus and brevis muscles neutralize the hand's flexion

Adduction or Ulnar Deviation

Prime movers: flexor carpi ulnaris, extensor carpi ulnaris muscles
Synergists: flexor digitorum superficialis, flexor digitorum profundus, extensor digitorum, ex tensor indicis, extensor digiti minimi muscles
Antagonists: extensor carpi radialis longus, extensor carpi radialis brevis muscles
Stabilizators: triceps brachii muscle stabilizes the flexors on the ulnar side at their origin from the medial epicondyle of humerus; 3rd interossei muscle stabilizes the 5th finger by preventing its separate abduction during ulnar deviation in the wrist joint
Neutralizers: flexor carpi ulnaris muscle neutralizes the extension of the hand during abduction in the wrist joint; extensor carpi ulnaris muscle neutralizes the hand's flexion

These complicated biomechanical relations change if one flexes or extends fingers simultaneously to the flexion or extension of the hand. Because the tendons of long flexors and extensors cross the wrist, metacarpophalangeal and interphalangeal joints, it is reasonable to expect that the fingers' flexion will simultaneously produce hand flexion, and vice versa. However, this does not occur, because the extensor digitorum muscle also contracts during flexion of the fingers to prevent hand flexion in the wrist joint. Thus, the extensor digitorum muscle in this case is both a muscle-antagonist and a neutralizer. It is the same for the relations between the long extensors and the long flexors during the fingers' extension.

Despite the complex anatomical structure of the forearm and hand, every movement is performed smoothly and precisely, thanks to great coordination between the different muscle groups as well as the muscles within the same group. Fig. 22 represents the physiological axis of movements in the wrist joint for different muscles. (The length of every line is inverse proportional to the work coefficient).

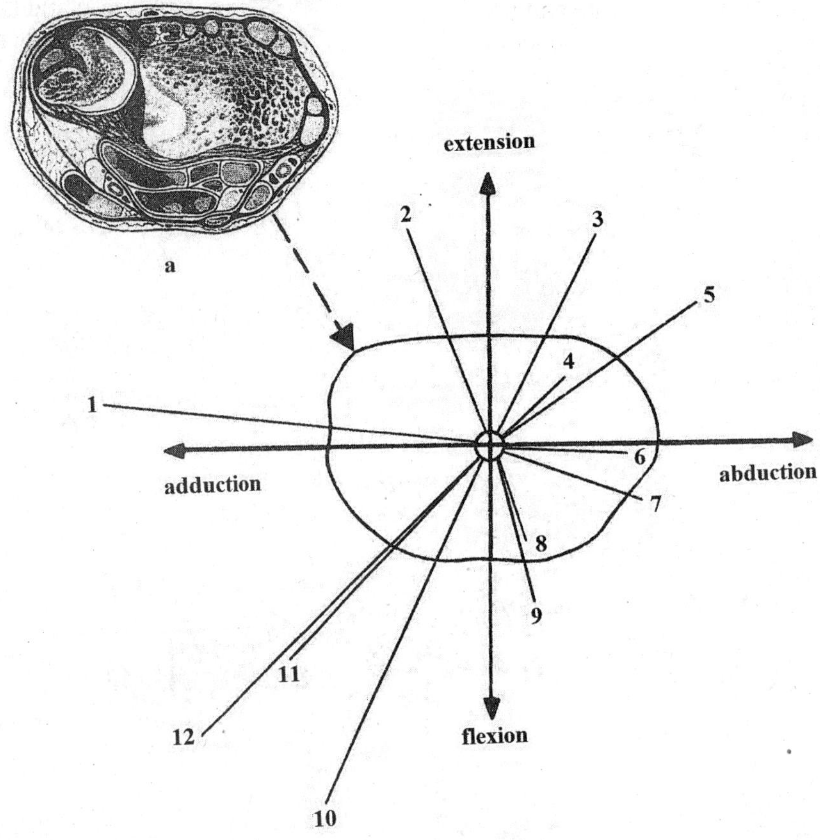

Fig. 22. The physiological axis of movements in the wrist by the forearm muscles (Steindler, 1964). a - cross section of the wrist joint

1 - extensor carpi ulnaris m.	**7** - m. abductor pollicis longus
2 - extensor digitorum m.	**8** - m. flexor pollicis longus
3 - extensor carpi radialis brevis m.	**9** - m. flexor carpi radialis
4 - extensor pollicis longus m.	**10** - m. flexor digitorum superficialis
5 - extensor carpi radialis longus m.	**11** - m. flexor carpi ulnaris
6 - extensor pollicis brevis m.	**12** - m. flexor digitorum profundus

In the normal wrist joint tension is developed by the flexors, is a larger than tension produced by extensors and tension by abductors is larger than adductors. This occurs because each muscle group has a different cross-sectional area. As was reported by Steindler, (1964), the total cross-sectional area of all hand flexors equals 33.4 cm , compared to 16.72 cm of extensors, and the total cross-sectional area of hand abductors equals 11.20 cm , compared to 10.20 cm of adductors. However, to obtain the optimal stability of the wrist (e.g., during compression), all muscle groups have to be under maximal tension.

b. Hand Prehensions

The human hand has several types of palmar, palmar-digital and digital prehensions. This allows us to perform extremely delicate and precise movements, as well as to grasp and hold objects with a force of more than 100 pounds. Generally, all massage techniques can be viewed as a combination of different hand prehensions. The number of prehensions varies in different publications. For example, Schlesinger (1919) recognized up to 12 different types of hand prehensions. I will refer to April (1990), who described 7 types of commonly accepted hand prehensions. Fig. 23 represents the prehensions of the human hand.

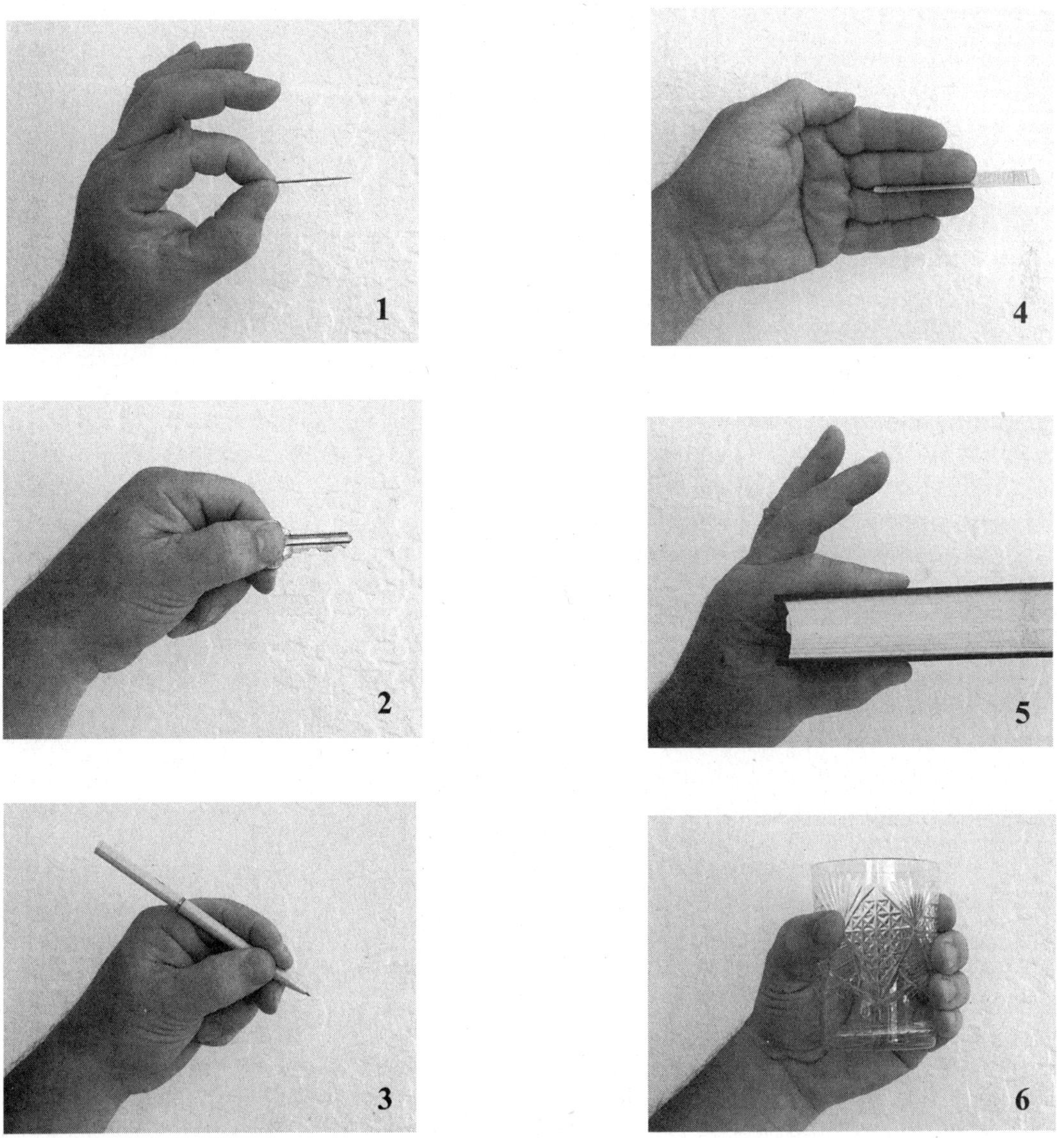

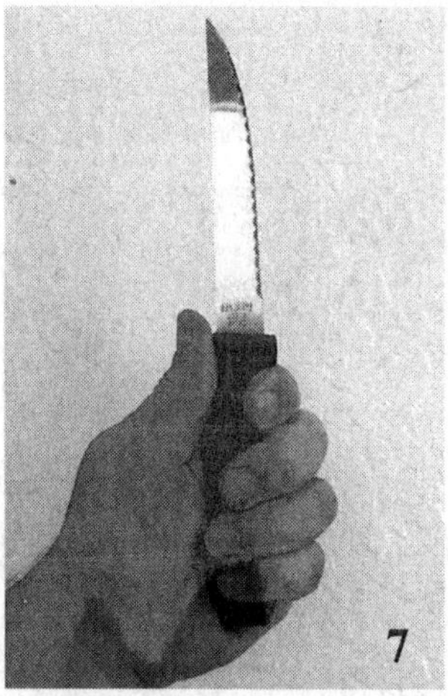

Fig. 23. Prehensions of the human hand

1 - digital prehension by terminal opposition
2 - digital prehension by subterminal opposition
3 - digital prehension by subterminal three-point opposition
4 - digital prehension by subterminal lateral opposition
5 - lateral digital opposition
6 - digital palmar prehension
7 - palmar prehension

All prehensions of the human hand can be performed in the **static** and **dynamic** regimes. The ability of the hand to execute dynamic grasp is one of its unique features (MacKenzie and Iberall, 1994). With dynamic prehension, we can grasp an object and simultaneously manipulate it. The dynamic grasp is a foundation of kneading technique. This function of the hand is supported by different muscle of the forearm and hand. However, I especially want to discuss the role of the following prime movers: flexor digitorum superficialis, flexor digitorum profundus and thenar muscles.

Flexor digitorum superficialis and profundus

The flexor digitorum superficialis originated from the medial epicondyle of the humerus, and inserts into the base of the 2nd phalanges of the 2nd through 5th fingers. The flexor digitorum profundus originated from the proximal 1/3 of ulna, and inserts into the base of the 3rd phalanges of the 2nd through 5th fingers. These muscles cross several joints between the place of their origin and insertion. As a matter of fact, the extensor digitorum profundus muscle crosses over 7 joints of the forearm and hand (see Fig. 20).

These muscles are prime movers for the flexion of fingers, and agonists for the flexion and slight adduction in the wrist joint. Thus, these muscles play the key roles in digital and palmar-digital prehension and, therefore, in massage treatment. Each finger has its individual level of strength and their ranking order is as follows: 3rd, 2nd, 1st, 4th, 5th (Scott, 1963).

A light extension of the hand in the wrist joint (approximately 15-20 degrees) is the most favorable hand position for the optimal contractile performance of both flexors and, consequently, for the strength of grip. The hand is placed in this position automatically as soon as fingers are flexed. If the therapist flexes fingers when the hand is placed in a neutral position or even slightly flexed in the wrist joint, the contractile performance of both muscles is significantly reduced and one looses the grip's power (Wells and Luttgens, 1976). Therefore, the hands quickly become exhausted from repetitive movements. Fig. 24 shows an example of hands in a positio unfavorable for both muscles. You can see in this photo that the operator's wrist is flexed, with simultaneous flexion of the fingers in the metacrpophalangeal joints as he works on the calf muscles.

Thus, the massage practitioner has to control this matter during treatment to use contractile potential of both digital and palmar flexors carefully, to be able to work longer and to prevent injuries.

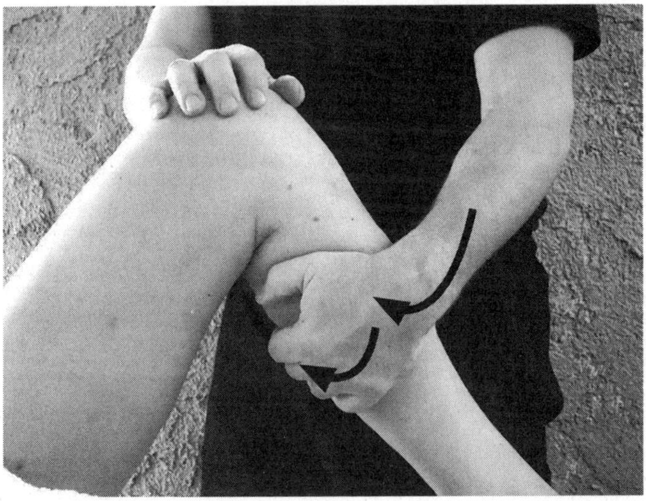

Fig. 24. Example of unfavorable position of the hand and fingers for muscle flexors

Thenar musculature

Effective palmar and palmar-digital prehension requires equal participation of the thumb. The anatomical opposition of the thumb creates the optimal conditions for effective counterpressure against the 2nd through 4th fingers by the thumb's flexion and adduction. This function is supported by the long thumb muscles (flexor pollicis longus, abductor pollicis and extensor pollicis muscles) and especially the thenar musculature.

The thenar is formed by the flexor pollicis brevis, the adductor pollicis, the opponens pollicis and abductor pollicis brevis muscles (see Fig. 21). The first three muscles play a critical role in the palmar and digital-palmar prehensions of the hand.

As was shown by Kapandji, (1970) the maximal stability of the thumb, in combination with maximal tension of the thenar muscles, is developed when the thumb is pressed in the direction of the index finger. Thus, in this thumb's position the thenar muscles become less exhausted during massage treatment.

c. Range of Mtoions in the Upper Extremity

The upper extremity is very movable. It has several degrees of freedom: three in the shoulder joint, two in the elbow joint, and three in the wrist joint. Besides this, the hand additionally has three degrees of freedom in every metacarpophalangeal joint and two degrees in each interphalangeal joint. Thus, by using all degrees of freedom, the human is capable of accomplishing the most precise and complex tasks. Fig. 25 represents the normal range of motions in the joints of upper extremity.

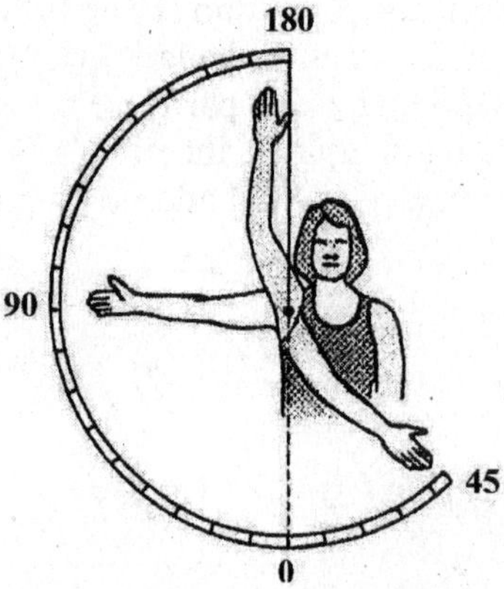

Shoulder joint: abduction/adduction

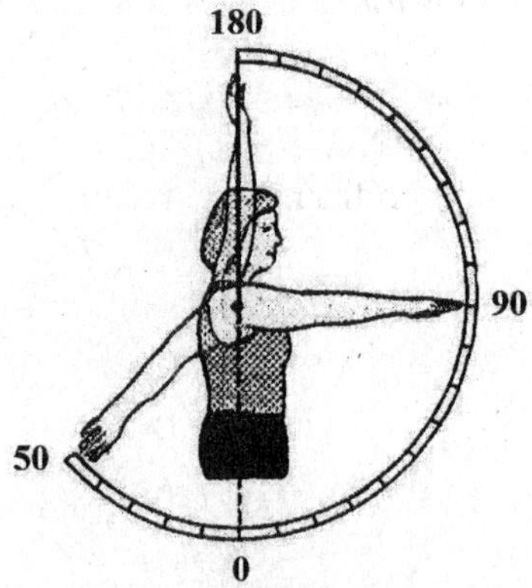

Shoulder Joint: flexion/extension

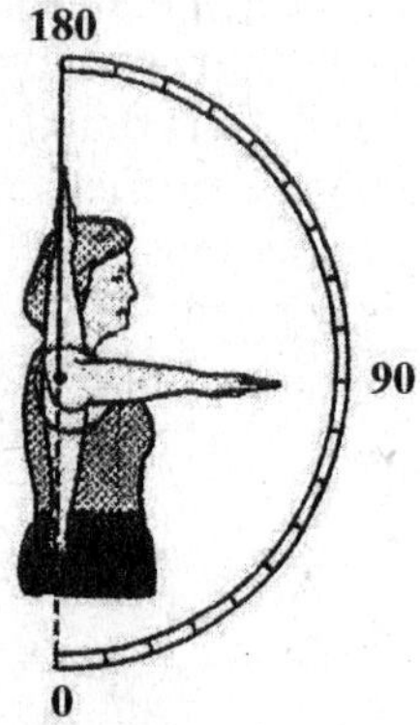

Shoulder joint: rotation

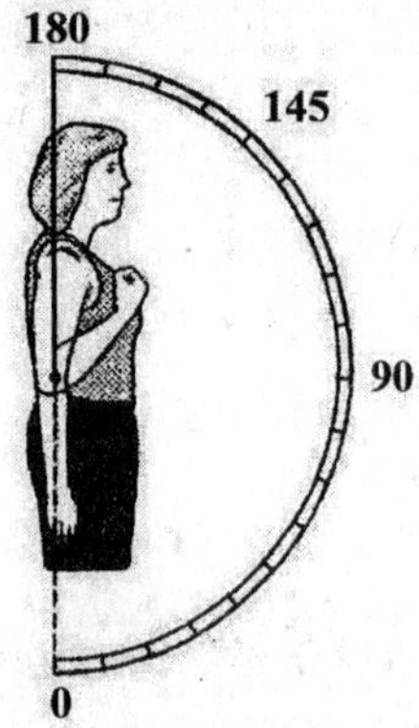

Elbow joint: flexion/extension

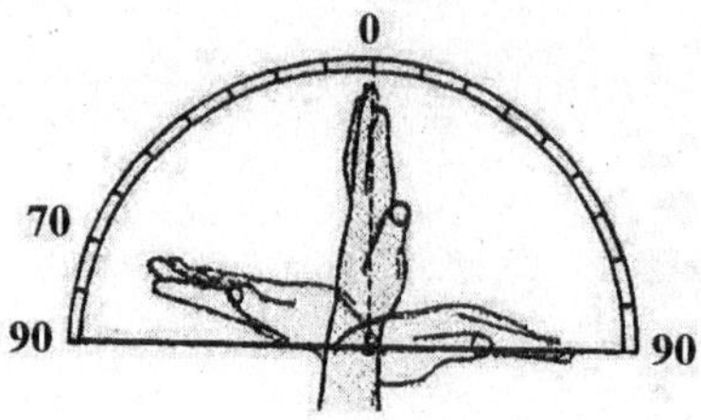

Wrist joint: flexion/extension

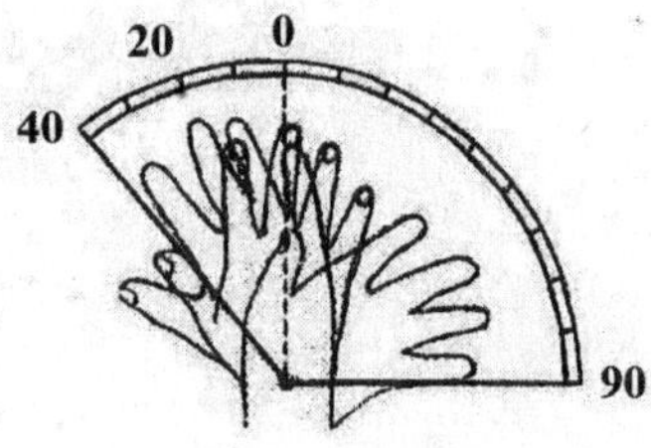

Wrist joint: deviation

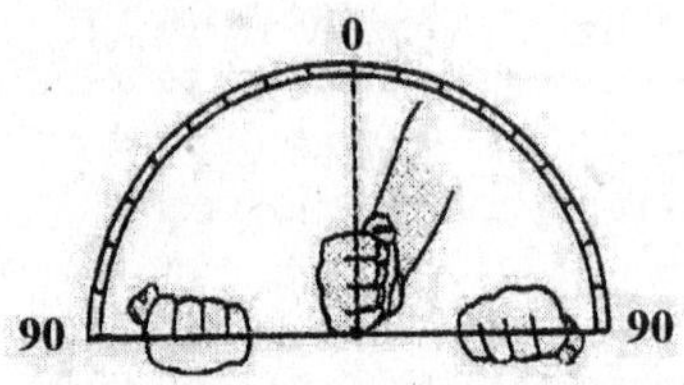

Wrist joint: pronation/supination

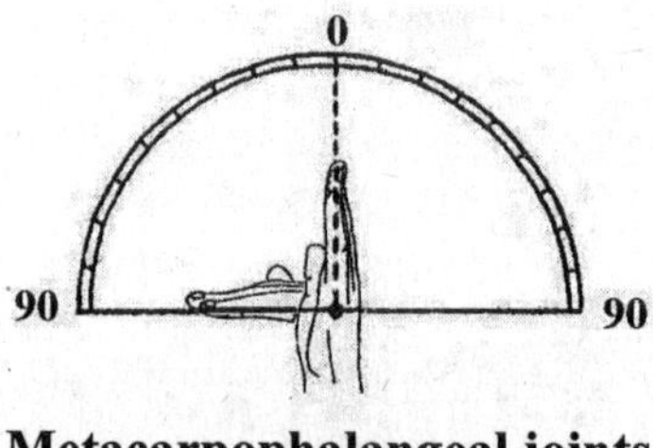

Metacarpophalangeal joints: flexion/extension

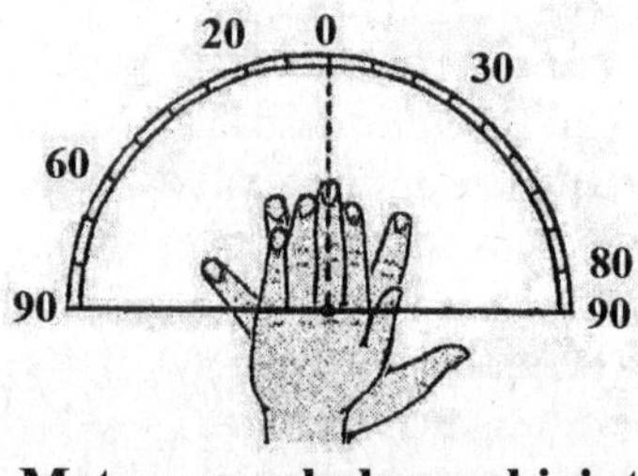

Metacarpophalangeal joints: abduction/adduction

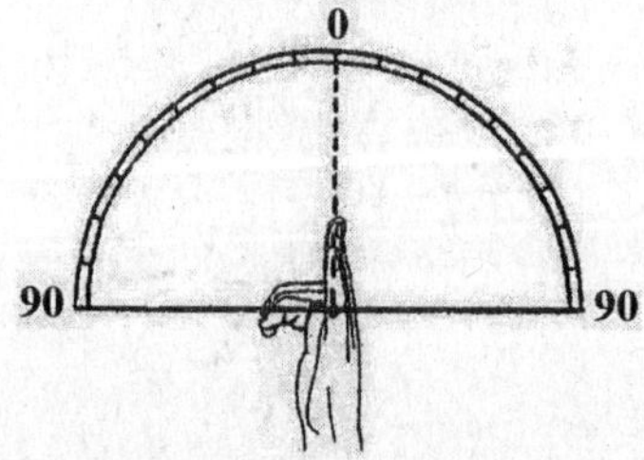

Interphalangeal joints: flexion/extension

Fig. 25. The range of motions in the joints of upper extremity

When the hand is in the physiological position, it has the greatest stability and strength for grasping. In this position the hand is extended about 20 degrees with a slight ulnar deviation in the wrist joint. The thumb is slightly flexed, abducted and opponed, and the fingers are partly flexed and abducted in the metacarpo-phalangeal joints (see Fig. 26). To prevent hand injuries, the massage practitioner must control any deviation from the physiological position, especially if additional pressure is applied.

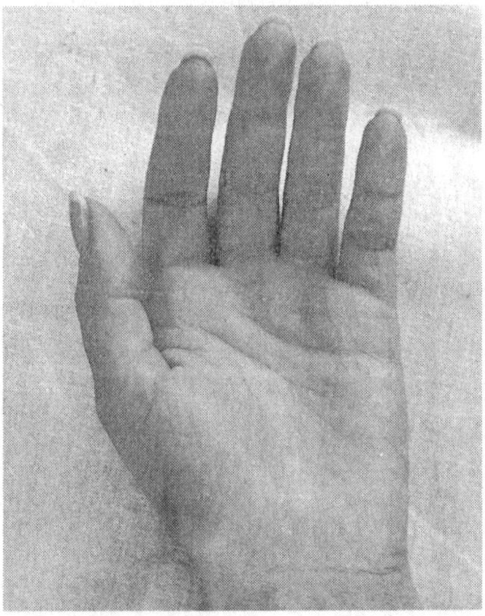

Fig. 26. Physiological position of the hand

d. Muscles of the Forearm and Hand from Massage Therapy Point of View

Everyone who practices massage worries about increasing forearm and hand muscle endurance and decreasing exhaustion. Another even more important problem is injury prevention. The muscles of the hand can provide effective isometric contractions for a long period of time if only 15% of maximal muscle strength is used. They are also able to provide long effective isotonic contractions only if 30% of their maximal strength is used. Of course, the reality is significantly different because massage treatment demands more energy, but these numbers give a basis from which to estimate and effectively use the personal potential. To reduce muscle exhaustion and prevent injuries, the massage therapist should use several basic principles:

1. Change the hands' position and posture as frequently as possible. Even the slightest change in arm or hand position during the massage significantly alters the biomechanical relations between different muscles, even within the same muscle group. As a result, the muscles' potential is used more efficiently, they can run longer and the operator is less exhausted.

2. As reported by Bankov (1977), the optimal distance between the opposed thumb and the other fingers is 4.5 cm, or approximately 2 inches (see Fig. 27). With this distance the operator's hand has the greatest strength for digital prehension. Further increasing the distance between fingers reduces the strength of digital prehension. If the character of strokes allows, try to keep the thumb in opposition within this range; i.e., grasp enough tissue to fulfill this 2 inches distance. In this case, the hand has more strength and becomes less tired during the massage treatment. It also reduces the possibility of professional injury.

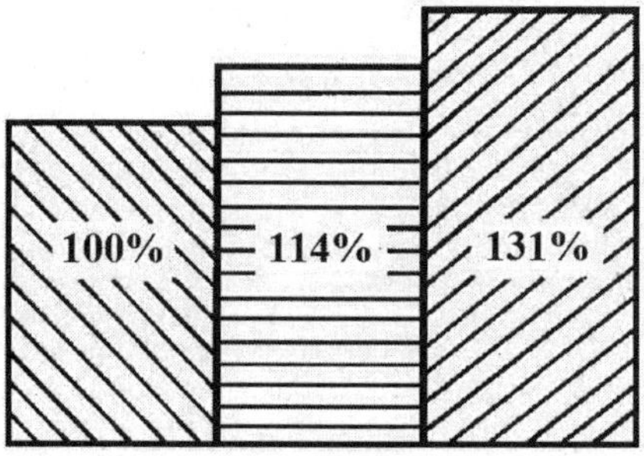

Fig. 27. Changes in the muscle strength with variation in distances between the thumb and 3rd finger during the digital prehension (Bankov, 1977)
100% - muscle strength of digital prehension with 1 cm distance between fingers
114% - muscle strength of digital prehension with 2.5 cm distance between fingers
131% - muscle strength of digital prehension with 4.5 cm distance between fingers

As correctly pointed out by MacKenzie and Iberall, (1994) the stability of a static and dynamic hand's prehension depends mostly from the distance between the opposed thumb and the 2nd-5th fingers. The distance is optimal if it is always "possible to increase the magnitude of the grasping force." If the distance between the 1st and the 2nd-5th fingers is too large, any further increase in the grip's power demands significantly more effort, or may even be impossible to achieve. These recommendations have an important practical meaning. For example, de Quervain's disease can be easily triggered during the wrong application of compression or deep friction. Fig. 28 'a' illustrates the secure position of the hand and fingers during the compression technique and Fig. 28 'b' presents the position of the hand that can cause de Quervain's disease.

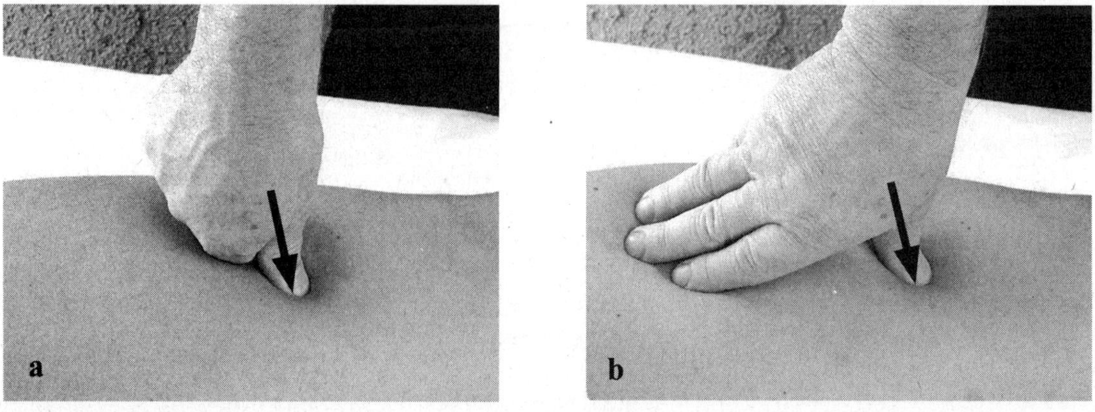

Fig. 28. Correct and incorrect positions of the hand during the application of the compression
a - correct position **b** - incorrect position

The operator can also save muscle energy and prevent injuries if he or she starts to use both hands, instead of the spread fingers of just one hand, when possible. Fig. 29 shows the combination of effleurage and compression techniques on the anterior surface of the thigh in one and two-hand applications. Muscles' exhaustion and the possibility of hand injury is lesser in the second variant.

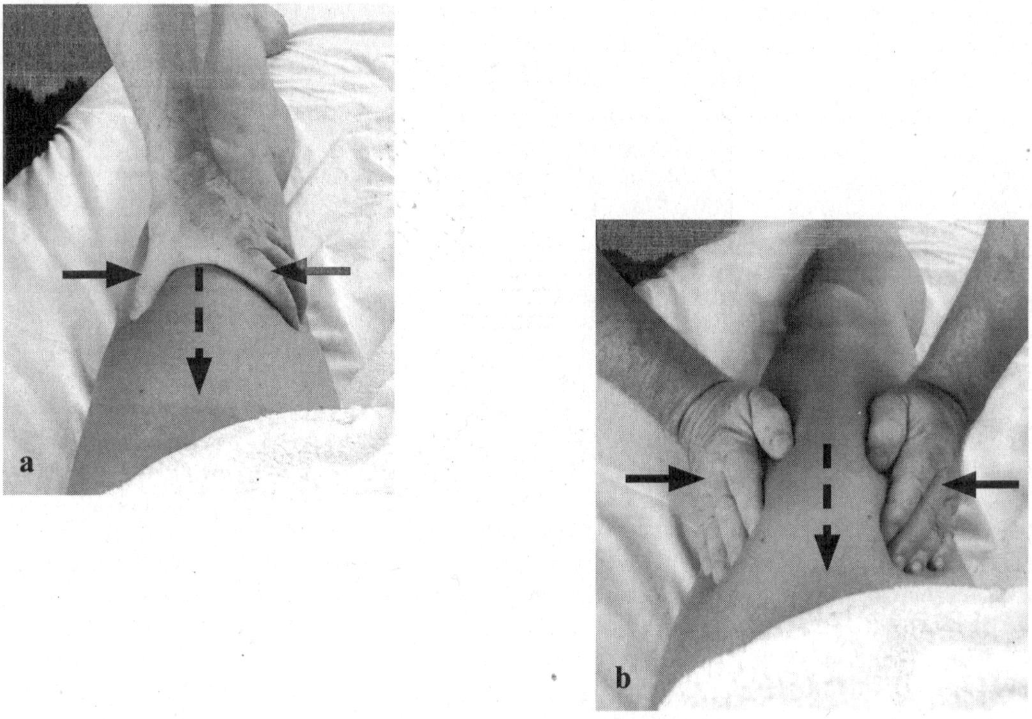

Fig. 29. The application of one and two-hand strong effleurage technique
Solid arrows - direction of compression
Dashed arrows - direction of the stroke
a - one-hand application
b - two-hand application

3. Change the rhythm of the strokes as frequently as is possible. This is also an important tool to prevent muscle exhaustion. At the same time, try to breath rhythmically.
4. Train yourself to use only the muscles that need to be involved in the completion of a particular technique, and relax the other muscle groups as much as possible. For example, flat superficial effleurage can be completed by the power of the hand(s) only. Thus, the arm and shoulder muscles should be maximally relaxed.
5. Every human has a dominant hand. The massage therapist has to be able to use both hands in equal degree. Before this becomes a habit, permanently control this matter.
6. Use a lot of isotonic and isometric exercises, especially if you have just begun to practice massage. Remember that exercises against the strong counterresistance build up muscle strength while prolonged, repetitive exercises with smaller counterresistance increase muscle endurance. Increase the amount of work gradually to give the hands time to adjust to new type of activity.

4. SKIN OF THE HAND

The skin on the palmar and dorsal hand is significantly different. The skin on the palmar surface of the hand is irreplaceable. This means it is so unique that actual loss of the palmar skin (e.g., after trauma or burn), cannot be adequately replaced by skin transplant from any other part of the body without losing some of its important features.

a. Skin on the Palmar and Dorsal Hand

The skin on the palmar hand has following unusual characteristics:

1. The palmar skin contains abundant nerve endings and receptors which detect pain, pressure, touch, vibration and temperature. The concentration of the receptors is the greatest, compared to any other part of the human body.
2. The skin on the fingertips has the greatest concentration of sweat glands. The moistened skin creates optimal conditions for the activation of tactile receptors and, therefore, intensifies tactile perception. Besides this, a hand with moistened skin grasps objects more securely. Palmar skin has 2.736 sweat glands per square inch of surface. The same parameter for the abdominal skin is 1.954 and for the skin on the lateral thigh only 554 (Rothman, 1954).
3. The skin on the palmar surface does not have hairs, sebaceous glands or pigment-forming cells. The absence of these structures, which are common to the skin on any other part of the body (except the soles of the feet), is a result of the hand's functional adaptation during evolution. This adaptation creates optimal conditions for tactile perception and grasping.
4. The thickness of the skin on the palmar surface is about 1.5-2 mm. Between 1/5 and 1/4 of the total amount of body dermis is located on the fingers and hand. Only the soles have thicker skin. The palmar skin is little movable and has a strong attachment to the three underlying anatomical structures: palmar aponeurosis, synovial tendon sheaths and bones (metacarpal and phalanges). This feature also support the hand's grasping and holding abilities.
5. The palmar skin, especially on the areas of the fingertips, has a special relief which is unique for every person. This special skin design is formed by an increased dermal papillae of papillary dermis. The dermal papillae form the epidermal ridges with grooves between them, and they contain a lot of tactile receptors. At the top of the epidermal ridges are the openings of the sweat glands. Thus, the epidermal ridges increase the hand's prehensions and support tactile perception.
6. The palmar hand has four deep creases, and the skin on each finger has three horizontal creases. The creases provide the ideal conditions for the optimal range of movements in the small joints. When the person makes a fist, up to 25% of the palmar skin goes into the creases.
7. The subcutaneous tissue on the palmar hand also has unusual characteristics. The subcutaneous tissue is separated on the lobes by fibrous fasciculi, which anchor the skin to the synovial tendon sheaths and bones. This structure of subcutaneous tissue also supports the grip of the hand.
8. The skin on the dorsal surface of the hand has the same characteristics as any other part of the body. Compared to the palmar skin, it is thinner, does not have a special design, is highly movable, has a thin layer of subcutaneous tissue and fewer receptors (except temperature receptors).

b. Skin of the Hand from Massage Therapy Point of View

Let's analyze the information from this section from the point of view of massage therapy:

1. Your hands are your main diagnostic and therapeutic tool. Be careful to protect your hands against any kind of trauma, especially on the palmar surface.
2. Take really good care of the skin. Avoid any activities which make the skin harder and form calluses, as this will significantly restrict your palpatory skills. For the same reason, use different types of softening hand lotions, and take weekly hot baths for the hands.
3. Maximally employ the tactile ability of your hands for diagnostic purposes. Numerous textbooks recommend a lot of different exercises to improve the individual level of tactile perception. Of course, individual tactile ability is important and should be built up. However, it is not the main component of palpatory examination. I strongly believe that the actual knowledge of what

abnormalities you are looking for, as well as where these abnormalities can be found, is the critical element to any successful diagnostic evaluation. Thus, as a first step in building your palpatory skills, you have to establish clear tactile distinction between the normal structure of every type of soft tissues (skin, fascia, skeletal muscles, etc.) and pathologically changed ones. This ability builds slowly with permanent self-education, everyday practice and constant communication with patients.

4. Strong attachment of the palmar skin to the underlying connective tissue structures and bones is an important feature for massage therapy. The hyperextension in the wrist, metacarpo-phalangeal and interphalangeal joints during massage causes microtraumas of the connective tissue structures, especially the palmar aponeurosis and flexor retinaculum. The constant micro-traumatization of palmar aponeurosis and flexor retinaculum can, finally, cause Carpal Tunnel Syndrome or Dupuyetrene's contracture (see below). Thus, be careful while placing hands in the position of hyperextension.

B. PROFESSIONAL INJURIES AND DISEASES OF THE HAND

A detailed discussion of injuries and diseases of the hand is not a subject of this book, but I think it is important to describe the more common ones at least briefly. The reader may find more detailed information about diagnostic evaluation and application of medical massage protocols in *Medical Massage* Volume I (**www.aesculapbooks.com**) and Video Library of **www.scienceofmassage.com** website.

1. TENDON SHEATH INJURY. TENDINITIS

Tendinitis is the one of most common types of professional injury. It can be a result of acute trauma (hyperflexion or hyperextension) as well as a result of excessive repetitive movements. Because of the specificity of massage work, the tendons of flexor muscles are usually affected more frequently, compared to the tendons of extensor muscles.

The main complaint is pain and crepitation during movement, especially if additional pressure is applied. By testing different movements in the wrist joint and fingers against resistance, it is possible to determine exactly which tendon(s) is affected. Another helpful test is compression along the tendon while the tested muscle is under tension.

One particular type of tendinitis is called de **Quervain's disease**, in honor of the author who described it for the first time in 1895. De Quervain's disease is also called stenosing tenosynovitis. It is a frequent type of hand injury for the massage therapist. In the case of de Quervain's disease, the abductor pollicis longus and extensor pollicis brevis tendons are affected at the level of styloid process of the radius where they are covered by the extensor retinaculum. Both tendons share a common synovial sheath.

Treatment: rest for at least 10 days; anti-inflammatory drugs; moist heat; paraffin; ultrasound; gentle massage along the affected tendon including Lymph Drainage Massage. As soon as symptoms become less acute, the duration and energy of massage treatment should be increased. Periostal massage in the area of the styloid process of the radius is the ultimate method of treatment of de Quervain's disease.

2. TRIGGER FINGER

Trigger finger is an unusual pathology. Due to trauma, chronic tendinitis, or excessive small repetitive movements, a small nodule forms and grows on the tendon. When the nodule is big enough it blocks the sliding of the tendon inside its tendon sheath. As a result, the patient feels the sudden snapping during the flexion or extension of the affected finger. In the advanced stages, a complete locking of the finger occurs. The more frequently affected tendons are flexors of thumb, 3rd and 4th fingers.

Treatment: anti-inflammatory drugs and injected; surgical removal of nodule. The main preventive measure for trigger finger is avoidance of tendon injuries.

3. PERIOSTITIS

Periostitis is an inflammation of the periosteum at the insertion of the ligaments or muscles into the bone. It is also a common type of professional massage injury. The more frequently affected areas are the 1st and 2nd metacarpal bones, the proximal phalanx of the thumb, and the 2nd and 3rd fingers. Periostitis in the areas of the ulna and radius is called **Styloiditis**. The same disorder in the areas of lateral and medial epicondyles of the humerus is called **Epicondylitis** (Tennis or Golfer's Elbow). The main complaint is local pain, which frequently has a burning character. It increases when the muscles which insert into the affected area of periosteum contract.

Treatment: anti-inflammatory drugs; complete rest for at least 2 weeks; moist heat (Jacuzzi); massage. The more effective method of treatment is periostal massage.

4. CARPAL TUNNEL SYNDROME

The compression of the median nerve in the carpal tunnel between the tendons of flexor muscles and transverse carpal ligament produces the variety of sensory and motor neurological abnormalities on the hand. Sanderland (1976) described two stages of median nerve compression in carpal tunnel:

1st stage: compression of interfascicular capillary network increases pressure inside the nerve; less oxygen and nutrition coming to the nerve and local hypoxia develops; venous drainage is blocked with following local edema formation. During this stage, appropriate conservative treatment prevents further median nerve compression.

2nd stage: with prolonged local hypoxia, the damage of the capillary endothelium occurs, along with an increase in local edema and intrafascicular pressure; fibroblasts start to proliferate in the ischemic areas of the nerve with following deposit of connective tissue, which makes the nerve damage irreversible.

Massage therapists are in the major risk group. During massage, the practitioner overloads the wrist joint and compresses the median nerve, as well as the synovial sheaths of the long flexors inside the carpal tunnel. The compression of synovial sheaths causes their inflammation and edema which, additionally, compresses the median nerve.

Females have smaller hands, and the pressure on the flexor retinaculum during the wrist flexion is 14% greater for females compared to males. As a result, women have Carpal Tunnel Syndrome an average of five times more frequently than man (Palastanga, et al., 1989). This is why regular self-massage or massage by colleague (see below), is a critical element in the prevention of carpal tunnel syndrome.

A very similar clinical picture can be detected if the Carpal Tunnel Syndrome is result of Anterior Scalen Muscle Syndrome, Pectoralis Minor Muscle Syndrome or Pronator Teres Muscle Syndrome. In all these cases, the massage therapist's professional capability is severely restricted.

Treatment: medical massage, stretching, and physical therapy are very helpful in the earlier stages of Carpal Tunnel Syndrome. In the cases of an advanced clinical stage, the surgical method of decompression is a priority.

5. DEGENERATIVE JOINT DISEASE

Massage therapists are at high risk for the early development of Osteoarthritis in the wrist and hand joints. The most commonplace is the 1st carpometacarpal joint, but the interphalangeal and metacarpo-phalangeal joints can be affected as well. Young females are more likely to develop early degenerative disease in these joints. Pain, stiffness, crepitation, sensitive subcutaneous nodules and the joint's deformation can severely affect the massage therapist's ability to work.

Treatment: regular rest; frequent therapeutic massages as a preventive measure; medical massage treatment, especially periostal massage; physiotherapy; anti-inflammatory medications.

C. GENERAL MEASURES FOR INJURY PREVENTION

1. The correct body mechanics is critical factor. When executing long massage strokes, try to follow your hands with your body (see Fig. 30). Do not lean forward into the direction of the stroke. If you follow your hands, you are in control of your hands and body position. This prevents possible injuries to the hands and lower back.

2. The therapist should use strong pressure (if needed), not only by the hand's prehension but also engaging body weight and hand's bony prominent parts as integrative part of each stroke.

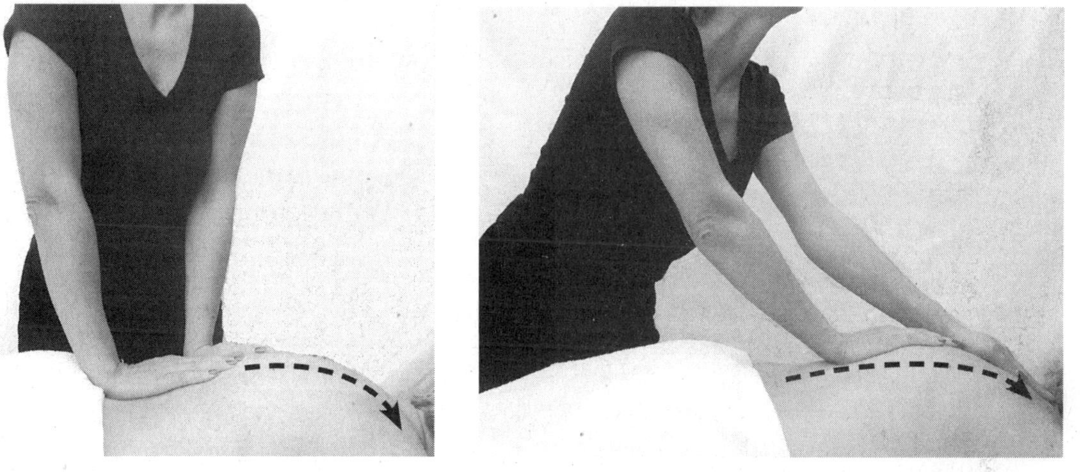

Fig. 30. Correct and incorrect execution of long massage strokes
a - correct position **b** - incorrect position
Dashed arrows - direction of strokes

The correct body mechanics is the foundation for a long successful career. To learn more about body mechanics during a massage session please visit the November/December Issue 2009 of the *Journal of Massage Science* where this information is presented in great detail in written and video format. Please visit: **www.scienceofmassage.com** and review this publication.

3. Apply as little lubricant as possible or remove it before kneading, ischemic compression or any deep tissue work. In this case you need much less muscle work to create the similar pressure, and it prevents practitioner's hand or fingers from sliding during the application of these techniques.

4. Do not use the same repeating strokes for a long time if it is not clinically necessary. A lot of practitioners restrict themselves to several basic techniques, which are used over and over again. The more technically rich arsenal the therapist has less exhausted he or she will become.

5. An inappropriate height in the massage table can cause muscle tension in the neck and upper back. Eventually it causes spinal and peripheral nerve irritation and compression and the development of neurological symptoms (i.e., pain, numbness, paraesthesia, etc.) in the hand. Always properly adjust the table height before treatment. The optimal table height (for a average size client) is equal to your extended upper extremity with the fist placed on the top of the table (see Fig. 31). Only in this case can you prevent the tension build up in the upper and lower back.

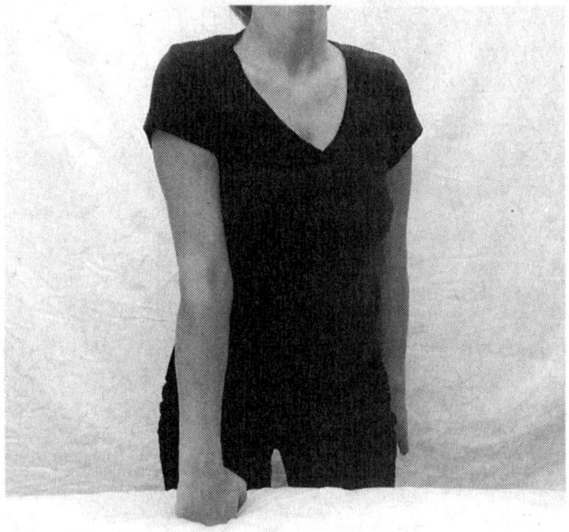

Fig. 31. Test for a proper table's height

6. Take any opportunity to give your hands a rest. Regular sessions of therapeutic massage and Jacuzzi prevent the build up of tension in the muscles and connective tissue structures. Always start the massage treatment on your colleague from the neck, arm and forearm. While doing self massage of the hand, or giving one to a colleague, one has to pay special attention to the following areas of the hand:

a. Wrist Joint

The wrist joint has only two areas where it can be directly accessed: the radial and medial sides of the joint under the styloid process of the ulna and radius. The palmar surface is covered by the retinaculum extensorum and tendons of flexors while dorsal surface is covered by tendons of extensors. After general massage, work carefully in the areas under the ulnar and radial styloid processes, as well as along the radial and ulnar collateral ligaments. Fig. 32 illistruates the location of these anatomical structures.

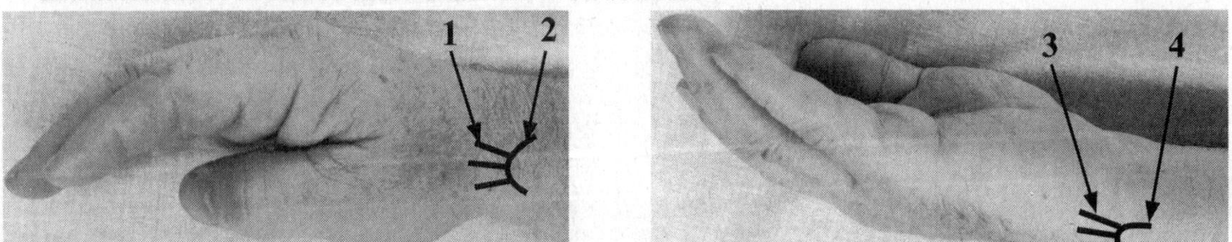

Fig. 32. Areas of styloulnar and styloradial processes of the hand

1 - radial collateral ligament

2 - styloid process of the radius

3 - ulnar collateral ligament

4 - styloid process of ulnar

After massage of the wrist joint, gently stretch the flexor retinaculum and proximal band of the transverse carpal ligament as shown in Fig. 33 'a.' The stretching of the distal band of the transverse carpal ligament is illustrated in Fig. 33 'b.' This stretch should be done after the massage of the palmar hand. These types of stretching are an important tool to prevent the development of Carpal Tunnel Syndrome.

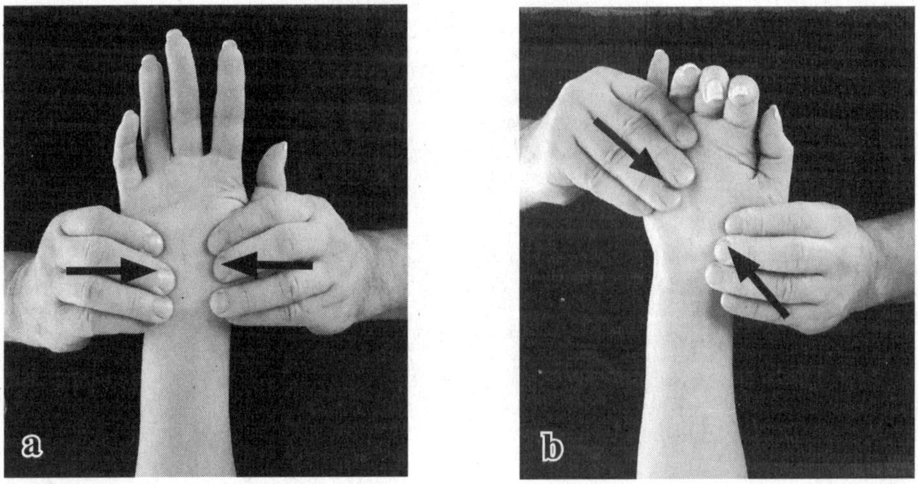

Fig. 33. Stretching of the flexor retinaculum
a - stretching of the flexor retinaculum and proximal band of the transverse carpal ligament
b - stretching of the distal band of the transverse carpal ligament
(Please note that the both thumbs create a conterpressure on the dorsal surface of the hand)

b. Capitate Bone and Transverse Arc

As discussed previously, the capitate bone is the biomechanical center of any movement in the wrist joint. Thus, any massage session has to include the mobilization of the capitate bone to reduce tension in the carpal ligaments and joints. Fig. 34 illustrates this mobilization. Please note that the operator's index fingers are placed on the capitate bone.

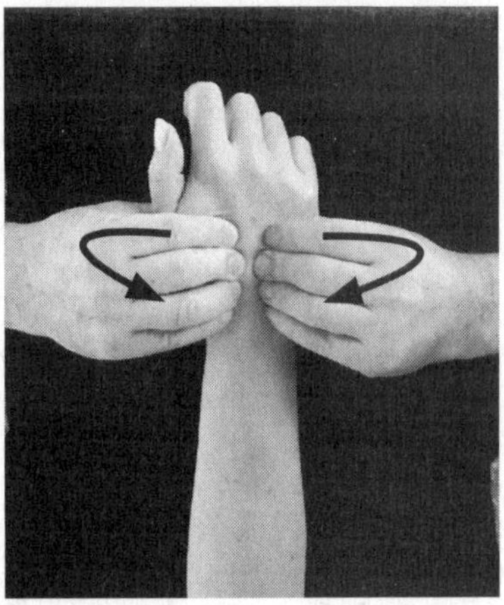

Fig. 34. Mobilization of the capitate bone

A transverse arc is formed by the 2nd-5th metacarpal bones, with the 3rd metacarpal bone as a higher point of the arc. To reduce tension in the transverse arc, stretch the palm across with the pressure applied on the head of the 3rd metacarpal bone (see Fig. 35).

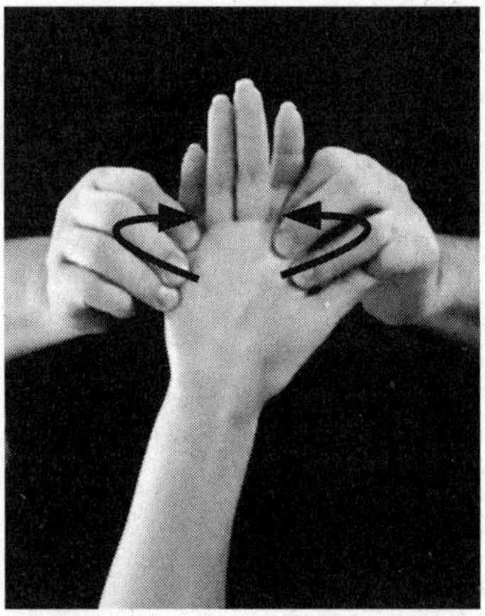

Fig. 35. Stretching of transverse arc

(Please note that both thumbs create a conterpressure on the head of the 3rd metacarpal bone on the dorsal surface of the hand.)

c. 1st Carpo-Metacarpal Joint

The 1st carpometacarpal joint is formed by the trapezium from the distal row and the 1st metacarpal bone (see Fig. 16). This joint carries a lot of pressure during massage and is very vulnerable to early degenerative changes. Periostal massage in the area of the 1st carpo-metacarpal joint is shown in Fig. 36.

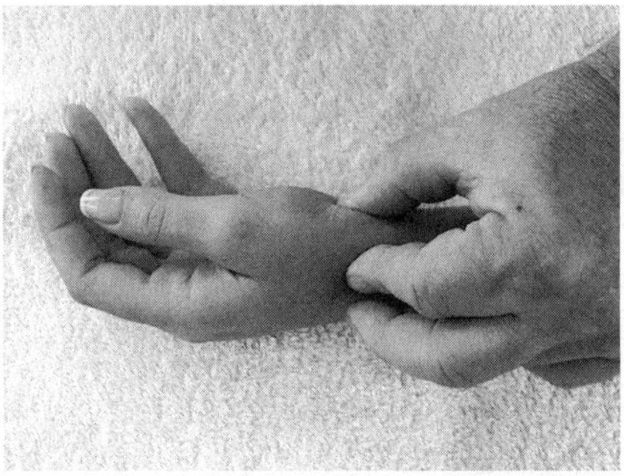

Fig. 36. Area of 1st carpo-metacarpal joint

d. Thenar

The thenar is the largest eminence of the hand which contains the biggest muscle mass. The thenar musculature plays a critical role in hand prehension. Thus, this area of the hand is under permanent pressure during massage and tension in the thenar muscles builds quickly.

During treatment, massage the whole thenar eminence and adductor pollicis muscle in the first metacarpal space (i.e., between thumb and index finger). Separately work along the attachments of the thenar musculature to the 1st metacarpal bone. Use periostal massage in this area, as shown in Fig. 37.

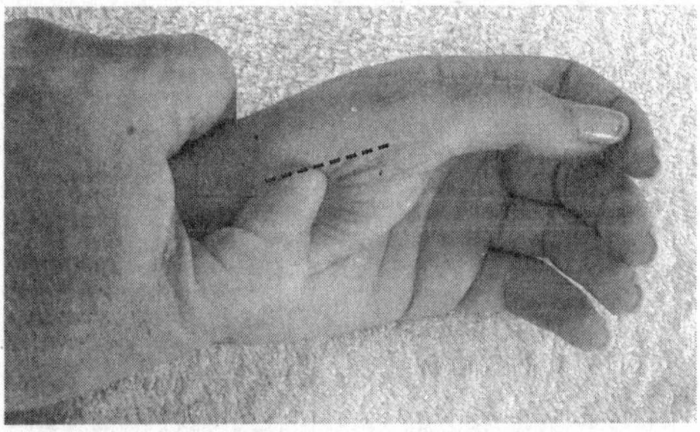

Fig. 37. Periostal massage in the area of insertion thenar muscles to the 1st metacarpal bone
Dashed line - edge of the 1st metacarpal bone

Another important area to work on is the site of median nerve bifurcation, where this nerve sends motor branches to the thenar musculature. This area is located about 2 inches below the distal transverse groove of the wrist joint on the palmar surface (see Fig. 38). In this area apply light, permanent and interruptive vibration.

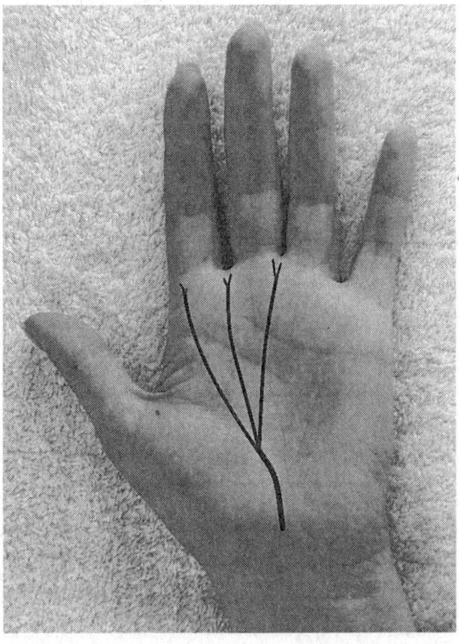

Fig. 38. The area of median nerve's bifurcation on the palmar hand

e. Hypothenar

The hypothenar is the second big eminence of the hand. It is formed by the flexor digiti minimi brevis, the abductor digiti minimi and the opponens digiti minimi muscles. These muscles also get tense quickly and should be worked on. Be sure that the ulnar edge of the hypothenar is addressed as well. After the massage of the thenar and hypothenar, carefully stretch the palmar aponeurosis, as shown in Fig. 39.

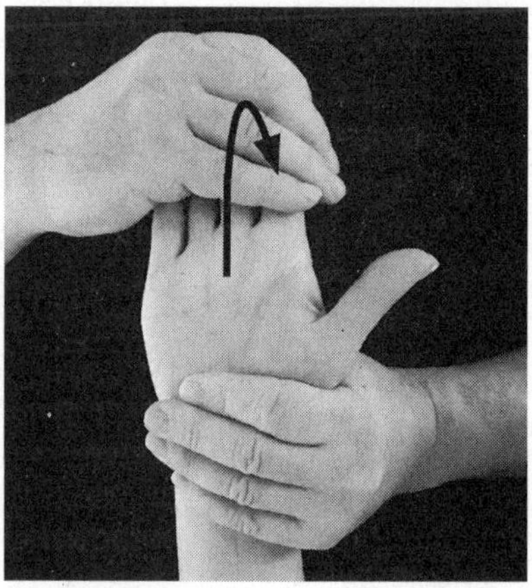

Fig. 39. The stretching of the palmar aponeurosis

f. Interossei Muscles

Three palmar and four dorsal interossei muscles provide the flexion-extension of the proximal phalanges in the metacarpo-phalangeal joints and abduction (dorsal interossei) as well as adduction (palmar interossei) in these joints. These small muscles are key players in the palmar prehension of the hand. Interossei muscles rotate each finger to different degrees to fit the grasping surface. They also strengthen the grip, stabilize the proximal phalanges and extensor digitorum muscle's tendons (Smith et al., 1966).

Interossei muscles are innervated by the ulnar nerve. The patients with ulnar nerve palsy lose about 50% of general palmar grip strength (Kovanov and Travin, 1983). Thus, the interossei muscles are very important for everyone who practices massage therapy.

The dorsal interossei muscles are easy to reach on the dorsal surface of the hand between the metacarpal bones. Try to additionally spread the two neighboring metacarpal bones as shown in Fig. 40 'a.' Also massage along the line of insertion of the interossei muscles into the meta-carpal bones (dashed line on Fig. 40 'b'). The palmar interossei muscles are difficult to reach since they are covered by the palmar aponeurosis and synovial sheaths. The pressure should be applied between the heads of metacarpal bones (see Fig. 40 'c').

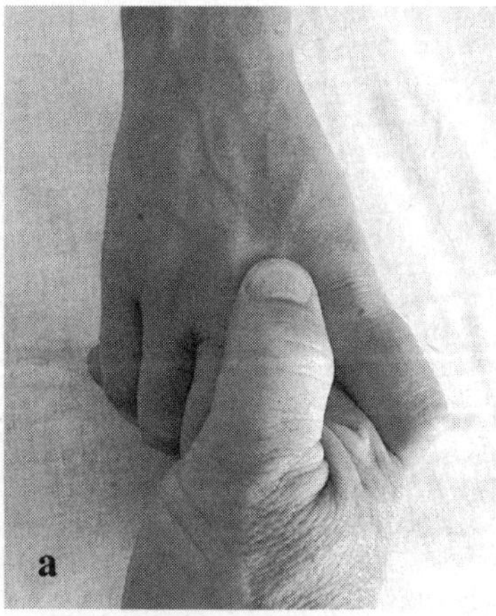

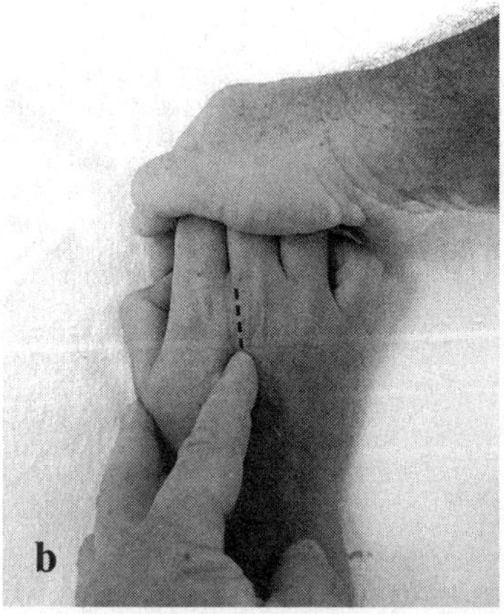

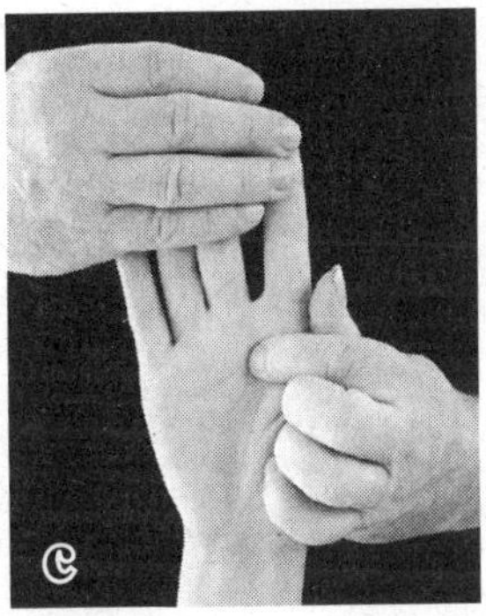

Fig. 40. Therapeutic approach to the dorsal and palmar interossei muscles
a - stretching between the metacarpal bones
b - periostal massage along the 3rd metacarpal bone
c - compression between the heads of the metacarpal bones on the palmar surface of the hand

g. Lumbrical Muscles

The four lumbrical muscles are located more superficially and have an unusual anatomy. They originate from the tendons of the flexor digitorum profundus muscle and insert to the extensor aponeurosis of each finger. Thus, they rum between two connective tissue structures. These muscles are very important for fine digital movements and strong digital grip. In fact, the lumbrical muscles have more muscle spindle receptors, compared to their mass, than any other muscle in the human body (Rabischong, 1967).

These muscles are also covered by the palmar aponeurosis, and it is practically impossible to directly massage them. To reduce tension in the lumbrical muscles it is best to stretch them (Travell and Simmons, 1983). This stretching also targets the interossei muscles. Place both hands with spread fingers opposite to each other as shown in Fig. 41 'a.' Be sure that both forearms form a straight line. Carefully push the hands against each other and simultaneously fully pronate both forearms (see Fig. 41'b'). Return to the neutral position and repeat this exercises 3-4 times.

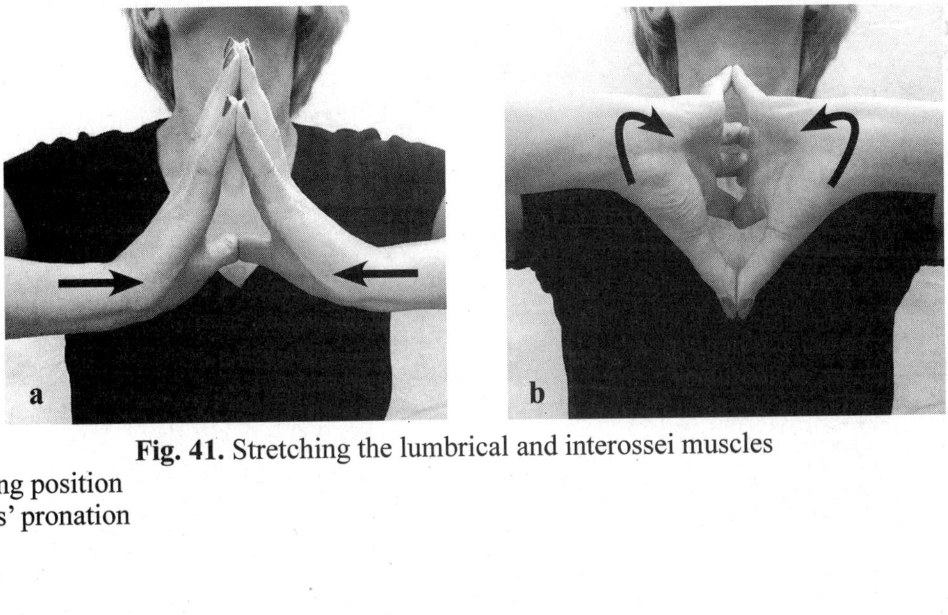

Fig. 41. Stretching the lumbrical and interossei muscles
a - starting position
b - hands' pronation

h. Massage Along the Major Nervous Pathways on the Upper Extremity

Periodically massage along the major nerves which innervate the hand: ulnar, radial, median. Be gentle, especially in the areas where nerves can be compressed against bone (see Fig 42). These areas for the **radial nerve** are: the lateral side of the arm on the border between the middle and lower 1/3, the head of the radius and the area of the styloid process of the radius.
For the **ulnar nerve**: behind the medial epicondyle of the humerus, along the distal end of the ulna and just below wrist joint (on the ulnar side).
For the **median nerve**: the anterior surface of elbow (area of pronator teres muscle), and the wrist (carpal tunnel) joints and thenar area.
For **all three nerves**: anterior surface of the shoulder in the area of the pectoralis minor m.

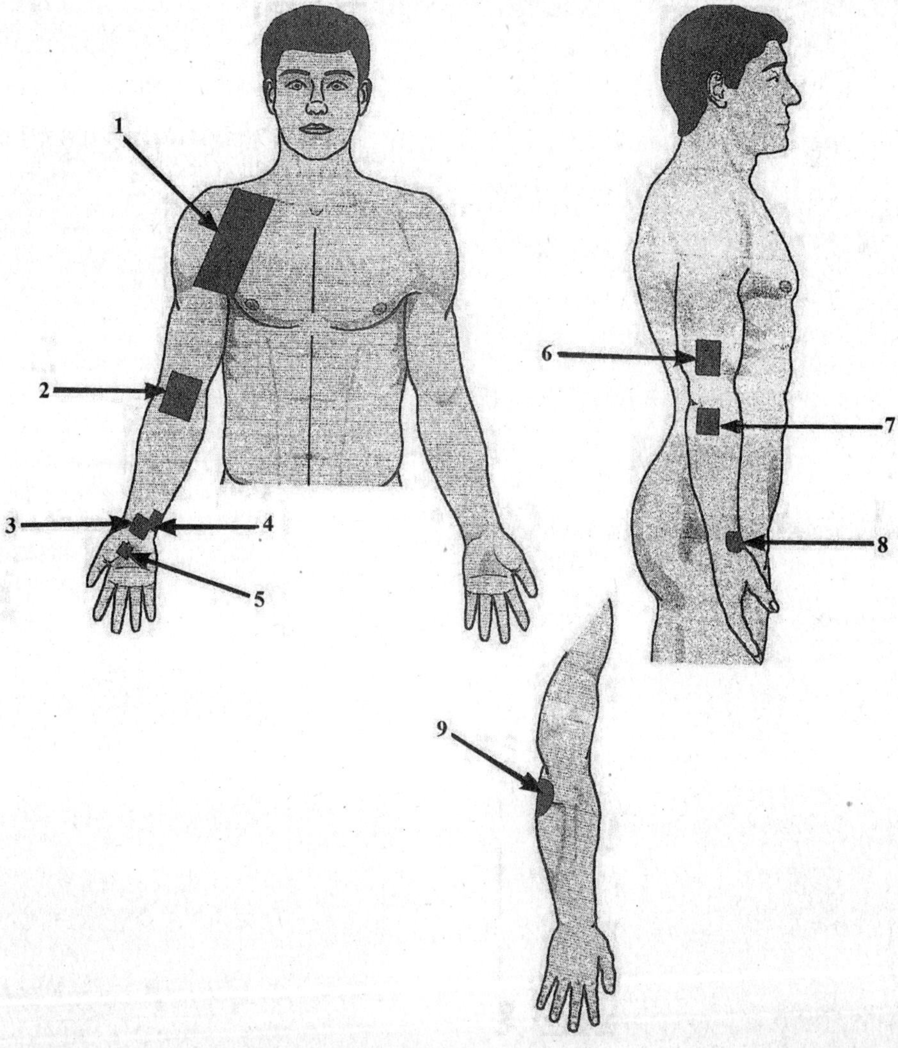

Fig. 42. Areas to be careful of during massage along the nerve pathways of the upper extremity

1 - all 3 nerves
2 - median nerve
3 - median nerve
4 - ulnar nerve
5 - median nerve
6 - radial nerve
7 - radial nerve
8 - radial nerve
9 - ulnar nerve

D. CONTACT AREAS OF THE HAND

The contact area is the part of the therapist's hand which makes contact with the client during each massage stroke. Fig. 43 presents the commonly used contact areas of the hand.

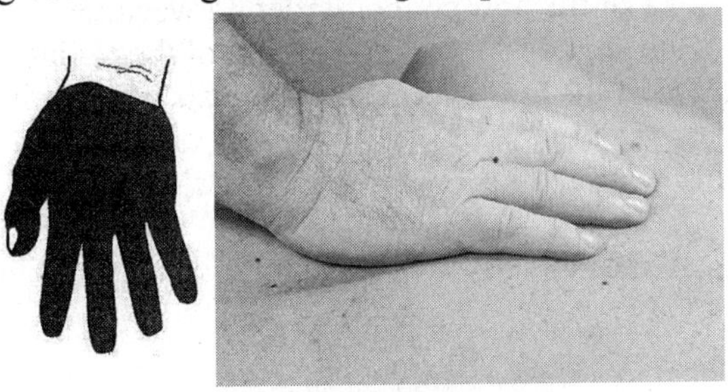

1. Whole palmar surface

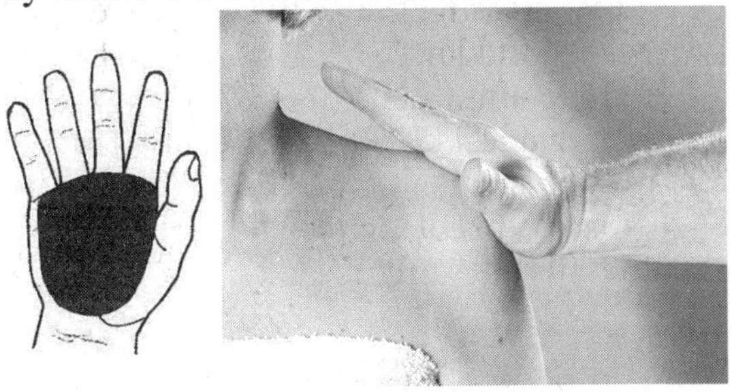

2. Palm only

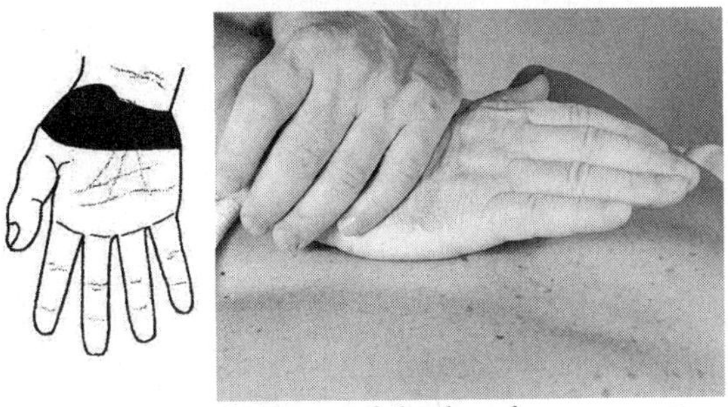

3. Base of the hand

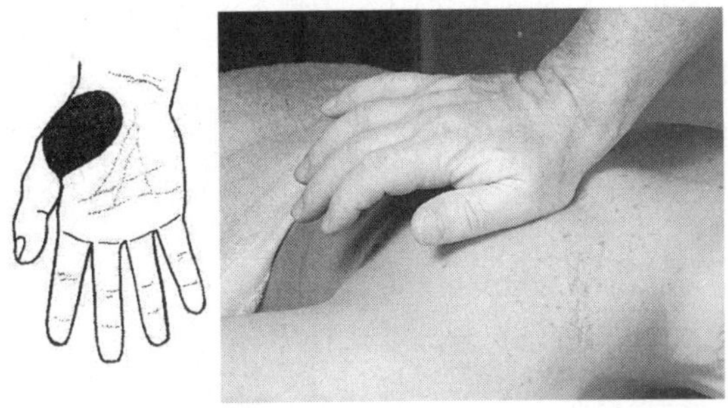

4. Thenar

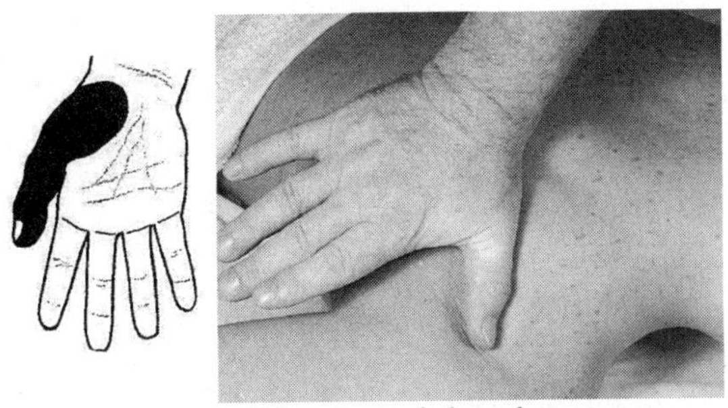

5. Thenar and thumb

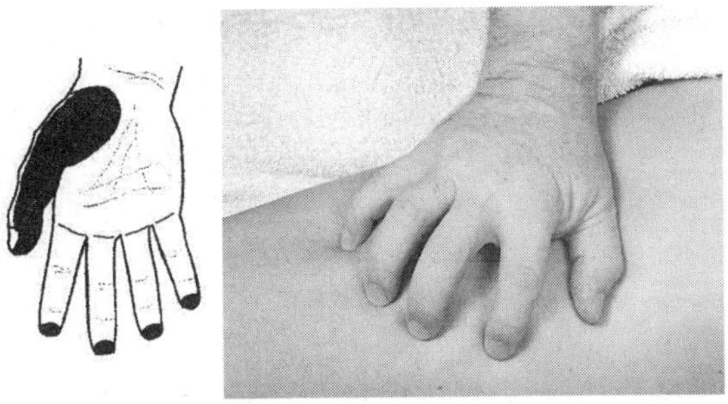

6. Thenar, thumb and fingertips

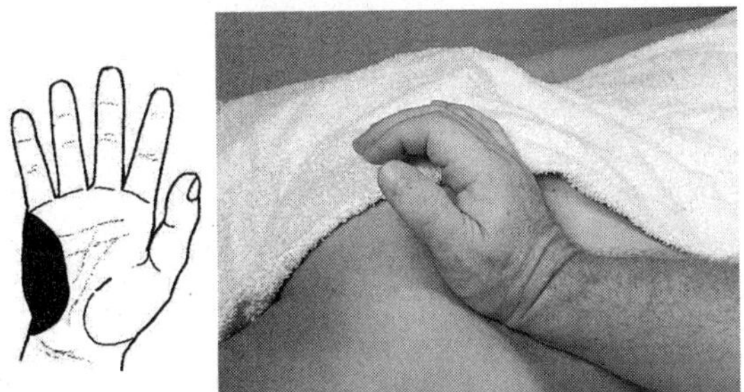

7. Hypothenar

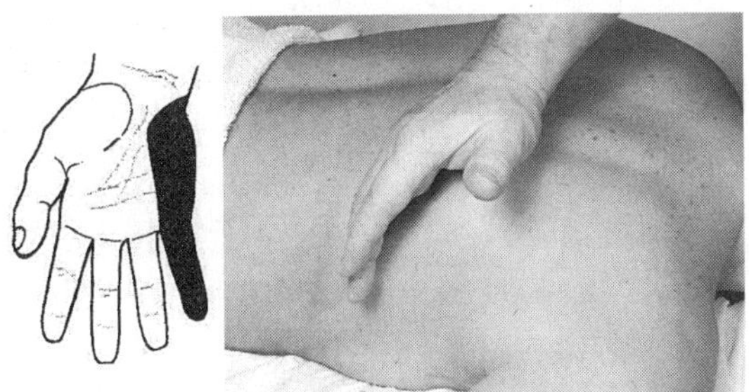

8. Hypothenar and 5th finger

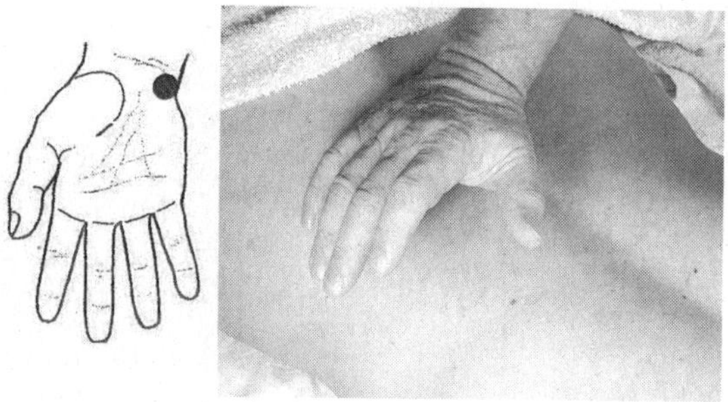

9. Pisiform bone

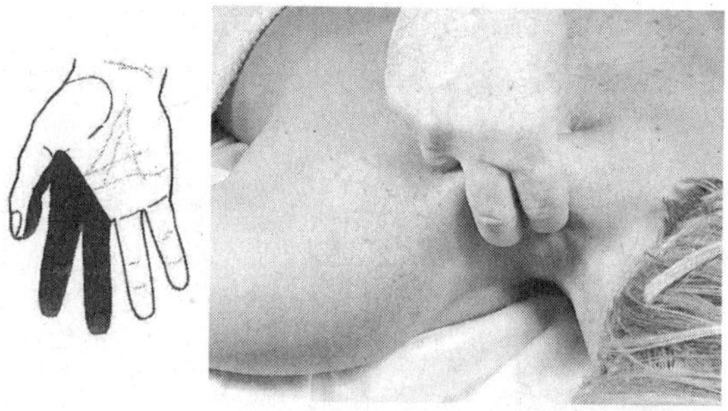

10. Palmar surfaces of 1st-3rd fingers

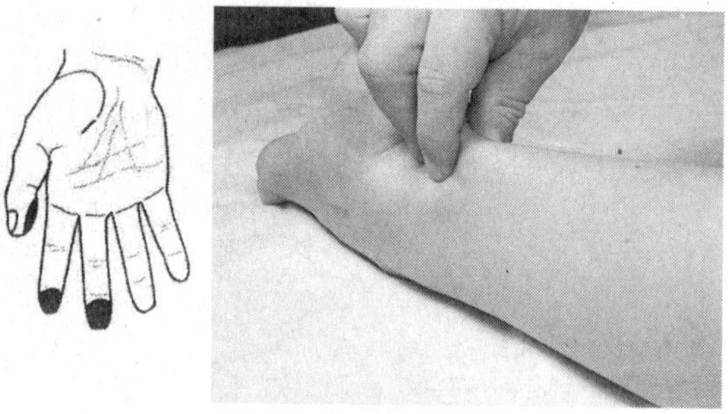

11. Three fingers prehension

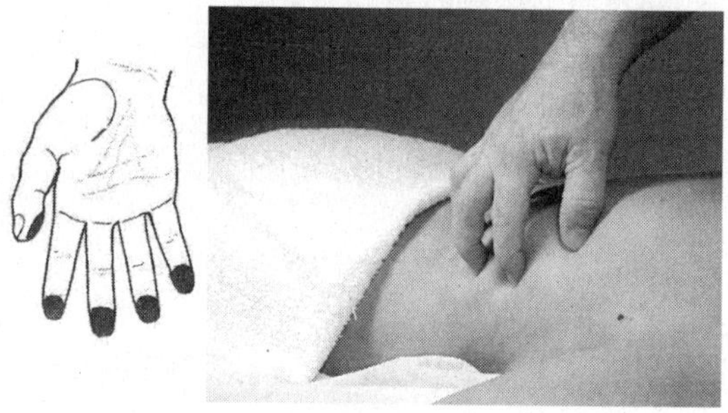

12. Fingertips of all fingers

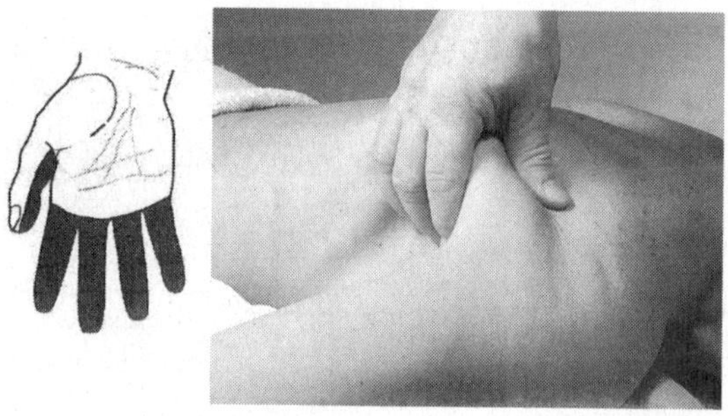

13. Palmar surfaces of all fingers

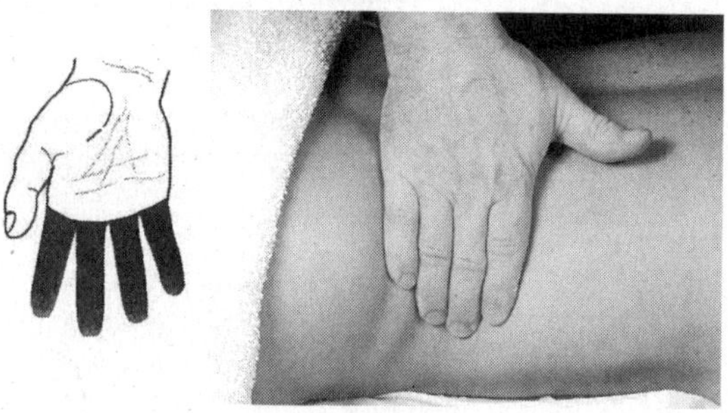

14. Palmar surfaces of 2nd-5th fingers

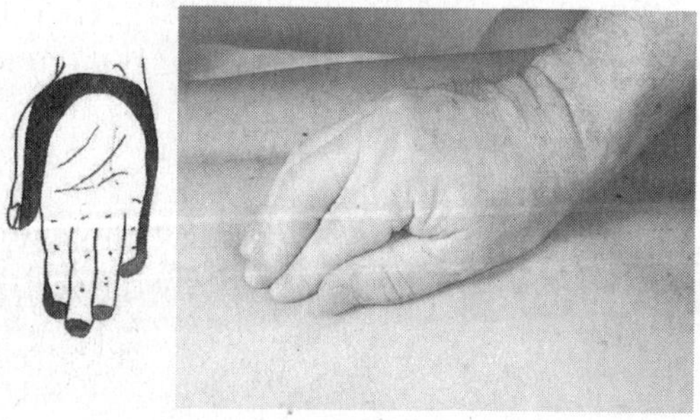

15. Cupping

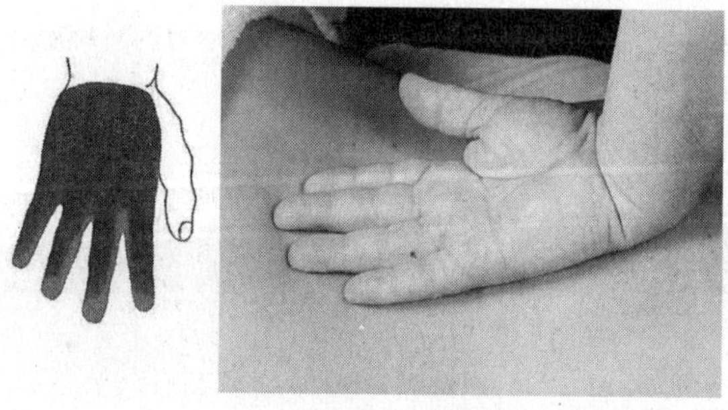

16. Dorsal surface of hand and fingers

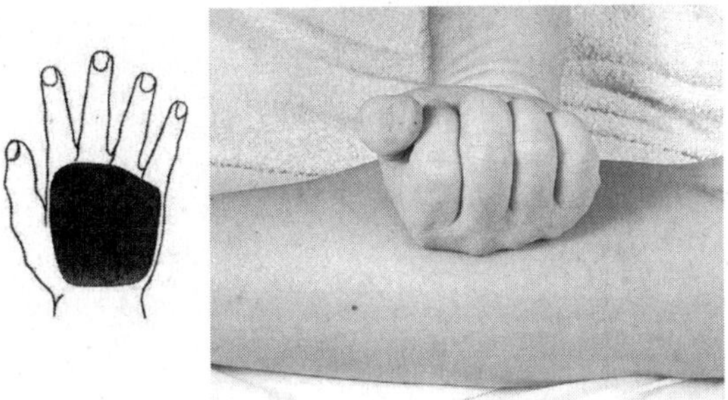

17. Dorsal surface of the hand/fist

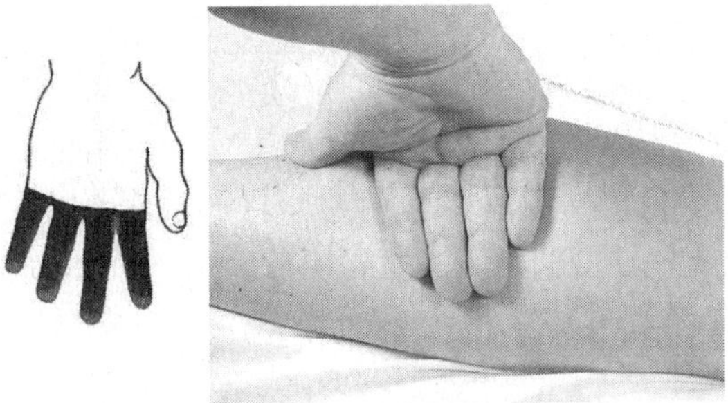

18. Dorsal surface of the fingers

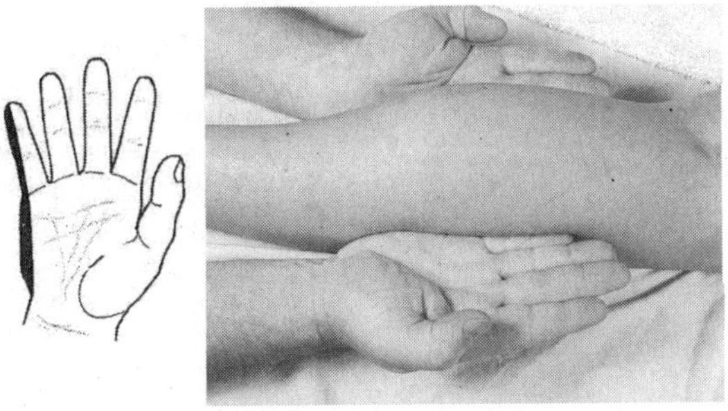

19. Ulnar edge of the hand

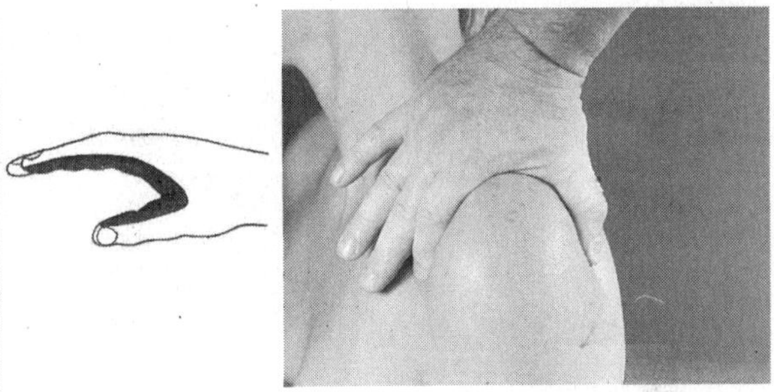

20. 1st interphalangeal space

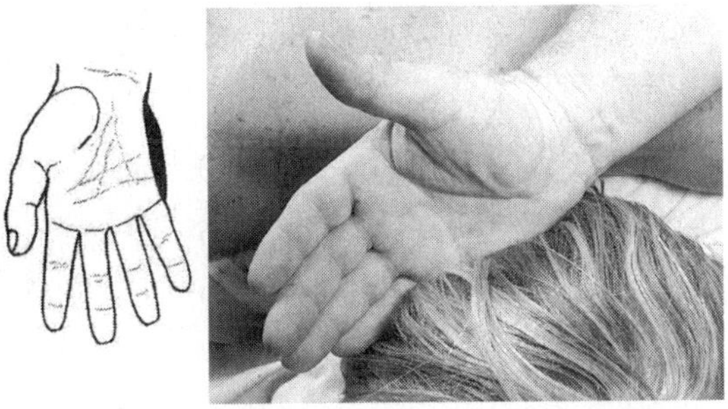

21. Ulnar edge of hypothenar

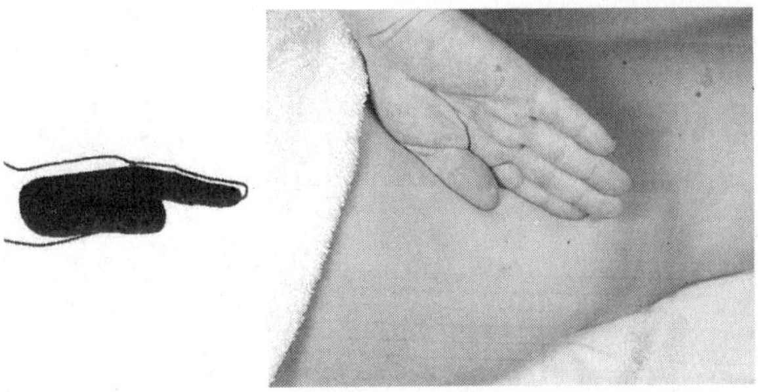

22. Radial edge of the hand

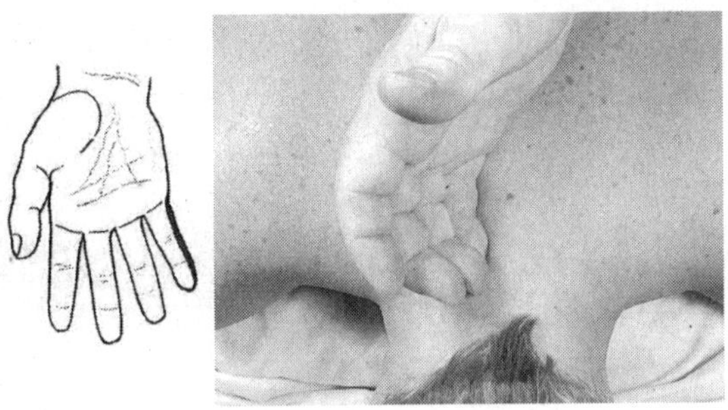

23. Ulnar edge of 5th finger

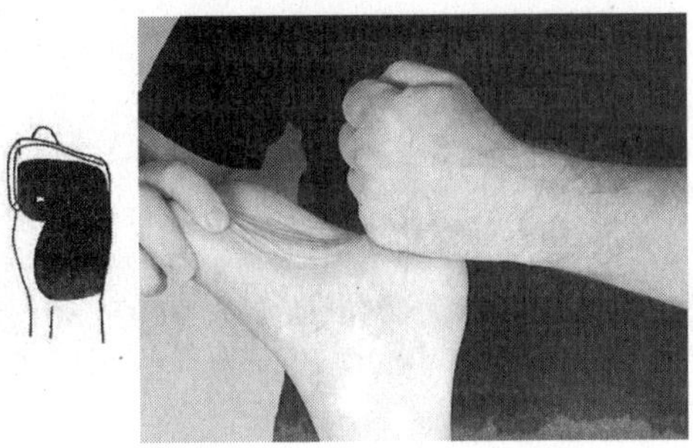

24. Ulnar edge of the fist

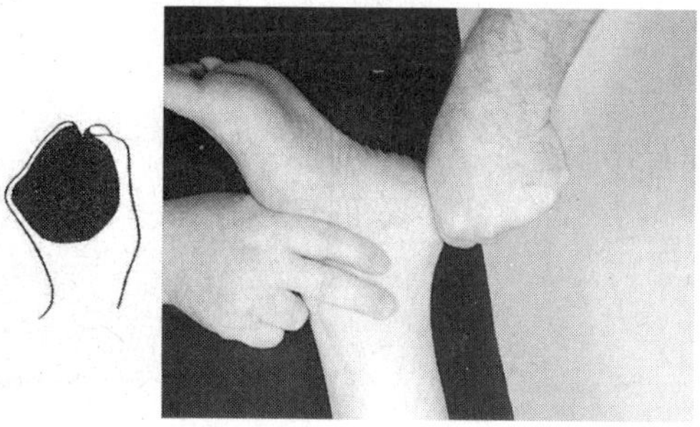

25. Radial edge of fist

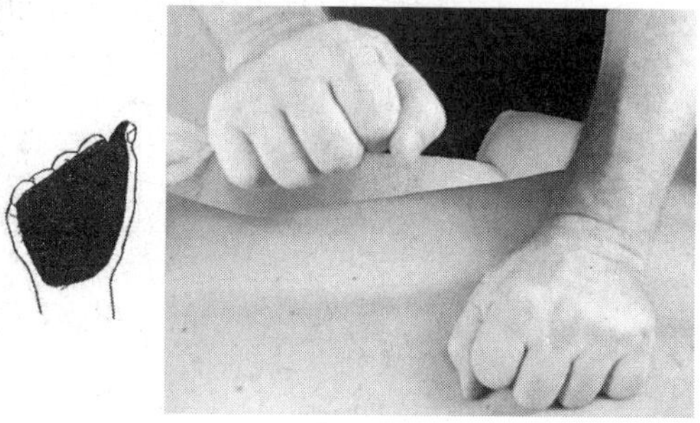

26. Palmar surface of fist

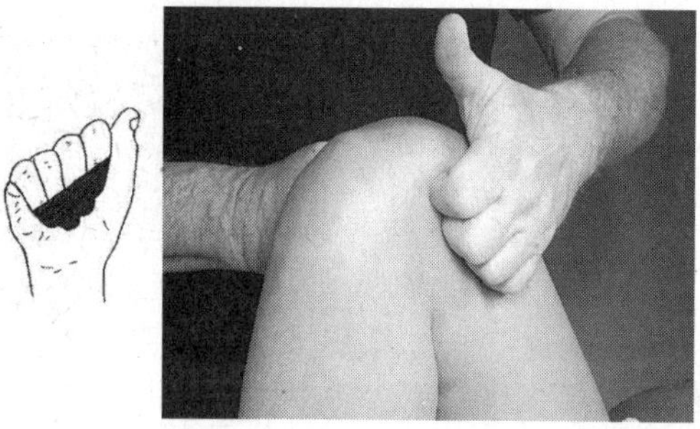

27. Dorsal surface of distal phalanges

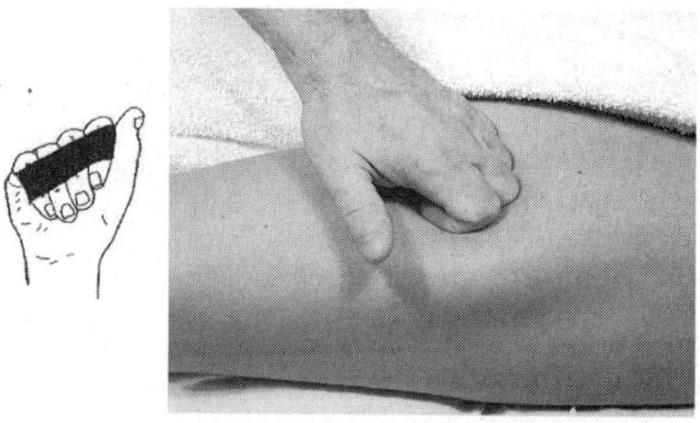

28. Dorsal surface of middle phalanges

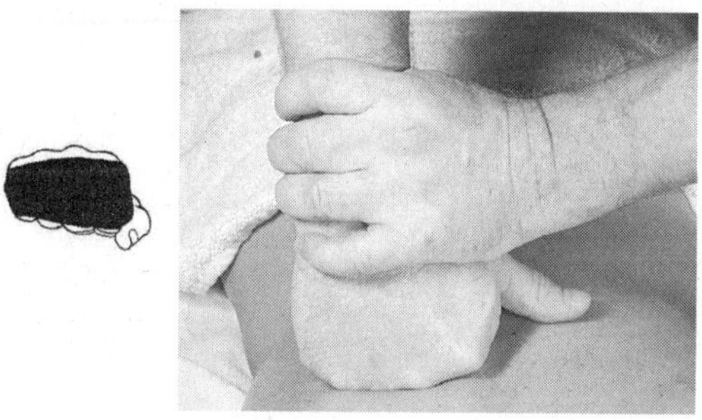

29. Dorsal surface of proximal phalanges

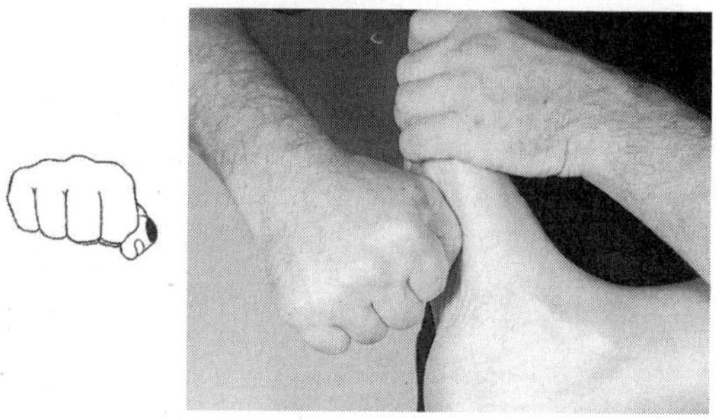

30. Knuckle of 1st interphalangeal joint

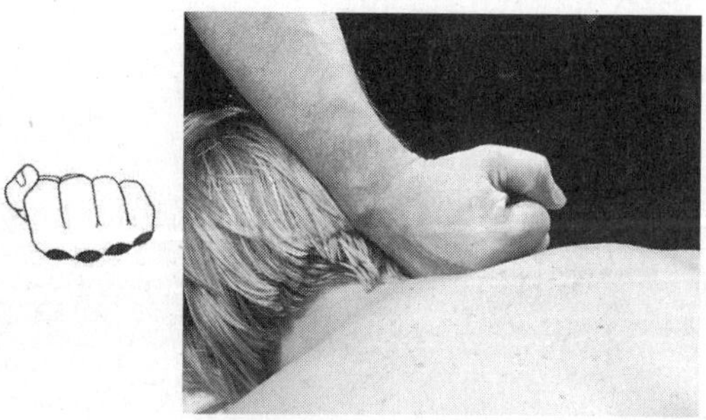

31. Knuckles of metacarpophalangeal joints

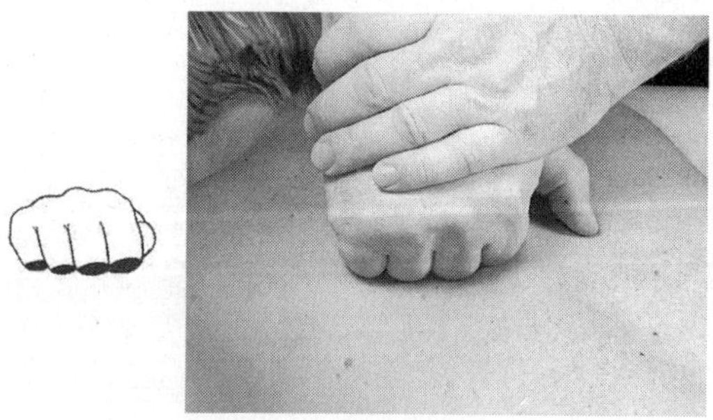

32. Knuckles of proximal interphalangeal joints

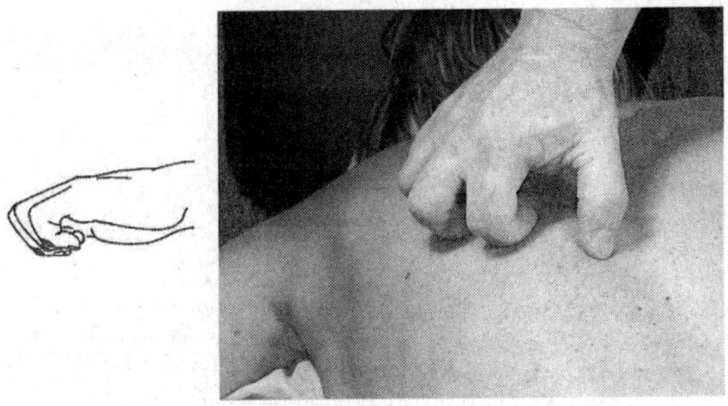

33. Knuckles of distal interphalangeal joints

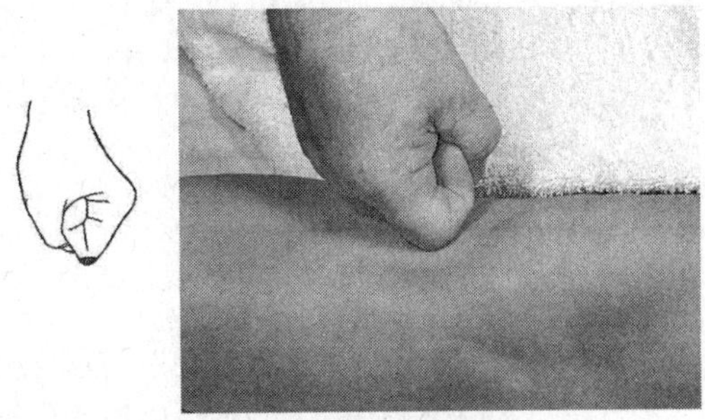

34. Knuckle of 2nd distal interphalangeal joint

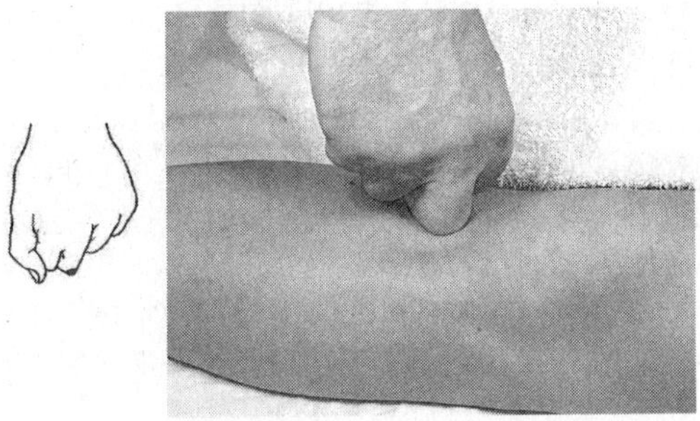

35. Knuckle of 3rd distal interphalangeal joint

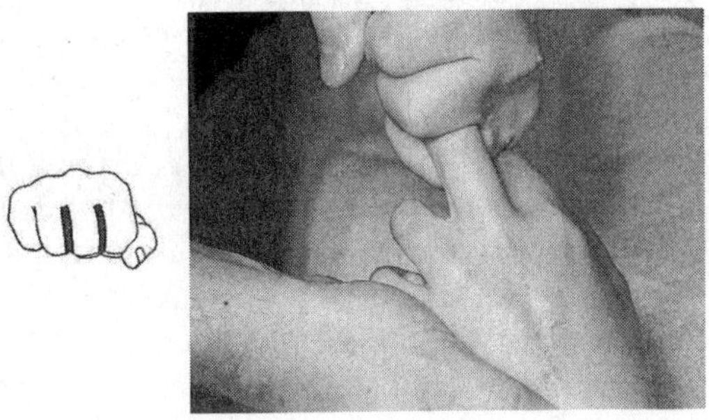

36. 2nd, 3rd or both interphalangeal spaces

Fig. 43. The contact areas of the hand

V. THERAPEUTIC MASSAGE TECHNIQUES

In this chapter we will discuss the variations of seven basic massage techniques: effleurage, friction, kneading, vibration, percussion, compression and passive stretching. This is attempt to summarize massage techniques used by Western school of therapeutic and stress reduction massage.

Every massage treatment is a combination of different techniques. They are not applied separately. I think everyone will agree with Dr. J. Dollinger, who wrote back in 1899 that massage techniques, like notes, never sound separately, but combine with each other to produce the perfect musical sound (Belaya, 1974).

PHENOMENON OF ADAPTATION

The level of a massage therapist's expertise completely depends on his or her ability to find the correct combination of massage techniques and adjust them for every client and for each new session. This brings us to the issue of **phenomenon of adaptation**.

Every massage practitioner will experience the situation when a regular client he or she has treated, sometimes for months, suddenly starts to go to a different massage place despite that this client has always praised and liked the work the practitioner did. This "disloyalty" has a physiological explanation in form of the phenomenon of adaptation or in other words, the practitioner's work is no longer considered by the client's body to be new and exciting.

What causes the phenomenon of adaptation? The majority of clients visit massage practitioners to maintain wellness and to reduce their level of stress. One's stress level is under the control of the autonomic nervous system, which manages all body functions without our conscious participation (as, for example, our heart rate or the flow of blood through our muscles). The autonomic nervous system consists of two divisions: the sympathetic and the parasympathetic nervous systems. Both divisions control the body's functions by constantly interacting with one another.

The sympathetic nervous system is the stress system. It is activated during emotionally or physically stressful situations, as well as generally during the waking hours. The parasympathetic nervous system has the opposite effects. It is more active during periods of relaxation, as well as generally during the sleeping hours.

In a healthy body, both divisions act upon the organs and tissues as a plus and minus, constantly balancing each other's effects, with the overall result of their interaction equaling zero. For example, if the sympathetic nervous system increases the heart rate, the parasympathetic system decreases it as soon as you stopped exercise. If the parasympathetic nervous system triggers bronchoconstriction, the sympathetic nervous system tries to produce bronchodilation.

When the relationship between the sympathetic and parasympathetic nervous systems becomes unbalanced, the sympathetic nervous system increases its activity, resulting in sensations of stress: physical tension, anxiety, morning stiffness, chronic mild pain, etc. This is the tipping point when a person under stress will decide to seek massage, or to practice yoga, meditation or aerobic exercise. These modalities will decrease the activity of the sympathetic nervous system, and thus in one's level of stress.

Modern medicine has come to understand chronic stress as a primary trigger of chronic disorders in the human body. Thus, owing to its effective stress-reduction impact, massage is an important tool of preventive medicine.

The practitioner works with soft tissue, which contains millions of sensory receptors that are activated during the massage. The peripheral receptors - receptors of touch, pressure, vibration, and temperature, as well as muscle spindle receptors and Golgi tendon organ receptors - all send sensory information to the spinal cord. This sensory information is primarily processed in the posterior horns of the spinal cord by spinal neurons. The spinal neurons are responsible for the further conduction of sensory information to other parts of the spinal cord and to the brain.

Massage impacts the central nervous system and restores the balance between the sympathetic and parasympathetic divisions through the activation of the peripheral receptors in the massaged area, and subsequently, activation of the spinal neurons located in the segment of the spinal cord responsible for the innervation of that area.

Each type of peripheral receptor has its own threshold of adaptation. A perfect example of this is the continuous application of each massage stroke in the same area. The client experiences the first strokes as sharper and more distinct, as compared with the same strokes in the same area conducted for one minute or more. Adaptation of the peripheral receptors (in this case, touch and pressure receptors) results in their desensitization.

The spinal neurons in the posterior horns of the spinal cord also have their own threshold of adaptation. After prolonged repetitive stimulation of peripheral receptors in the soft tissues, the spinal neurons reach their own threshold of adaptation due to the consistent flow of (harmless) sensory information they receive from the peripheral receptors in the massaged area. Thus, the desensitization (that is, the attaining of the threshold of adaptation) of the spinal neurons occurs secondarily to the desensitization of the peripheral receptors brought about by the practitioner's strokes.

The peripheral receptors and spinal neurons are able to overcome adaptation but it happens differently. Whereas peripheral receptors are able to shake off their adaptation and restore their full working potential very quickly after a repetitive stimulation has ceased (the moment therapist stopped the application of effleurage, for instance), spinal neurons, on the other hand, stay adapted for a while after sensory information has ceased to flow to them from the peripheral receptors. When spinal neurons reach their threshold of adaptation, they allow less sensory signls to reach other parts of the spinal cord and the brain itself. As a result, the balancing impact of massage strokes on the relation between the sympathetic and parasympathetic divisions of client's autonomic nervous system is now lessened. At this point, the client the practitioner has been treating starts to feel that he or she is getting a lesser benefit from the regular massage sessions despite the fact that the therapist is using the **same routine** which the client really liked 3-4 months ago.

How do we control, and thus prevent, the phenomenon of adaptation? The best solution to successfully building a practice that will keep clients interested and coming back is a richer, more varied technical repertoire. There are more than 60 variations of 7 basic massage techniques which are discussed in this publication, but when practitioners compose their massage routine, they often use only a very limited number of these variations, applied over and over again. A limited technical repertoire and a never-changing massage routine are two major factors which contribute to the adaptation of clients' spinal neurons and thus, their further lack of interest. It undermines the therapist's practice. Conversely, by investing in a variety of techniques and routines, a massage therapist ensures that their clients will remain fascinated with their work and, just as importantly, that the therapist's own level of interest in and excitement for what they do will continue to grow.

Variety doesn't mean that practitioner needs to use all 60 variations each time he or she works on regular clients. The solution is much simpler. So let's discuss in practical terms how to control, and thus prevent, the unwelcome phenomenon of adaptation.

Let's say practitioner has developed an hour-long (or 1.5 hour-long) massage routine. This is his or her foundation of successful practice. To control the phenomenon of adaptation, practitioner simply needs to incorporate one or two new variations into each day's massage routine, switching these around daily with other variations, or combinations of variations. For example, practitioner decides that for all clients today he or she will incorporate into massage routine ridging friction and scrolling kneading. In such a case, practitioner adds both techniques to the massage of each segment of the body. Tomorrow, within regular routine, all clients will receive two different variations from the previous day: for example, stretching friction and mobile kneading. If practitioner has 5 to 7 such gourmet sets of massage techniques, he or she can incorporate them into routine and constantly rotate their application on a daily basis. In this way, regular clients will never reach the threshold of adaptation and feel bored; each time they visit the practitioner he or she will be surprising their peripheral receptors and spinal neurons in some different way.

This is why the main goal of this chapter is to provide a comprehensive collection of therapeutic massage techniques developed by the Western School of Massage Therapy. The greater the technical arsenal the practitioner has, the more successful practice he or she will build. Also, readers may study the application of massage techniques presented in this publication in video format in the Video Library at **www.scienceofmassage.com**.

For some massage techniques developed in the Eastern Europe that are also presented in this chapter, I tried to find the closest English translation. Thus, the results reflect only the author's opinion, and a professional translator may find more precise analogies in English.

EFFLEURAGE

A. GENERAL CHARACTERISTICS

Effleurage is one of the most ancient massage techniques. Even Homer mentioned it in his poems as early as 800 B.C. According to Bear (1952), in the *Odyssey* the beautiful women gently rubbed war-wom heroes with oil to restore and refresh them after the battle.

Effleurage is a very important technique. It seems so technically simple that sometimes even experienced therapists underestimate the importance of its correct application. Massage of any segment of the body starts and finishes with effleurage. Consequently, this is a stroke which the patient feels as the first and the last one. The first impression is extremely important because it builds the client's confidence and creates a bond of trust between the practitioner and the client. Effleurage is also the last touch the client feels after the session for a period of time.

Effleurage also is used at the beginning to spread lubricant over the massaged area. While doing that, the therapist determines the contour of the body surface and superficially tests the soft tissues. Effleurage also creates a kind of massage basis. This means that effleurage is used as the **transition stroke** between every new, sometimes more complex, massage technique.

Thus, effleurage links all applied techniques into one sophisticated procedure of the therapeutic massage. Besides these general features of effleurage, some techniques have unique therapeutic meaning. For example, effleurage with unequally distributed pressure is the best technique for draining lymph and venous blood on the upper and lower extremities (see below p.126).

B. TECHNICAL DISTINCTIONS

1. CONTACT AREAS

Effleurage is a superficial gliding stroke along the skin, without stretching it significantly. It is usually applied over large areas. The hand must follow the contours of the massaged segment. The proper amount of lubricant is important for the correct application of effleurage.

2. DIRECTION OF THE STROKES

The hand must follow the contours of the massaged segment throughout the entire stroke. This is an important tip for correct completion of effleurage. Different placement of the hands or fingers lets the practitioner to apply different types of effleurage.

The operator can use this technique in different directions. Effleurage may have a crossing, longitudinal, circular, spiral or Z-shaped direction. The right direction should be chosen according to the contour of the massaged segment, or in accordance with the anatomy of muscles in massaged area. Long effleurage strokes are mostly directed along the venous and lymph drainage.

The proper application of an effleurage stroke from start to finish is another important subject which should be discussed. Let's take as an example the effleurage stroke on the forearm. Fig. 44 illustrates the correct application of effleurage, and Fig. 45 shows the incorrect sequence. If you compare these pictures, you will notice some important differences. The correct execution of effleurage (see Fig. 44) starts with the radial edge of the therapists's hand. With further proximal advancement, the whole palmar surface makes contact with the forearm. At the final point, below the elbow joint, the ulnar edge of the hand and the 5th finger are the last areas in contact with the forearm before the therapist's hand is completely released. In contrast, the practitioner who executes effleurage incorrectly (see Fig. 44) places the hand flat in full contact with the forearm just above the wrist joint, flatly advances it forward and withdraws it just below the elbow joint. In such a case, the therapist cuts each effleurage stroke short at the distance which equals double the width of the therapist's hand.

The correct application of effleurage allows the practitioner to increase the length of the stroke and prolong actual contact with the massaged segment. This is especially important in cases where the therapist has large hands and the massaged area is small. Long, flowing effleurage strokes are also one of the key components of every stress-reducing massage treatment.

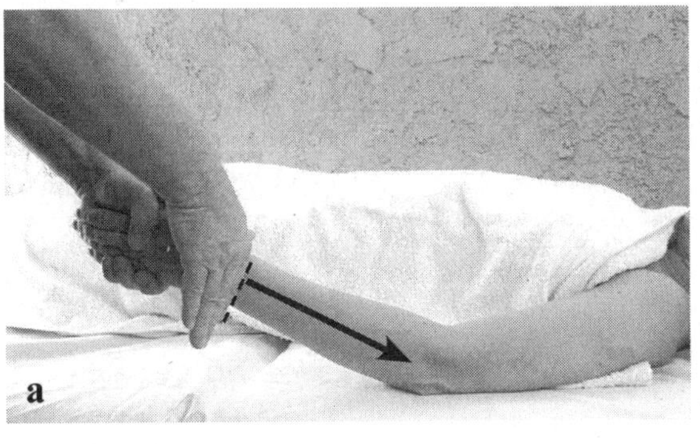

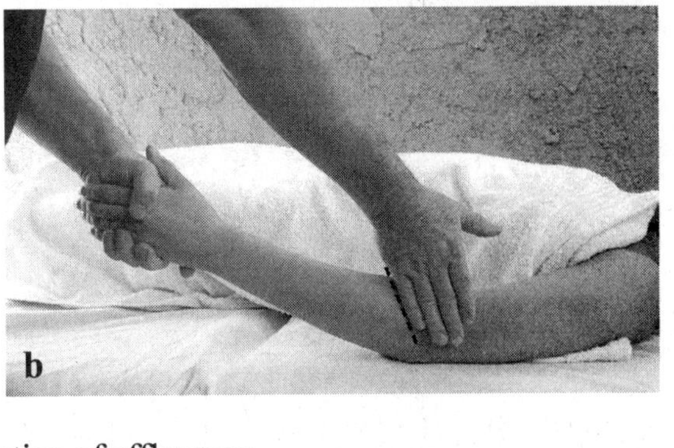

Fig. 44. Correct application of effleurage

a - starting position of the hand
b - position of the hand at the end of the stroke
Dashed lines - first and last contact areas

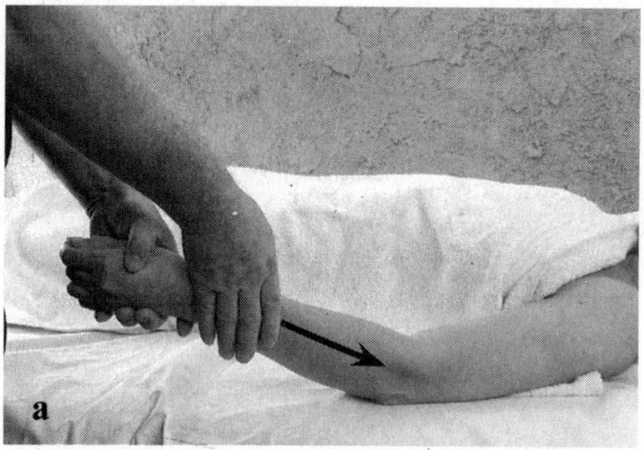

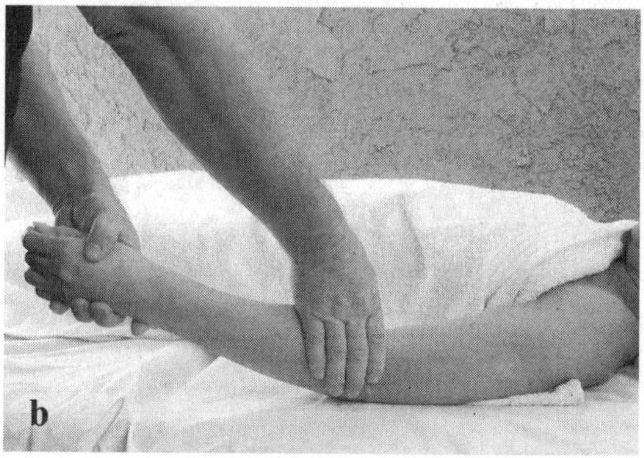

Fig. 45. Incorrect application of effleurage
a - starting position of the hand
b - position of the hand at the end of the stoke

3. SPEED AND PRESSURE

Effleurage has a low to moderate speed of execution. It is generally about 35-40 strokes per minute. A lower speed should be used in stress-reducing massage sessions, with a much higher speed (around 80-100 strokes per minute) used in sports massage. It is best if the applied strokes have a rhythmic character.

As it was already mentioned, effleurage is a superficial stroke and the hand(s) has to be relaxed during its execution. The applied pressure has a horizontal direction. It can be increased by tightening the hand and fingers or by increasing the vertical pressure on the massaged area. The pressure has to be equally spread throughout the contact area. The operator has to maintain constant pressure during the massage stroke. All effleurage techniques that are discussed below can be applied with light or medium to-strong pressure. In the case of stronger pressure, the appropriate amount of lubricant has to be used, to prevent the skin from excessive stretching.

The massage therapist can employ different types of effleurage even during the same stroke by changing the position of the hand(s) or fingers, by applying different degree of pressure or by alternating contact areas.

C. TYPES OF EFFLEURAGE

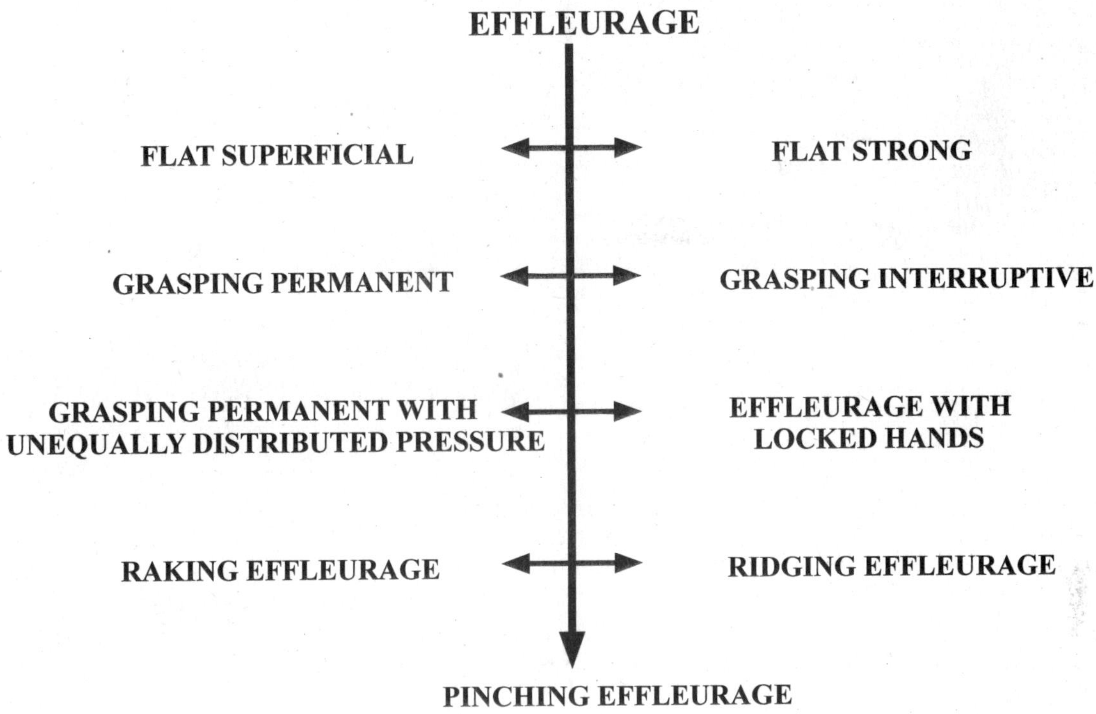

Fig. 46. Classification of effleurage techniques

1. FLAT SUPERFICIAL EFFLEURAGE

This type of effleurage is a light stroke which can be directed along the venous and lymphatic circulation as well as against it. Flat superficial effleurage is best performed by the palmar surface of the hand with adducted thumb (see Fig. 47). The hand should be placed flat and follow the body's contour.

Another variant of this technique is performed with the dorsal surfaces of the 2nd through 5th fingers pressed together. Both variants can be combined. For example, the stroke from the lower part of the massaged segment to its upper part can be done by the dorsal surfaces of the fingers, but the return to the starting position can be done by the palmar surface of the hand.

Flat superficial effleurage is a one- or two-handed technique. In the latter case the hands stroke the massaged area in parallel or follow each other.

The primary target of flat superficial effleurage is the skin. This technique stimulates local circulation, body's metabolism and increases skin elasticity. Rhythmic and repetitive application of this stroke also has a sedative effect on the central nervous system and is also used as a part of inhibitory massage treatment during medical massage session. Flat superficial effleurage is also an introductory stroke which is frequently used to spread the lubricant, examination of the superficial soft tissues, and definition of the massaged segment contour.

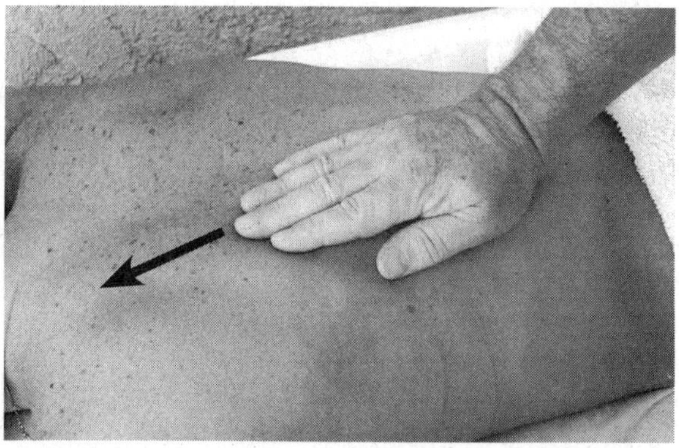

Fig. 47. Flat superficial effleurage on the back

2. FLAT STRONG EFFLEURAGE

Generally, flat strong effleurage follows the flat superficial one. Strokes are directed along venous and lymph drainage only. Similarly to flat superficial effleurage the application of strong effleurage, requires that the pressure is spread equally throughout the contact area. To increase it, the operator may add vertical pressure on the hand or place one hand over another and use them as one tool. The lubricant does not allow this type of effleurage to become the friction technique.

This technique is used during abdominal massage. The operator presses the hand into abdomen and slowly pushes hand forward. The patient must be comfortable with the applied pressure. Fig. 48 illustrates flat strong effleurage in the abdomen with different contact areas.

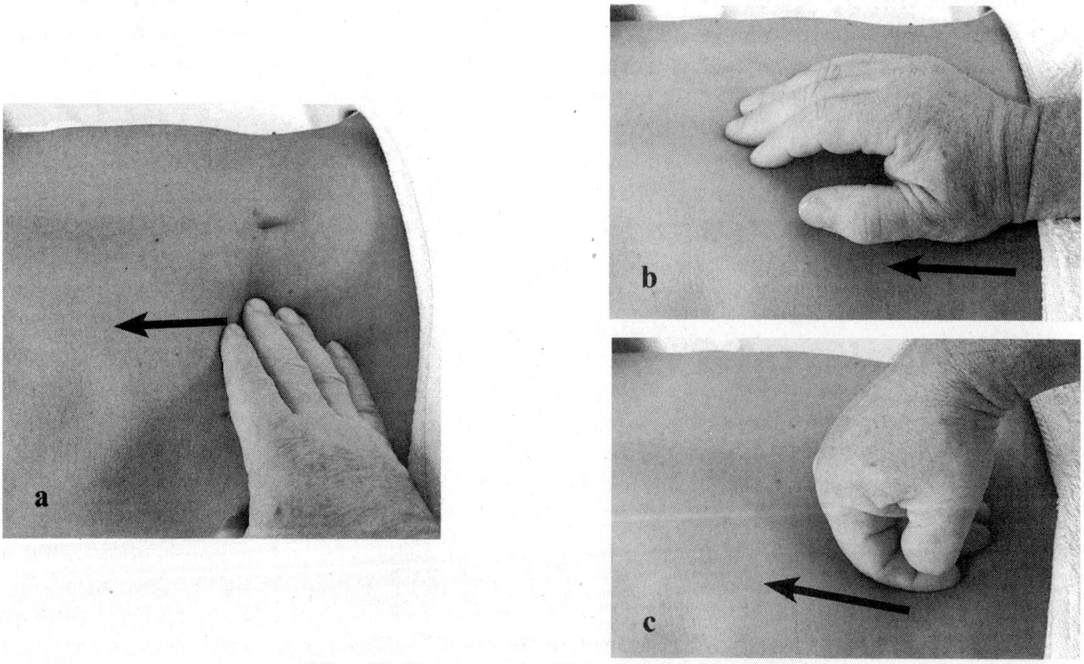

Fig. 48. Flat strong effleurage on the abdomen

a - palmar surfaces of 2nd-5th fingers
b - base of the hand
c - dorsal surfaces of 2nd-5th fingers

During flat strong effleurage, connective tissue structures and superficially located muscles are also targeted. The skin is more deeply affected. The exfoliation of old epithelium during this stroke stimulates the growth and renewal of the epithelial and epidermal cells.

This type of the effleurage also enchances the drainage of extracellular fluid from subcutaneous tissue. Sarkisov-Sirasini, (1957) and later Kunichev, (1985) reported that flat strong effleurage increases the drainage of extracellular fluid by 16-58%.

3. GRASPING PERMANENT EFFLEURAGE

Grasping permanent effleurage can be performed on the neck, upper shoulders, lateral surfaces of the thoracic cage and abdomen, and the upper and lower extremities. The operator compresses the 2nd through 5th fingers together and abducts the thumb. In this position, the hand(s) embraces the massaged segment (see Fig. 49).

Grasping permanent effleurage is a one- or two-handed technique. The entire palmar surface of the hand(s) must be in contact with the body. The hand(s) must move along the massaged segment from its lower to upper parts with consistent speed and pressure as it follows the body's contour. along the venous and lymph drainage.

The massage therapist can also add pressure by compressing soft tissues between the 2nd through 5th fingers on one side and the thumb on the other, and/or by compressing the hands against each other if the two-handed variant is performed on the upper or lower extremity. When the two-handed variant is used try to add your body weight into the stroke to decrease the pressure on the hands.

This type of effleurage supports venous and lymphatic circulation. With the rhythmic, repetitive application of grasping permanent effleurage, the practitioner can also expect significant inhibition of the nervous system because the large area of sensory receptors is stimulated. It increases their adaptation with simultaneous decrease of the afferent (i.e., ascending) discharge to the spinal cord and the brain. Thus, this type of effleurage is especially valuable in cases of stress-reducing massage and medical massage treatment in the inhibitory regime.

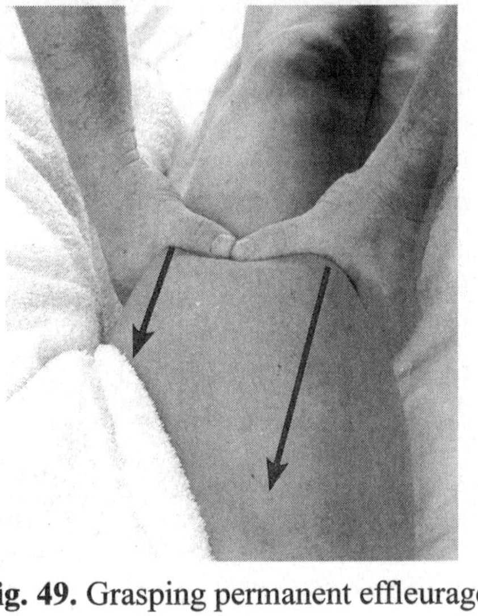

Fig. 49. Grasping permanent effleurage

4. GRASPING PERMANENT EFFLEURAGE WITH UNEQUALLY DISTRIBUTED PRESSURE

The grasping permanent effleurage with unequally distributed pressure has unique impact on the drainage in the extremities. In this type of effleurage, the pressure is unequally distributed through the palmar part of the hand. In such case effleurage drains the afferent veins and lymphatic vessels which are located in intermuscular septas. These septas are parts of the deep fascia and run between and around muscle groups and neurovascular bundles. Fig. 50 illustrates the intermuscular septas on the cross-section of the thigh.

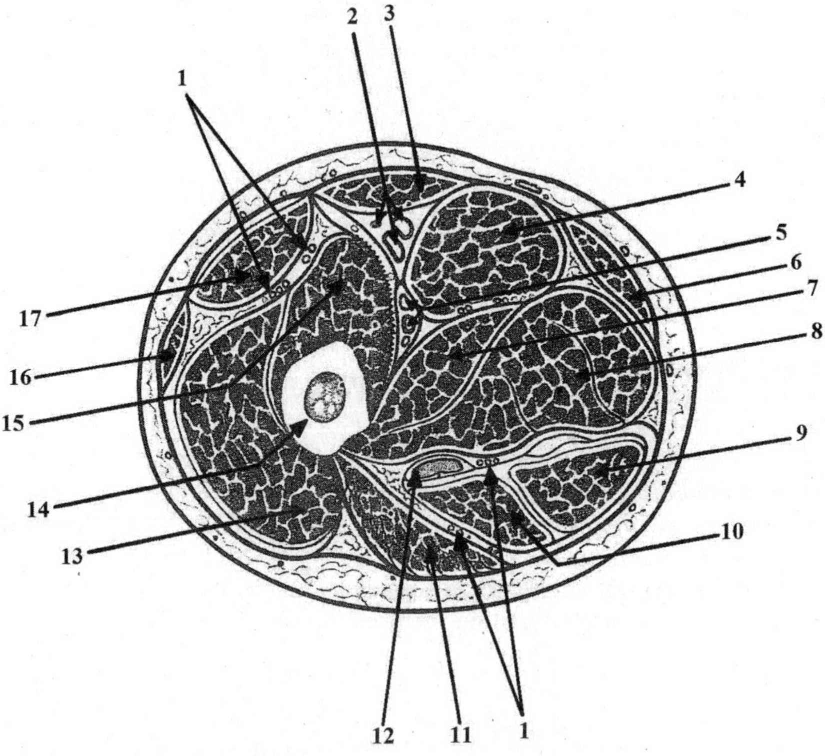

Fig. 50. Transverse cut through the upper 1/3 of the right thigh

1 - arteries and veins of large intermuscular septas
2 - femoral artery, vein and saphenous nerve
3 - sartorius muscle
4 - adductor longus muscle
5 - deep femoral artery and vein
6 - gracilis muscle
7 - adductor longus muscle
8 - adductor magnus muscle
9 - semitendinosus muscle
10 - long head of m. biceps femoris
11 - gluteus maximus muscle
12 - sciatic nerve
13 - vastus intermedius of m. quadriceps
14 - femur
15 - vastus medialis of m. quadriceps
16 - tensor fasciae lata muscle
17 - rectus femoris muscle

This two-handed technique is used on the large segments of the upper and lower extremities like thigh (see Fig. 51), and the one handed technique can be used on smaller parts, like the forearm.

To perform this technique correctly, the operator must compress the soft tissue between the thumbs and the index fingers. With each hand form a half circle using your thumb and index finger, encircle the body segment by connecting the fingers together (thumb to thumb, index to index). This forms a "ring" of strongest pressure. The palms and remaining fingers should tightly press the soft tissues against the bone but only using about 50% of pressure compared to the 100% of pressure that is used along the thumb-index ring. While maintaining steady pressure, the hand slowly moves up (proximally) through the massaged part of the extremity to the area of the nearest lymph nodes.

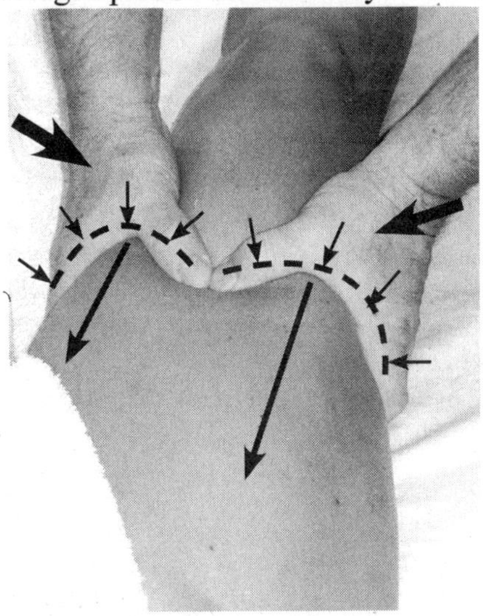

Fig. 51. Grasping permanent effleurage with unequally distributed pressure on the left thigh
Dashed lines with the small arrows - line of strongest pressure
Wide short arrows - compression of soft tissues against the bone by both palms
Narrow long arrows - general direction of the stroke

Kramarenko, (1953) showed that only this technique can efficiently drain fluid from the afferent veins and lymph vessels located in the large intermuscular septas. In a series of experiments, the author injected ink into the muscles of a dog, then applied the different types of massage strokes. Only after grasping permanent effleurage with unequally distributed pressure did almost all of the ink disappear from the muscle as well as from the deep interseptal veins. After every other type of massage stroke, the ink was drained from the muscle but was detectable in the lumen of the interseptal veins and lymphatic vessels.

Compression of the soft tissues between the thumb and index fingers pushes the fluid from the muscles and interseptal vessels into the mainstream of the afferent vessels. The rest of the hand compresses the muscles against the bone long enough to prevent the return of fluid into the lumen of interseptal veins after the stroke is over.

This type of the effleurage is very helpful in cases of the peripheral edemas and in the sports massage. During vigorous exercise or sports competitions the amount of blood that circulates through the muscles increases dramatically. Because arterial circulation is more powerful and compared to venous circulation, the amount of blood delivered to the muscles exceeds the capability of venous and lymphatic drainage. In such cases, more and more reserve capillaries are open and blood circulation throughout rhythmically contracting muscles is increased by up to 30 fold (Ganong, 1993). The main goal of this increase is the adequate delivery of O_2 to the working muscles. In fact, the oxygen consumption of contracting muscle increases up to 100 fold during vigorous exercise.

Despite these positive effects, the increase in blood circulation through the muscles has a negative outcome on the athlete's performance because it increases muscle mass. This is one of several reasons why contractile ability of muscles decreases during sport competitions. Thus, grasping effleurage with unequally distributed pressure should be performed during the breaks of sport competitions or afterward to stimulate the drainage and accelerate the athlete's recovery.

5. GRASPING INTERRUPTIVE EFFLEURAGE

With grasping interruptive effleurage, the practitioner's hand(s) has same position on the massaged segment as during grasping permanent effleurage (see Fig. 49). The main difference is advancement of the hand(s) throughout the massaged area. The therapist has to move the hand(s) by short strokes. It is very useful to imagine dividing the massaged segment into equal parts and moving the hand(s) from one segment to another in a short, powerful propulsion.

The dimensions of each segment depend on the general size of the massaged area and the operator's hand. Generally 2-3 segments are enough to properly complete this technique. After every propulsion, the hand(s) remains in contact with the massaged area, or they can be removed and immediately reapplied on the same area in the same position. In the last case, the stimulating effect of grasping interruptive effleurage is significantly increased. Fig. 52 shows the patient's thigh with imaginary lines forming the massage segments.

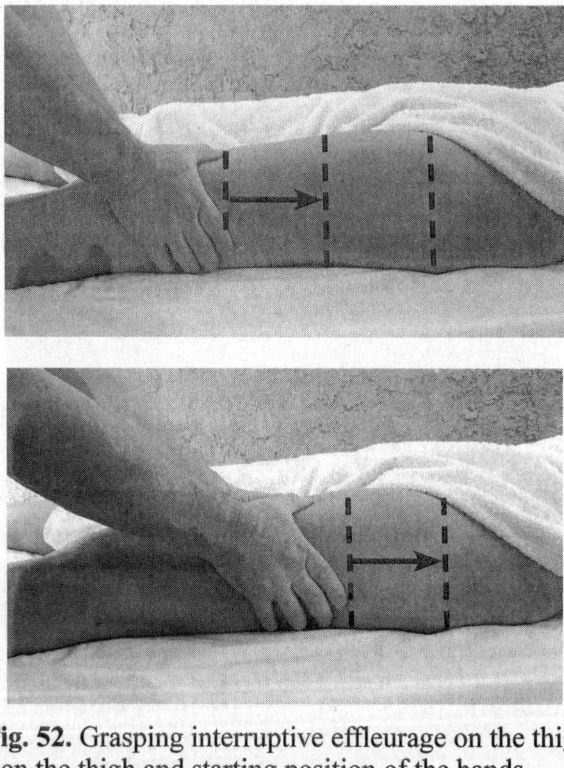

Fig. 52. Grasping interruptive effleurage on the thigh
a - imaginary segments on the thigh and starting position of the hands
b - final position of the hands at the end of the first segment

In bi-manual variant of this technique, both hands simulateneosly apply the same stroke in the opposite direction on each side of the massaged segment (see Fig. 53).

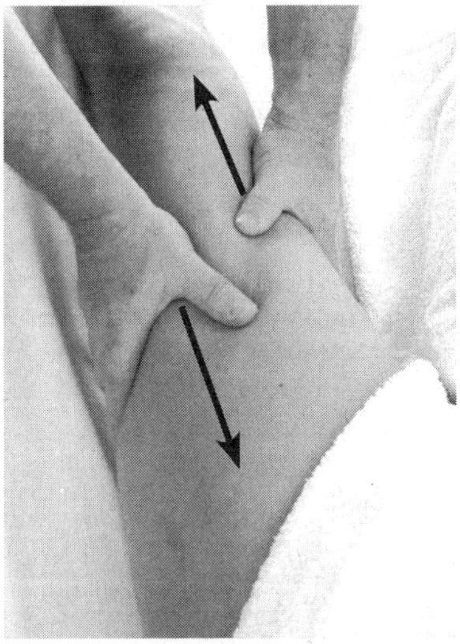

Fig. 53. Grasping interruptive effleurage with oppositely directed hands

The grasping interruptive effleurage affects the skin and skeletal muscles by producing local vasodilation, stimulating venous and lymph circulation and increasing local temperature. Another important outcome of this technique is stimulation of the nervous system by the increased flow of afferent (i.e. ascending) sensory impulses to the spinal cord and brain. As a result, the upper and lower motor centers send the motor, efferent (i.e., descending) impulses back to the skeletal muscles to support their tonus and contractile ability.

This type of effleurage is very helpful for athletes before sporting competitions, as it prepares muscles for optimal performance. In such a case, the speed of these strokes must be increased. Grasping interruptive effleurage is beneficial for the treatment of patients with hypotension (i.e., low blood pressure).

Belaya, (1974) recommended the application of grasping interruptive effleurage with oppositely directed strokes in the area of the pseudoarthrosis for the stimulation of callus formation.

6. RIDGING EFFLEURAGE

This ridging effleurage is performed by the knuckles of the metacarpo-phalangeal, proximal or distal interphalangeal joints. Ridging effleurage can be completed by one hand, both hands moving through the massage segment in the parallel or opposite manner with some distance in between, or by two hands acting as one tool. In the last case, one hand tightly grasps the thumb of the other, as shown in Fig. 54. Please notice that both hands are acting as one tool and the thumb of the left hand is grasped by the right hand.

During ridging effleurage, the applied pressure is more significant, especially if this technique is performed by the knuckles of the proximal interphalangeal joints. Thus, the massage practitioner has to be careful on sensitive areas. This stroke is very helpful if the therapist works on large muscle groups or on the areas with strong fascial support; for example, palms, soles, or lateral surface of the thigh.

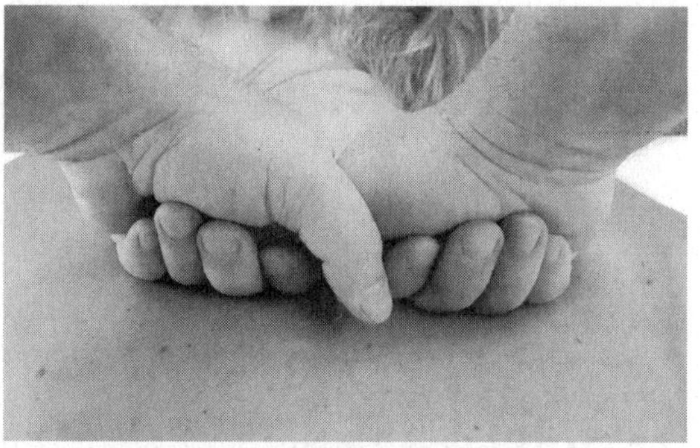

Fig. 54. Ridging effleurage performed by the knuckles of proximal interphalangeal joints

7. RAKING EFFLEURAGE

Usually raking effleurage is used on large areas. The practitioner has to keep the hand flat and spread the fingers. If raking effleurage is linear direct strokes toward the operator (see Fig. 55). If the hand moves in a spiral manner direct the strokes from the operator. This effleurage is performed by one or two hands and in the latter case hands can be either parallel or follow each other.

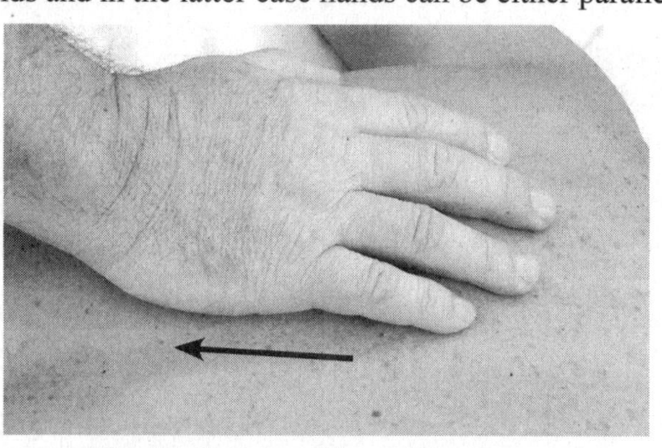

Fig. 55. Simple raking effleurage

The operator can increase the pressure by slightly bending the distal phalanxes (see Fig. 56 'a'). In this case, the pressure is spread throughout the thenar, hypothenar and all fingertips. To further increase the pressure, one hand can be placed over another. To increase the effectiveness of raking, the fingers of one hand can be placed between the spread fingers the other (see Fig. 56 'b').

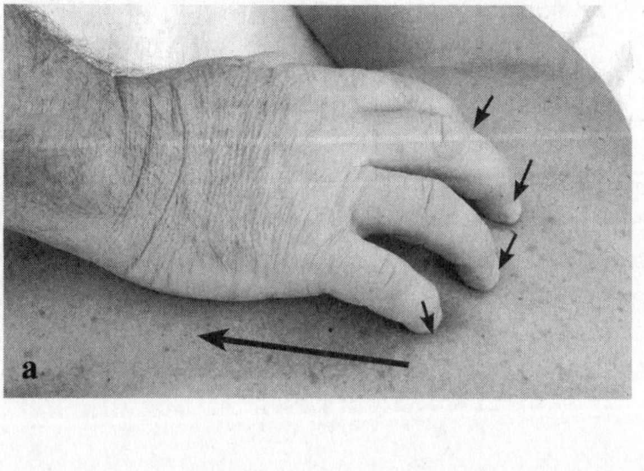

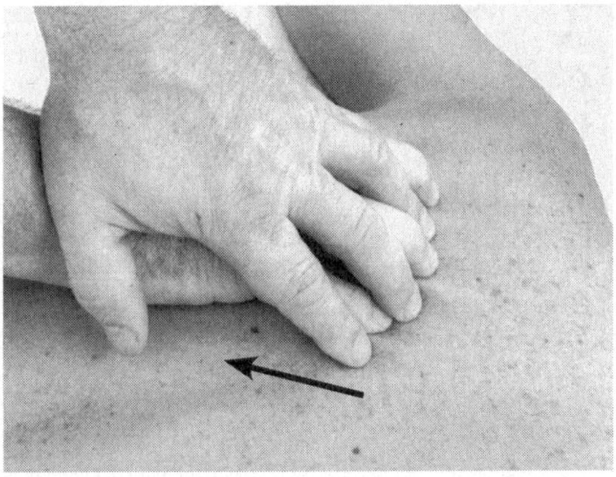

Fig. 56. Raking effleurage with increased pressure
a - raking effleurage with bend distal phalanges
b - raking effleurage with both hands acting as one tool

Another variant of this technique is raking effleurage in combination with stretching of the skin. To perform it, place the hand with spread and flexed fingers, as shown in Fig. 57 'a'. During the stroke, extend the fingers and try simultaneously to stretch the skin between the thenar-hypothenar area and the fingertips until the hand becomes completely flat (see Fig. 57 'b'). As soon as the hand is flat, again flex the metacarpo-phalangeal joints and repeat the cycle while moving forward.

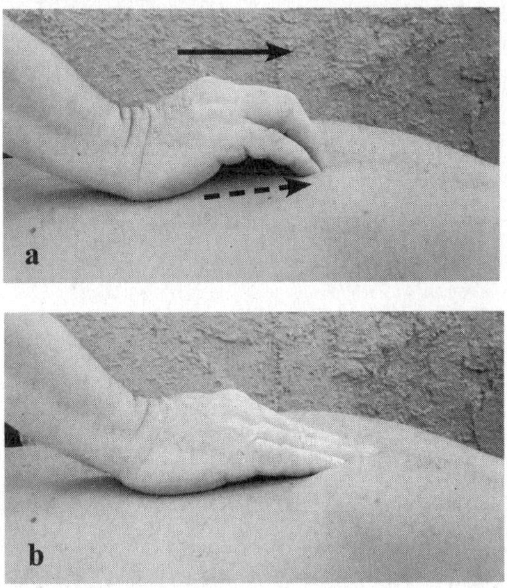

Fig. 57. Raking effleurage in combination with stretching of the skin
a - starting position **b** - final position
Solid arrow - direction of the massage stroke
Dotted arrow - direction of the skin's stretching during the massage stroke

Raking effleurage is useful when the therapist works on the ribs and along the intercostal spaces. Sarkisov-Sirasini, (1963) achieved a reduction of tachypnea (i.e., fast, shallow breathing) in patients with emphysema using raking effleurage. In his opinion, this effect is the result of the inhibition of the CNS and the suppression of the respiratory center located in the brain steam.

This technique is also used in the abdominal area. It stimulates the gastric and intestinal peristalsis and mechanically helps to mix the intestinal contents. Technique is also used in the areas of skin which can not be massaged (i.e., rash, varicose veins). Raking effleurage with simultaneous skin stretching is used in medical massage for the treatment of reflex zones in the skin.

8. EFFLEURAGE WITH LOCKED HANDS

This type of the effleurage is bi-manual technique with interlocked fingers. It is used mostly on the large joints. The main contact areas are both palms. The fingers are not in direct contact with massaged segment, but they hold the hands together during the strokes. If the therapist wants to target a smaller area, he or she may use only the thenar or hypothenar areas of both hands. To increase the pressure, both hands can be pressed against each other.

This technique is the best way to work on the joints and very effective approach to prepare a joint affected by Osteoarthritis, for the medical massage. Effleurage with locked hands increases circulation in the capsule, periosteum and subchondral bone. It also has an analgesic effect.

The effleurage with locked hands can be done in different directions: parallel longitudinal, opposite longitudinal, parallel circular and opposite circular (see Fig. 58).

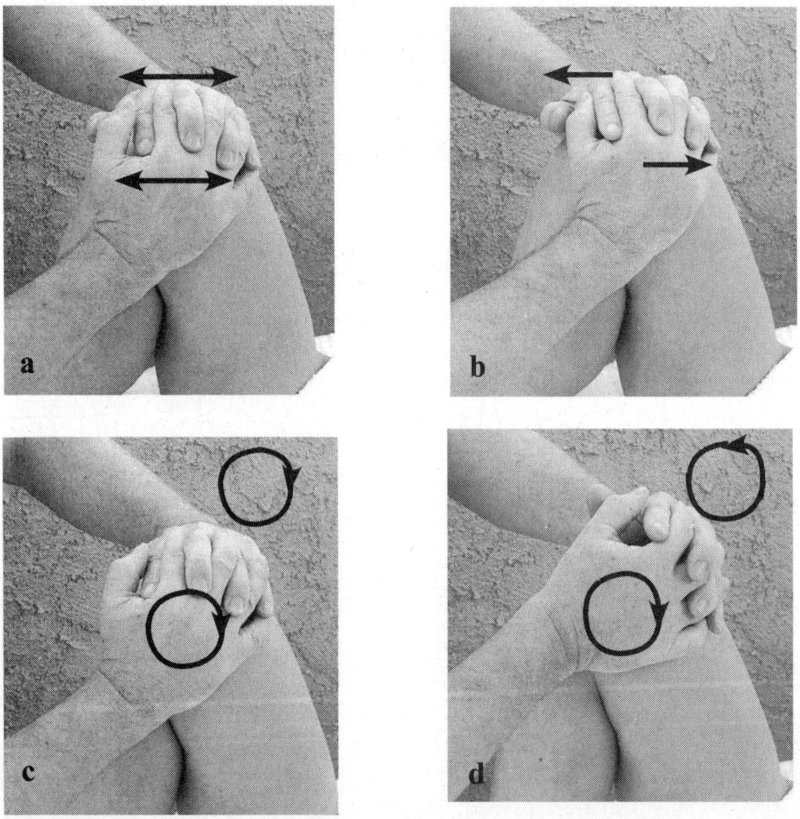

Fig. 58. Effleurage with locked hands on the knee joint

a - parallel longitudinal

b - opposite longitudinal

c - parallel circular

d - opposite circular

9. PINCHING EFFLEURAGE

Pinching effleurage is used on small areas of the forearms, hands and feet. This type of effleurage is conducted by the thumb on one side and the 2nd to 3rd fingers on the other side, or by the thumb and index fingers only. Thus, the massaged segment is slightly pinched between fingers. The contact areas can be restricted to the fingertips, or can include the palmar surfaces of all phalanxes of the 1st through 3rd fingers, and also the surface of the 1st interphalangeal space.

Pinching effleurage along the finger or toe can be ended with gentle stretch of the small joints to loosen capsule, ligaments and tendons. It is especially important on the feet where the vertical load spreads unequally and, therefore, causes additional tension in the skin, fascia, plantar aponeurosis and muscles. Fig. 59 illustrates the application of pinching effleurage on the foot.

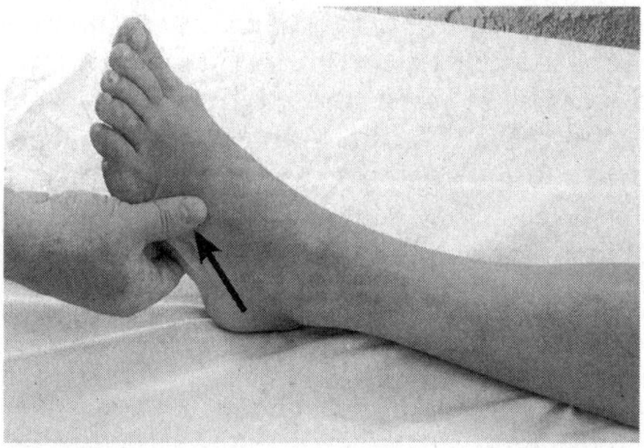

Fig. 59. Pinching effleurage on the foot

...

FRICTION

A. GENERAL CHARACTERISTICS

Hippocrates was the first author who described the friction technique and the basic rules of its clinical application. However, it was the Roman physician Galen (131-201 A.D.) who developed a detailed system of treatment by the friction technique. Working as a doctor in the gladiator school of Pergamum, Galen developed the practical concept of preparatory friction, or *frictio praeparatoria*, which was used to prepare gladiators before a fight, and therapeutic friction, or *frictio apoterapia*, which was used as a treatment procedure for the rehabilitation of injured gladiators.

Friction has a different technical approach compared to effleurage. The main difference is in the level of application. In the case of effleurage, the skin is affected most. When the practitioner applies friction, he or she targets the connective tissue structures (i.e., fascia, aponeurosis, periosteum) and skeletal muscles as well. Thus, the massage practitioner has to apply enough pressure to 'pass' the skin's level to achieve the correct application of friction. Another difference is the increased speed of strokes to cause the local hyperemia. When combined with applied pressure, a very powerful stimulation of the soft tissue is created.

Friction is a local technique and does not affect large areas at once. Thus, the friction can be done in the direction of venous and lymphatic drainage as well as against it. Friction causes many local and general effects. First of all, friction triggers a local hyperemia in the skin and underlying soft tissues. During the intensive friction, the temperature between the contact area of the hand and massaged soft tissues can rise on additional 36 C (96.8 F) degrees (Sarkisov-Sirasini, 1963). This increased of local temperature, in combination with applied pressure, causes local **controlled inflammation**. As we discussed earlier, this inflammation stimulates oxygenation and, consequently the metabolism of the soft tissues in the massaged area and activates fibroblasts.

According to Jacob, (1960), friction releases the largest amount of **histamine** from the tissues than any other massage technique. The release of histamine causes local capillary dilation in the massaged area and increased its level in blood produces general vasodilation of arterioles. Thus, blood circulation increases through the whole body, including the internal organs. This is a great example of a viscero-somatic relationship in the human body. The increased histamine concentration is a messenger which attracts fibroblasts and they start the healing process.

Friction is a very important method of elimination in the reflex zones in the skin during medical massage. Friction with moderate pressure increases the contractile response of the muscles. This effect is widely used in sports massage to prepare athletes directly before competition.

This type of massage stroke has a very unusual effect on the nervous system. From one side, friction has a stimulating impact on the central nervous system. From the other, it has the strongest analgesic effect compared to any other massage stroke. The unusual combination of touch, pressure, vibration and increased local temperature activates C nervous fibers. This helps to keep the 'gates' in the closed position and inhibits the transmission of pain stimuli to the central nervous system. Friction also increases the adaptation of the peripheral receptors and their inhibition. All these events are responsible for the great analgesic effect of friction.

Another important effect of friction is the stretching or elimination of fibrotic connections between the skin and the fascia, aponeurosis, tendons, ligaments or periosteum. Friction is the best way to deal with these abnormalities because of its detailed approach the massaged tissues. This is why the friction is successfully used in scar and cellulite treatment. In such a case, the main benefit of friction can be obtained by detailed work in the affected area. Friction with moderate pressure is also the best way to prepare muscles for the subsequent application of the kneading technique.

B. TECHNICAL DISTINCTIONS

1. CONTACT AREAS

Friction is a deeper stroke then effleurage. Thus, the therapist has to apply moderate vertical pressure first to 'pass' the skin level, and only after this strat the friction in the horizontal direction.

Friction can be applied with or without stabilizing the skin. In the first variant, the operator tightens the skin in the massaged area with the one hand while applying friction with other. If the therapist uses the second variant of friction, the skin moves with the contact area of the hand; e.g., Cyriax's friction.

2. DIRECTION OF THE STROKES

Friction can be directed longitudinally or across: to the lines of cleavage in the skin, to the direction of muscle fibers, or to the fascial planes. The lines of cleavage reflect the predominant orientation of collagen fibers in the skin. To find the direction of these lines in any part of the body, slightly pinch the fold of skin. The folds of skin is created more easily in one direction than in another (compare see Fig. 60 'a' and 'b').

Friction strokes across the lines of cleavage are helpful in cases of fibrotic adhesions between the skin and fascia. Friction strokes along the muscle fibers are valuable for warming up the entire muscle that has hypertonic pathology (i.e., hypertonus, trigger point or myogelosis). In any case, cross friction has to alternate with longitudinal friction. Friction can be also done in a spiral or circular manner, as well as in the opposite direction when two hands are used.

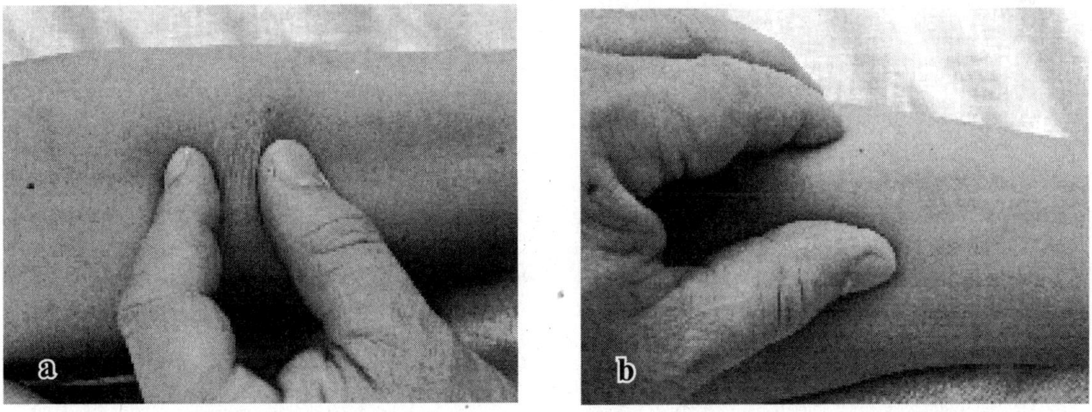

Fig. 60. Detection of the lines of cleavage on the inner surface of forearm
a - several small folds form along the lines of cleavage
b - one fold of skin is formed if pinch is across the lines of cleavage

3. SPEED AND PRESSURE

The speed of friction has to be significant to produce beneficial therapeutic effects. It can range between 80 and 120 strokes per minute. The amount of applied pressure is another important factor. Quick strokes with light pressure affect the skin mostly. We will discuss this subject below in the section on superficial friction on page 147. Friction with moderate pressure affects the skin also, but the main targets are the connective tissue structures and superficial skeletal muscles. Deeper friction targets the deep fascia and deep skeletal muscles. Thus, to perform friction correctly, the practitioner first has to press the contact area into the soft tissues, 'pass' the skin level, and only after this start the application of friction.

During friction the practitioner can use constant pressure or slightly change it during the application of technique. One has to remember that friction using the knuckles creates much more pressure compared to any other contact area. Another important tip: When less lubricant is applied to the massaged area, less energy is consumed to produce the same therapeutic effect, and at the same time the friction strokes become more effective.

C. TYPES OF FRICTION

The same techniques as grasping permanent effleurage, effleurage with locked hands, ridging, raking, and pinching effleurage, which we discussed previously, can be used for friction as well. Of course, the speed and pressure have to be adjusted for the friction purposes. In this section we will discuss special friction techniques (see Fig. 61).

FRICTION

SAWING FRICTION	**ALIGNED FRICTION**
STRETCHING FRICTION	**PLANING FRICTION**
CROSSING FRICTION	**RIDGING FRICTION**
CYRIAX'S FRICTION	**SUPERFICIAL FRICTION**
SARKISOV-SIRASINI'S FRICTION	**FRICTION -KNEADING FRICTION**
GRASPING PERMANENT FRICTION	**FRICTION WITH LOCKED HANDS**
RAKING FRICTION	**PINCHING FRICTION**

Fig. 61. Classification of friction techniques

1. SAWING FRICTION

This type of friction should be used on any flat part of the body especially in areas close to bone structures (e. g., along the medial edge of the scapula or between spinous processes). Sawing friction should be conducted by the ulnar edge of one or both hands. In the latter case, the hands placed about 1 inch apart, with the palms facing each other. The therapist presses hands into the tissue and moves them in the same or cpposite direction (see Fig. 62-63).

Friction with both hands also can be done **with** or **without** a fold of skin between them. This is an essential detail because the fold of skin increases the hands' mobility and allows to use friction with larger range of strokes (see Fig. 62). This is important in the cases of fibrotic connections between the skin and connective tissue structures (i.e. fascia, aponeurosis, tendons, ligaments or periosteum). If the therapist does not have a fold of skin between the hands, sawing friction affects the skin mostly by stretching it in the opposite direction between the two hands (see Fig. 63) and it is used during a medical massage of the cutaneous reflex zones.

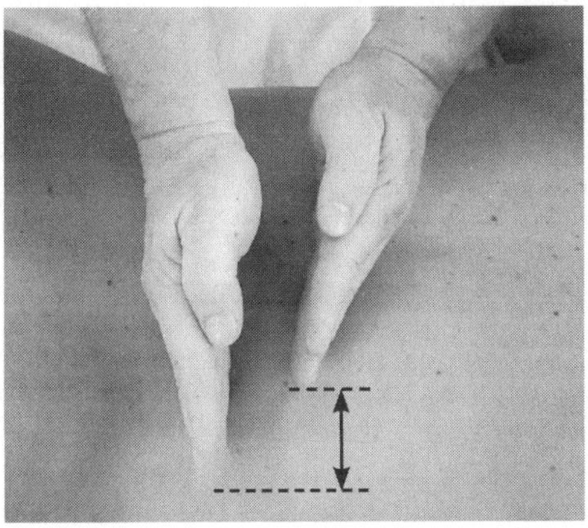

Fig. 62. Sawing friction with two hands in the opposite direction **with** a fold of skin in between
Two **dashed lines** and **arrow** indicate range of friction strokes

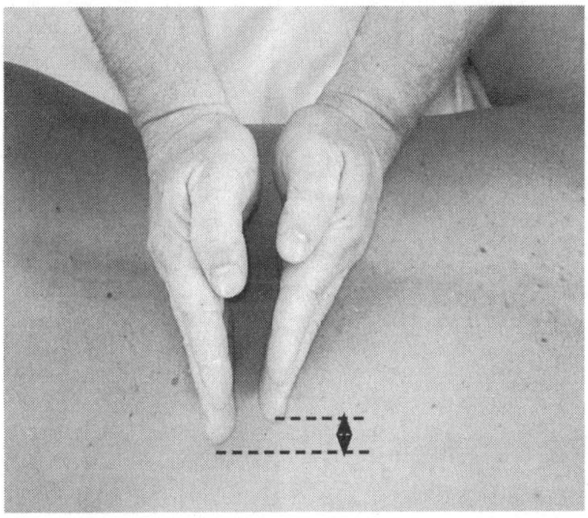

Fig. 63. Sawing friction with two hands in the opposite direction **without** a fold of skin in between
Two **dashed lines** and **arrow** indicate range of friction strokes

2. ALIGNED FRICTION

This type of the friction is performed using the fingertips of 2nd-3rd, 3rd-4th or 2nd-5th fingers. It depends on the size of massaged area. The practitioner has to bend fingers in the meta-carpo-phalangeal joints, compress them together, and arrange the fingertips in one line at an angle of about 40-50 degrees to the body surface. To apply additional pressure, increase the angle between the fingers and the body surface. The fingertips are the main contact areas. Fig. 64 shows an example of aligned friction.

Aligned friction targets the skeletal muscles and can be applied in the direction along and across to the main orientation of fibers in the muscle belly. Aligned friction is very effective in the areas of fibrotic adhesions between the skin and fascia or aponeurosis. This technique also lets the practitioner perform a lot of detailed work on the postsurgical scars to loosen and stretch the sot tissue in these areas.

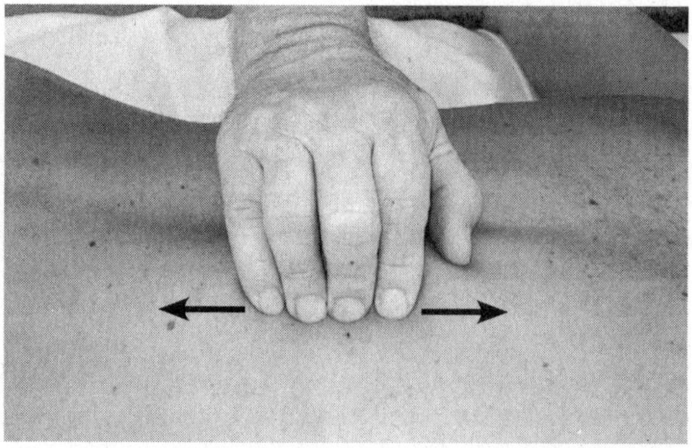

a - using the fingertips of the 2nd-5th fingertips

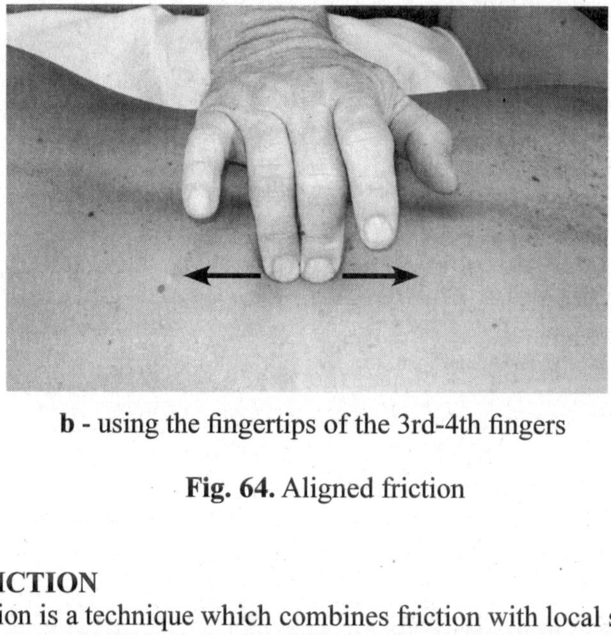

b - using the fingertips of the 3rd-4th fingers

Fig. 64. Aligned friction

3. STRETCHING FRICTION

Stretching friction is a technique which combines friction with local stretching of the skin, superficial fascia or aponeurosis. This type of friction is a local technique which employs the whole hand. Thus, it should be performed on the large flat parts of the body; e.g., the back.

Start with pressing the base of the hand (i.e., thenar-hypothenar area) into the soft tissue. Next, press the fingertips of the flexed fingers into the skin (see Fig. 65'a'). Thus there are two contact areas: the thenar-hypothenar and the fingertips of the 2nd through 5th fingers. Now, slide and push the fingertips forward until the hand becomes completely flat. While doing that try to stretch skin and fascia between base of the hand and fingertips (see Fig. 65 'b'). Try to keep the fingers together. Bring the hand to the starting position by flexing the fingers back and repeat the stroke on the same area. The therapist can move fingers in a longitudinal or spiral pattern while sliding them forward during the stroke. To move to the neighboring segment, relocate the base of the hand first.

To reduce the strain on the hand place the other hand on top of the active hand to reinforce the movement of fingertips forward. During this stroke, the threapist performs the classical friction and, at the same time, stretches the skin and fascia between the fingertips and the base of the hand.

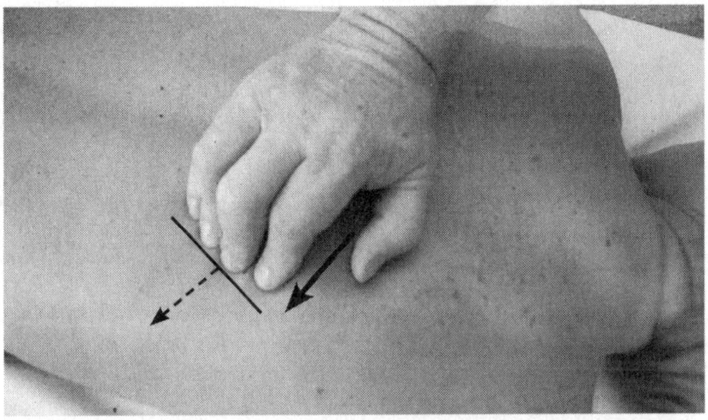

a - position of the hand at the beginning of the stroke

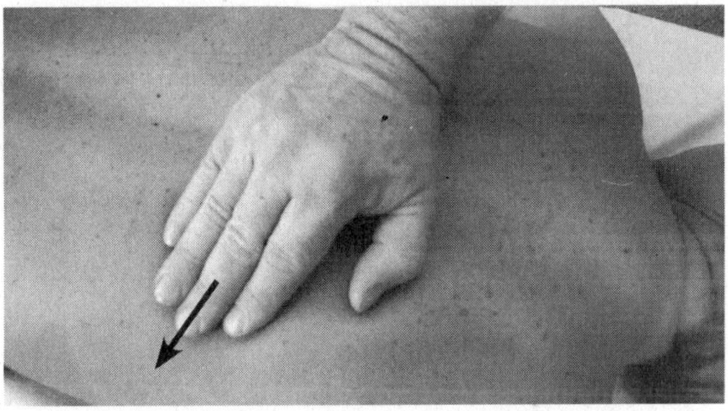

b - position of the hand at the end of the stroke

Fig. 65. Stretching friction in the longitudinal pattern

Dashed arrow - direction of the stroke **Solid arrow** - direction of the stretching

Another variant of stretching friction is to widely spread the fingers while pushing them forward. In this case, the larger area is covered (see Fig. 66). This technique can be done bi-manually when hands are placed on the top of each other and they act as one tool.

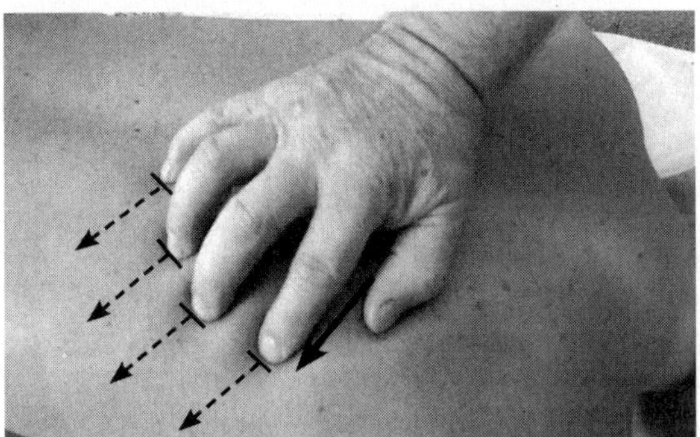

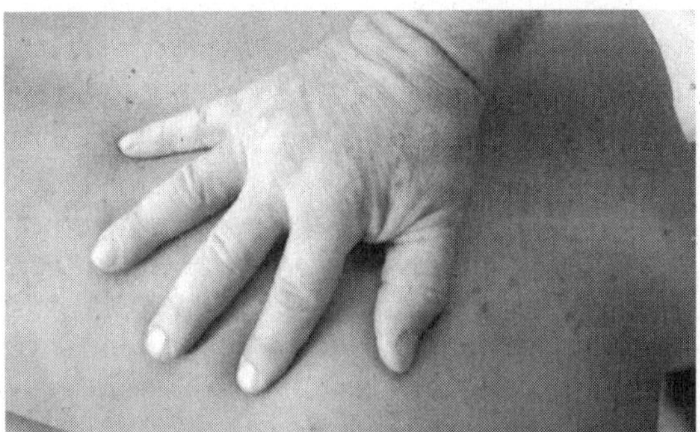

a - hand at the beginning of the stroke **b** - hand at the end of the stroke

Fig. 66. Stretching friction with spread fingers

Dashed arrow - direction of the stroke **Solid arrow** - direction of the stretching

4. PLANING FRICTION

Planing friction is performed using one or both hands, which follow each other. This technique is a combination of friction and percussion. The practitioner has to completely extend the hand and fingers and press them together. The contact areas are the fingertips of the 2nd through 5th fingers. The hand(s) has to be placed at an angle of 30-45 degrees to the massaged area.

Press the fingertips of one hand into the soft tissue, 'passing' the skin level and push the skin forward. Immediately release the hand and replace it with your other hand which is supposed to hit the same area. Repeat the application 3-4 times alternating hands before moving to the neighboring area. When done correctly, a fold of skin is formed up to the fingertips (see Fig. 67). Arrange hands in a parallel manner to let them follow each other during the application of the stroke. Arrows indicate the movement of hands from the current position which is shown in the photo.

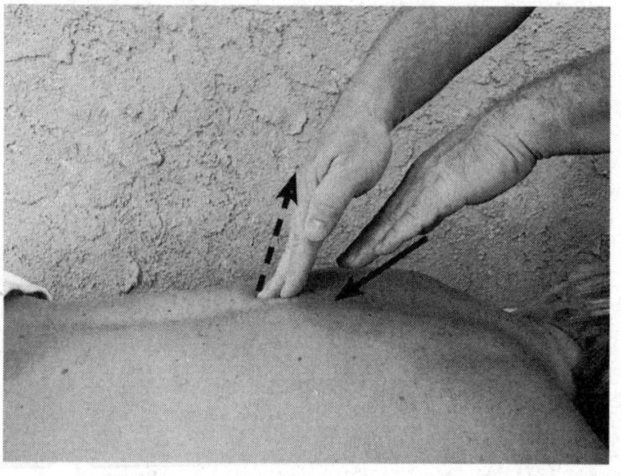

Fig. 67. Two-hand planed friction

Because of the combination of friction and percussion, this technique is effective in the areas of fibrotic connections between the skin and fascia and scars. It also stimulates the nervous system and muscles. As a result of planned friction, the muscle tone increases and contractile response accelerates. This technique is useful in cases of chronic pulmonary disorders to accelerate sputum drainage. A very light variant can be applied on the abdomen to stimulate gastro-intestinal motility.

5. SARKISOV-SIRASINI'S FRICTION

In 1963, Dr. I.M. Sarkisov-Sirasini father of Russian Sports Massage School offered combination of deep pressure and simultaneous friction in the longitudinal or circular pattern. This technique must be used on the large, flat areas of the body; e.g., along the vertebral column.

The contact areas are the thenar, the palmar surface of the thumb, and the fingertips of the 2nd through 5th fingers. The thenar and thumb of the operating hand are placed on the massaged area. The supportive hand is placed on top of the active hand to produce additional pressure. Using supportive hand the practitioner presses the thenar and thumb of the active hand into the soft tissue and move both hands **together** along the massaged segment. The actual movement of both hands along the massaged segment is result of the upper hand pushing lower hand forward while the fingertips of the 2nd through 5th fingers of the lower hand simultaneously perform circular friction.

This friction targets the skeletal muscles as well as the fascia and aponeurosis. Because of the significant pressure, all muscle layers are affected. However, clients do not feel strong pain because the contact area is large and the pressure spreads equally.

Sarkisov-Sirasini's technique is very effective as a preparation of the muscle with hypertonic pathology to the medical massage especially to ischemic compression. To do so, place the thenar of the operating hand on the area of the trigger point and compress the tissue. However, do not move through the massaged area; stay still. In this case, moderate ischemic compression is achieved and it is combined with the friction on surrounding tissues. This is very helpful when the client has a very pain-sensitive area of the trigger point or hypertonus. This technique is also effective as a final transition to the kneading. Fig. 68 shows an example of this technique from two points of view.

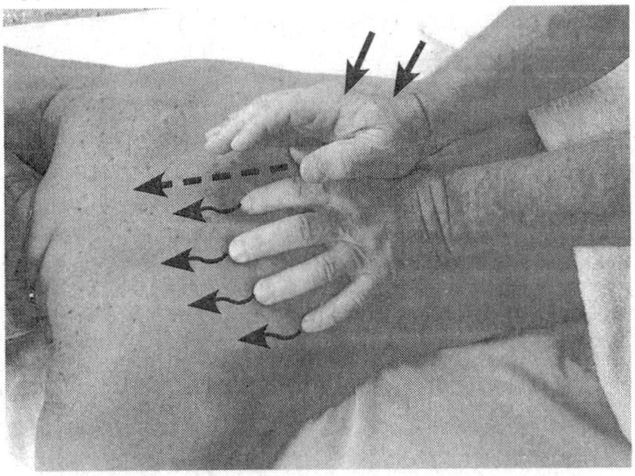

Fig. 68. Sarkisov-Sirasini's friction

Solid arrows - vertical pressure by the supportive hand
Waved arrows - direction of circular friction by the fingertips of the 2nd through 5th fingers
Dashed arrow - general direction of stroke by the operating hand

6. CROSSING FRICTION

Crossing friction is used on the round-edged areas; i.e., shoulders, legs. The operator has to use the radial edge of the hand between the thumb and index finger; i.e., the 1st metacarpal space. These parts of the hands perfectly match the rounded edges of the arms or legs. If two hands are used two hands moving in the same or opposite direction. The therapist has to be sure that the fold of skin is formed between the hands. If there is no fold of skin, crossing friction mostly affects the skin. Fig. 69 illustrates crossing friction with two hands moving in the opposite direction.

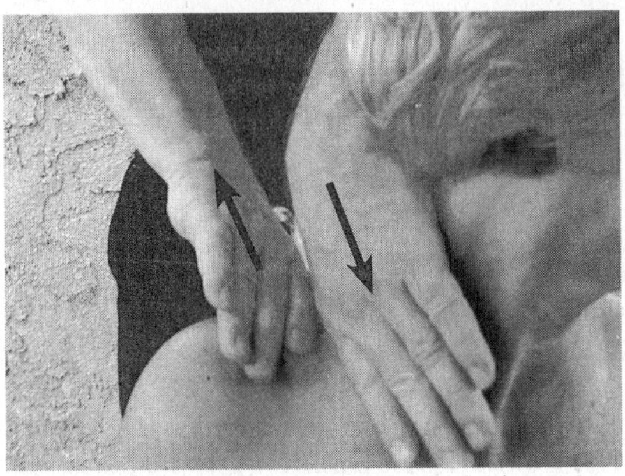

Fig. 69. Crossing friction with two hands moving in the opposite direction

7. CYRIAX'S FRICTION

Dr. J. Cyriax developed technique of strong friction in a direction perpendicular to the predominant orientation of collagen fibers in the tendon or myofibrils in the muscles. The main target of Cyriax's friction is connective tissue structures where tension developed as a tight fibrotic bridges between skin and the fascia, aponeurosis, tendon or periosteum. By stroking the skin against fascia the therapist stretches fibrotic bridges and restores the normal function of the connective tissue. As a result, tension in the underlying skeletal muscles is decreased as well.

Use the fingertips of the 1st, 2nd or lst-2nd fingers. Friction has to be strong enough to move the finger with the skin over the underlying tissues. The therapist should slowly increase the speed of the strokes. Dr. Cyriax (1976) formulated five conditions for the correct application of cross-fiber friction: accurate diagnosis, exact knowledge of the main orientation of fibers in the tissue, perpendicular direction of strokes, movement of the finger with the skin, sweep of the strokes.

This friction is used in cases of Tendinitis, ligamental injuries and periostal abnormalities (e.g. Tennis Elbow). Fig. 70 illustrates Cyriax's friction on the Achilles tendon.

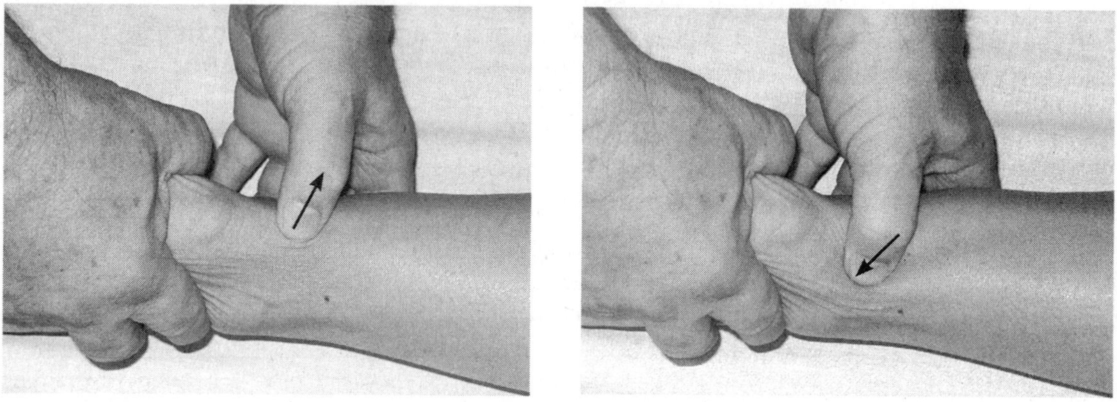

Fig. 70. Cyriax's friction on the area of the Achilles tendon

8. RIDGING FRICTION

Ridging friction is used on any part of the body with one or both hands and it has three subtypes: ridging friction using the knuckles of the distal interphalangeal joints, ridging friction using the knuckles of the proximal interphalangeal joints, and ridging friction with ischemic compression.

Ridging friction can be fixed or mobile. In the case of fixed ridging friction, the hand(s) stays on the same massaged area. If mobile ridging friction is used, the hand(s) moves along the massaged segment. In the latter case, the operator has two choices: Continue to stroke the massaged area using the fingers or hold them still. For the best effect, use as little lubricant as possible.

a. Ridging Friction Using the Knuckles of the Distal Interphalangeal Joints

Make a fist(s) and place the knuckles of the distal interphalangeal joints of 2nd through 5th fingers on the massaged area. Slightly spread the flexed fingers. Stabilize the thenar-hypothenar area (i.e., base of the hand) by pushing it against the body, and start to move each finger separately, one after another. In some way the movement should resemble playing the piano when each finger moves independently. Each finger can be moved back and forth or form small ovals.

Fig. 71 illustrates fixed, circular ridging friction using the knuckles of the distal interphalangeal joints which create oval shaped movements. The contact areas can be seen on Fig. 43 '33'.

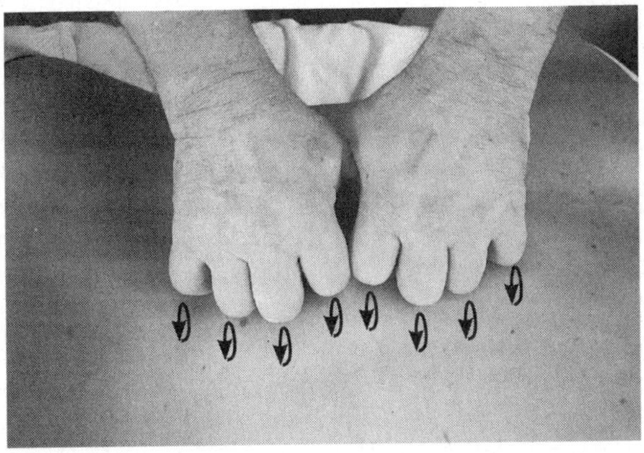

Fig. 71. Circular, ridging friction using the knuckles of the distal interphalangeal joints

b. Ridging Friction Using the Knuckles of the Proximal Interphalangeal Joints

This type of ridging friction creates the strongest pressure. Therefore, the operator has to be more careful. The contact area is the knuckles of the proximal interphalangeal joints of the 2nd through 5th fingers (for contact areas see Fig. 43 '32'). Make a fist(s), press the knuckles into the soft tissue, 'pass' the skin level, and move the hand(s) through the massaged segment. This type of ridging friction is performed in the mobile regime only. If this technique is conducted bi-manually, the hands can move in a parallel manner or follow each other.

In another variant of bi-manual performance, the hands act as one tool. In this case, one hand tightly grasps the thumb of the other. This technique is similar to ridging effleurage, as shown in Fig. 53 but with stronger pressure application. The practitioner should use the weight of the body to enhance vertical pressure during the application of ridging friction. Finally, both hands can be placed on opposite sides of the extremity and compress the soft tissue against the bone during the stroke. Fig. 72 illustrates this example of ridging friction conducted on the thigh.

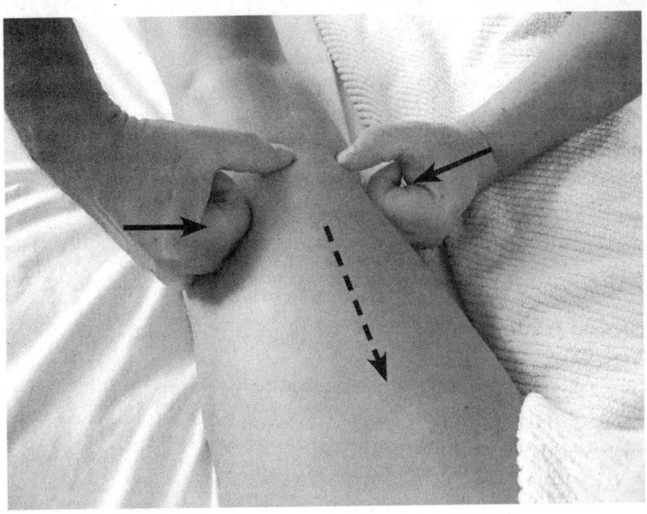

Fig. 72. Ridging friction using both hands placed on the opposite sides of the thigh
Solid arrows - direction of compression
Dashed arrow - direction of stroke

c. Combination of Ridging Friction and Ischemic Compression

Another important variant of ridging friction is used in the medical massage treatment of the hypertonus and trigger point. This technique combines ischemic compression and friction. For more information about ischemic compression, see below in the"Compression" section.

After the trigger point is located, place the thumb into it. The knuckles of the proximal interphalangeal joints of the 2nd-5th fingers should stroke the surrounding area with small circular strokes while the thumb maintains vertical compression. Continue to slowly increase direct pressure into the trigger point until a desirable depth of submergence is reached. During compression, continue to stroke the surrounding trigger point tissues using the 2nd-5th fingers.

This type of friction also can be done in a mobile way. To do that, the thumb stays in the area of the trigger point to create and maintain ischemic compression. The contact areas of the 2nd-5th fingers move around the thumb. Thus, the whole hand makes a half circle around the thumb, which continues to press into the trigger point. The practitioner has to change hands to stroke the tissue on the other side and create a full circle around the thumb which is pressed into the trigger point. The mobile variant of the treatment is more helpful.

This type of ridging friction is very effective because it allows the practitioner to work on the trigger points directly and simultaneously reduce tension in the surrounding soft tissue. At the same time, ridging friction of the surrounding area significantly reduces the pain felt by the client during ischemic compression by activating the mechanism of counter irritation. In this case, the C nervous fibers are activated and it shifts the balance from a fast to slow pain system. As a result, the flow of afferent (i.e. ascending) pain stimuli to the central nervous system is partly blocked. Fig. 73 illustrates an example of this technique.

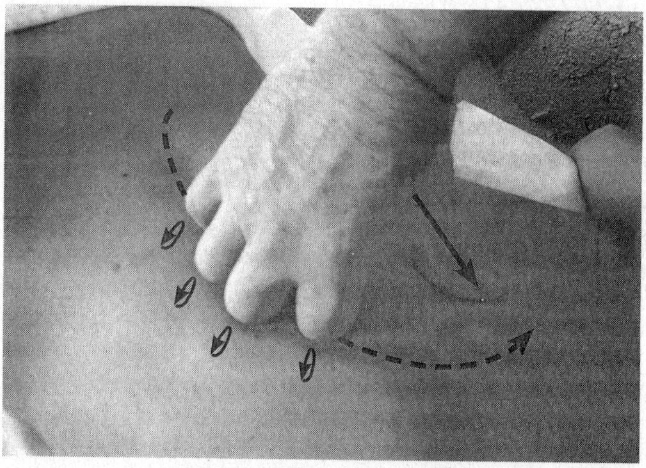

Fig. 73. Combination of ridging friction and ischemic compression in a mobile mode of application
Solid arrow - direction of ischemic compression
Small circular arrows - circular friction using the 2nd-5th fingers
Dashed arrow - direction of a half circular stroke by the hand around a fixed thumb

9. FRICTION-KNEADING TECHNIQUE

The author developed this technique for massage on large areas with significant muscle mass (e. g., paravertebral regions, thigh, etc.). This is a two-handed technique, with one hand playing the leading role and the other hand having supportive role (see Fig. 74).

The leading hand makes a fist and is placed on the massaged area on the dorsal surface of the proximal phalanges of the 2nd-5th fingers (see Fig. 43 '29'). The supportive hand is placed on the ulnar edge, creates fold of skin and loosely embraces the fist of the leading hand to allow its circular strokes. To perform the friction-kneading the operator must press the ulnar edge of the supportive hand into the tissue, and 'pass' the skin's level (see Fig. 74). After this, the leading hand starts to make circular strokes in the wrist joint with simultaneous application of vertical pressure.

If the circular strokes have a small radius the actual contact area is the dorsal surfaces of the 2nd-5th phalanges, and the operator creates friction only. If the therapist increases the radius of circular motions and uses the knuckles of the metacarpophalangeal and proximal interphalangeal joints of the 2nd-5th fingers as the main contact areas (see Fig. 44 '31' and '32') with a simultaneous increasing of vertical pressure, the therapist combines the therapeutic impact of friction and kneading at the same time. The operator achieves the kneading effect by displacing the muscle layers in the horizontal direction using knuckles of the metacarpophalangeal and proximal interphalangeal joints of the 2nd-5th fingers during each part of circular stroke conducted by the leading hand.

I want to discuss the role of the supportive hand separately. First of all, the supportive hand tightens the skin and creates fold of skin in the massaged area. Secondly, the supportive hand stabilizes the leading hand and, what is more important, prevents wrist injury. During this friction, the wrist joint is vulnerable to injury because of the combination of circular motions and vertical pressure. Thus, the supportive hand is a guarantee of safety during the application of friction-kneading.

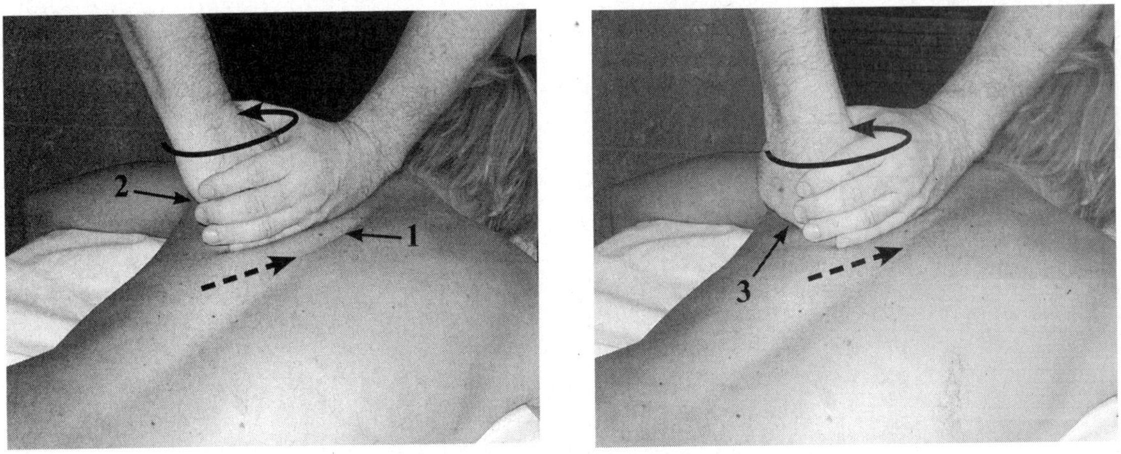

Fig. 74. Friction-kneading technique

1 - fold of skin
2 - part of circular stroke using the knuckles of proximal interphalangeal joints of the right hand
3 - the contact area is switched to the knuckles of metacarpophalangeal joints of the right hand
Dashed arrow - direction of stroke
Solid arrow - direction of circular motion in the wrist joint

Friction-kneading technique has mobile variant when both hands move through the massaged area as a single tool. An important practical tip to increase the therapeutic impact of this technique is the constant maintenance of the skin's fold up to the ulnar edge of the supportive hand.

In such a case, the supportive hand pushes the active hand forward while it continues its circular strokes but at the same time the ulnar edge of the supportive hand pushes the fold of skin forward as well. Thus, the operator employs the unique combination of friction, kneading, and connective tissue massage at the same time. We recommend friction-kneading in mobile regime as a transitional element to the kneading technique especially in the segments with large muscle mass. Friction-kneading is also helpful during medical massage when it is used just before the application of connective tissue massage.

10. SUPERFICIAL FRICTION

Superficial friction is not a classical type of friction technique. As we discussed above, during friction, the practitioner has to press contact area of the hand into the soft tissue, 'pass' the skin level and then perform the friction. In the case of superficial friction, the main target is the skin itself and it changes rules of the game.

To perform this technique the skin has to be tightened by the other hand first. After fixing the skin, use the following contacts areas: whole palm, thenar-hypothenar, dorsal surfaces of the proximal or middle phalanges, ulnar side of the hand or fist, or figertip(s) (see Fig. 43; ## 2; 4; 7; 12;19; 24; 27; 28; 29).

The hand has to slide superficially along the massaged area with great speed in a forward-backward direction. The feeling of heat or even burning has to be created between the contact area of the therapist's hand and the patient's skin. Do not move the skin against the fascia and superficial muscles otherwise you will apply regular friction, hand must to slide along the skin. Fig. 75 illustrates superficial friction; the thumb of the right hand tightens the skin, while the proximal phalanges of the 2nd-5th fingers of the left hand stroke the skin.

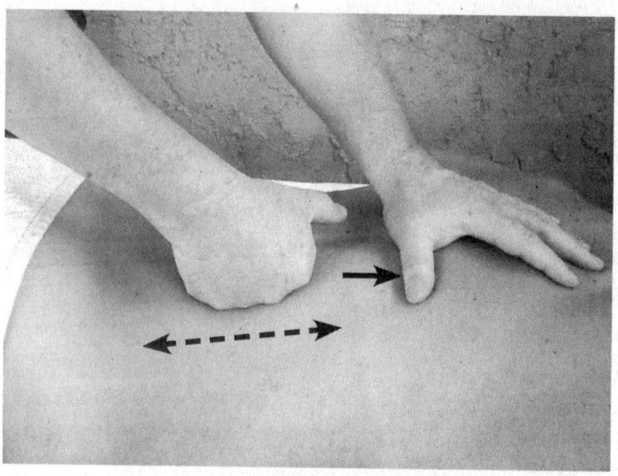

Fig. 75. Superficial friction
Solid arrow - direction of skin tighten by the right hand
Dashed arrow - direction of superficial friction conducted by the left hand

Superficial friction is a very important technique of medical massage which is used in the areas of cutaneous reflex zones and cutaneous trigger points. The increase in local temperature and vasodilation stimulate the circulation and metabolism in these areas. At the same time, the level of adaptation of peripheral sensory receptors is reached quickly. All these events help to eliminate the cutaneous reflex zones completely, sometimes even after one application.

KNEADING

A. GENERAL CHARACTERISTICS

Kneading is the latest massage technique. According to Bear, (1952), this term appeared for the first time in the works of the Italian physician Fabricus of Aquapedente (1537-1619). Kneading is a very important and highly effective technique of therapeutic massage. I agree with Dr. Kramarenko, who wrote in 1953: "One can estimate the level of a massage therapist's expertise by testing the kneading technique only."

The development of the various kneading techniques is important contribution of the Russian Massage School. All authors agreed that the massage therapist has to spend at least 50% of time of each massage session on kneading techniques (Kramarenko, 1953; Belaya, 1974; Kunichev, 1985; Vasichkin, 1991; Turin, 1992; Dubrovsky, 1995; Fokin, 1997).

The main target of kneading is the skeletal muscles, but the skin and connective tissue structures are affected as well. During kneading, the practitioner grasps the muscles and soft tissues, lifts, rolls, stretches and compresses them between the hands and bone structures. Kneading can also be applied to the skin only. In this case, the therapist grasps a fold of skin along and later perpendicular to the lines of cleavage and performs the kneading using the fingers as contact areas.

Every kneading technique consists of several components, which must follow and flow into each other. To properly apply a kneading, the practitioner has to practice to perform these complicated techniques smoothly with as less as possible hands' strain. Every part of the applied technique has to "flow" into another. If several kneading techniques are used they also have to follow each other smoothly.

Let's discuss the physiological effects of kneading on muscles in the order of this technique application. Kneading usually starts on the distal areas of a transition muscle to the tendon, or insertion muscle to the bone structure with progressive proximal advance along a muscle or group of muscles. In these areas, the therapist should use a lot of lifting and lifting/stretching. In this case, the Golgi tendon organ receptors are activated. Their sensory output inhibits the lower motor centers in the spinal cord. As a result, the amount of efferent (i.e., descending) motor stimuli to the muscles decreases and they start to relax.

The next part of kneading involves working on the muscle's belly. In this area, compression and local stretching in opposite directions should be predominant. As a result of compression and stretching, the muscle spindle receptors in the skeletal muscles are activated. Because the stretching of the muscle belly is not significant during the kneading, the slow parts of the muscle spindle receptors (i.e., nuclear chain fibers) are stimulated. They form the ascending flow of sensory impulses, which has a slightly stimulating effect on the lower motor centers in the anterior horns of the spinal cord. Thus, this part of kneading helps to support normal muscle tone and activates the contractile apparatus of massaged muscles.

Thus, kneading has an alternately stimulating and relaxing effect on the skeletal muscles. Because of this dual effect of kneading, Dr. Sarkisov-Sirasini called the kneading techniques "passive exercises for the skeletal muscles."

Massage treatment on any part of the body shouldn't start with kneading. The practitioner must warm up and prepare the muscles by other massage techniques: effleurage to stimulate drainage; moderate friction to loose attachments of the fascia to the muscle tissue and so on.

One of the key elements of proper execution of all kneading techniques is complete muscle relaxation. It allows the operator to grasp enough muscle tissue in hand(s). This is very difficult to achieve if the muscles are under even the slightest tension. A state of complete muscle relaxation includes two equally important components: a voluntary effort on the client's side and a biomechanically correct positioning of client's body or segment of the body chosen for massage.

The first component is obvious and does not need any special discussion. However, the second component is frequently missed, which significantly reduces the effectiveness of kneading. Let's discuss this matter with the help of Fig. 76. If, for example, the practitioner wants to effectively use kneading techniques on the posterior thigh muscles, he or she must flex the knee to an approximate angle of 90 degrees. In this case, the massaged muscles will be relaxed because the distance between the points of their origins and insertions got shorter. Compare the amount of muscle tissue that the therapist has in the hand with knee flexed (see Fig. 76, 'a') and with knee extended (see Fig. 76, 'b'). In another example, kneading is applied to the latissimus dorsi and teres major muscles when the arm is adducted to the body (see Fig. 76, 'c') and with abducted arm (see Fig. 76, 'd').

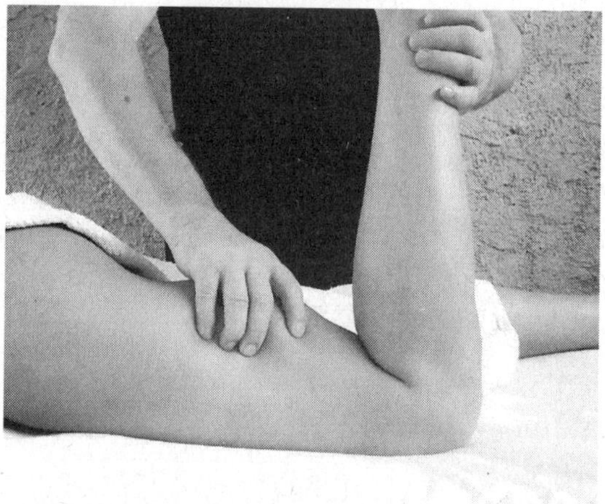

a - kneading of thigh muscles with flexed knee

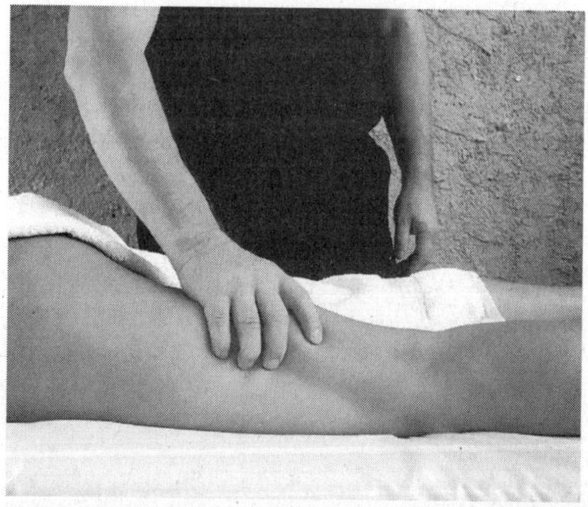

b - kneading of thigh muscles with extended knee

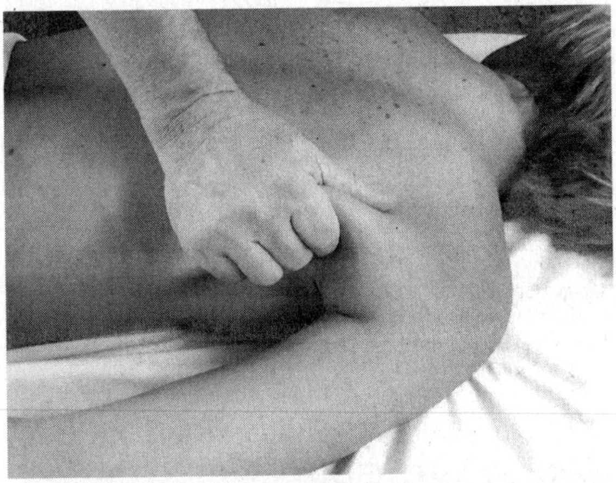

c - kneading of latissimuss dorsi and teres major muscles with adducted arm

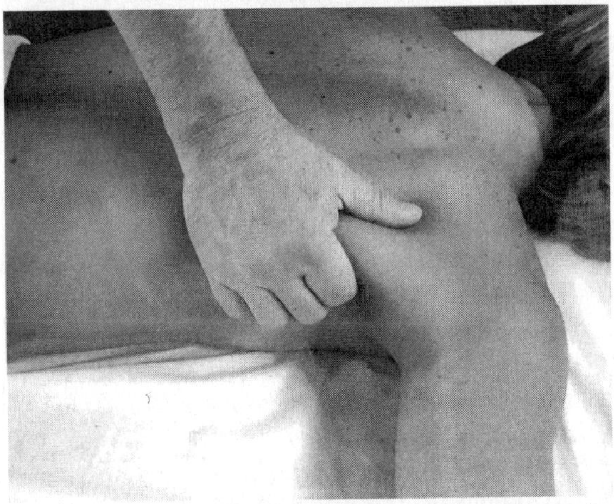

d - kneading of latissimuss dorsi and teres major muscles with abducted arm

Fig. 76. Biomechanically optimal position for kneading of a body segment

Because kneading combines and alternates different types of stimulation (pressing, stretching, rolling, etc.), the various receptors are permanently stimulated. Thus, during kneading a tremendous amount of afferent sensory impulses is generated by the receptors in the skin, connective tissue structures and skeletal muscles. As a result, the afferent sensory or ascending flow to the central nervous system is formed. Clients feel more energetic and optimistic, with simultaneous decrease of the anxiety and mood swings.

Another important benefit of this technique is its effect on peripheral circulation. During the kneading, the practitioner rhythmically compresses large bulk of soft tissue, especially skeletal muscles. From one side, it stimulates arterial circulation by producing the vasodilation, and from other side, the kneading acts as a pump which supports the venous and lymphatic drainage.

Kneading has a profound effect on the functions of the pulmonary system. As reported by Sucharev, et al. (1965), during kneading on the anterior and posterior surfaces of the thoracic cage, alveolar ventilation increased up to 24.2% and oxygen consumption increased up to 33%. After a session of kneading, these parameters of pulmonary function remained increased up to 10.4% and

19.3%, correspondingly. Turin, (1995) also reported similar influence of kneading on blood oxygenation. All these effects make kneading one of the most powerful and effective techniques of therapeutic and medical massage.

B. TECHNICAL DISTINCTIONS

1. CONTACT AREAS

The main contact areas for kneading techniques are the therapist's palms and fingers, the entire palmar surfaces of the fingers or the fingertips only. In some variants of kneading, one hand is used as a main therapeutic tool and the plays a supportive role by helping to additionally mobilize the soft tissue. For this supportive role, the other parts of the hand can be used as contact areas as well; for example the fist.

2. DIRECTION OF STROKES

The efficiency of kneading techniques strongly depends on the order and direction of the strokes. The order of treatment depends on the treatment goal. If muscles in the massaged area have to be stimulated, the following order of treatment must be applied: Start the massage from the distal part of muscle in the place of the tendinous part inserts into the bone. Next, use the same treatment on the proximal end of the muscle. Finally, work on the muscle's belly in the middle of the massaged segment.

If the muscles have to be relaxed, start treatment on the distal part of the muscle, then move to the middle part (i.e., muscle belly), and then finish work on the proximal part of the muscle. With this order, the final impact of the treatment is muscle relaxation. Repeat this sequence 2-3 times to get proper response and reset peripheral receptors.

3. SPEED AND PRESSURE

The speed of kneading should be moderate to low, because the operator has to have enough time to work with the muscles. Thus, the speed of the strokes should vary between 30-50 per minute. It depends on the type of kneading. Some kneading techniques are complex strokes, and therefore require more time to execute.

The right degree of applied pressure is another important issue. Kneading does not imply ischemic compression. Thus, the operator has to apply enough pressure to lit and stretch the muscles. Do not use excessive pressure during kneading. Because of the special character of the kneading techniques, the applied pressure is intermittent.

For the proper execution of kneading techniques, the matter of lubricant should be discussed. To achieve maximal therapeutic effect with kneading techniques, use as little lubricant as possible. I personally think it is best to completely remove the lubricant from the massaged area (e.g. by alcohol) or even use a thin cotton fabric to grasp the tissues more tightly. Also, the practitioner uses much less energy during kneading if he or she removes the lubricant from the skin before treatment started.

The effortless and fluid execution of each kneading technique requires the correct **body mechanics**. This is an important topic which requires a separate discussion. The reader may find a detailed article on this subject in the November/December 2009 issue of the *Journal of Massage Science* (please visit: **www.scienceofmassage.com**)

C. TYPES OF KNEADING

KNEADING

LONGITUDINAL PERMANENT KNEADING — **TRANSVERSE PERMANENT KNEADING**

LONGITUDINAL & TRANSVERSE INTERRUPTIVE KNEADING — **SINGULAR & DOUBLE SCROLLING KNEADING**

SIMPLE KNEADING — **DIGITAL KNEADING**

DOUBLE CIRCULAR KNEADING — **STRETCHING KNEADING**

MOBILE KNEADING — **PINCHING KNEADING**

ROLLING KNEADING — **WAVE KNEADING**

TISSUE DISPLACEMENT KNEADING

Fig. 77. Classification of kneading techniques

1. LONGITUDINAL PERMANENT KNEADING

This technique is performed using one or both hands, which follow each other. The hand(s) is located along the axis of extremity, or to the anatomical direction of the muscle in the large flat area (i.e., back). The thumb and thenar areas are placed on one side of the massaged muscle(s), and the 2nd-5th fingers and the hypothenar area are placed on the other (see Fig. 78 'a'). The operator has to grasp enough soft tissue to fill the hand. Now, compress and lift the grasped muscle (see Fig. 78'b') while pressing base of the hand into the soft tissue to create counterpressure.

At the peak of lilting, add a local stretch by slightly rotating the 2nd-5th fingers and the hypothenar using the thumb as a turning point . While doing so, very slightly decrease the pressure generated by the thumb (see Fig. 79 'a'). The next step is to rotate tissue in the opposite direction around the 2nd-5th fingers pushing by the thumb and thenar area (see Fig. 79 'b'). While doing so, slightly decrease the pressure generated by the 2nd-5th fingers and the hypothenar. Put the tissue back, but do not release the hand's grip, and repeat the strokes 3-4 times on the same area. The therapist can concentrate on one area, or move along the massaged segment.

The practitioner can combine longitudinal permanent kneading with simultaneous digital kneading (see below Fig. 82). This technique is helpful for kneading in places of transition muscles into the tendons or the insertion of tendons to the bone structures.

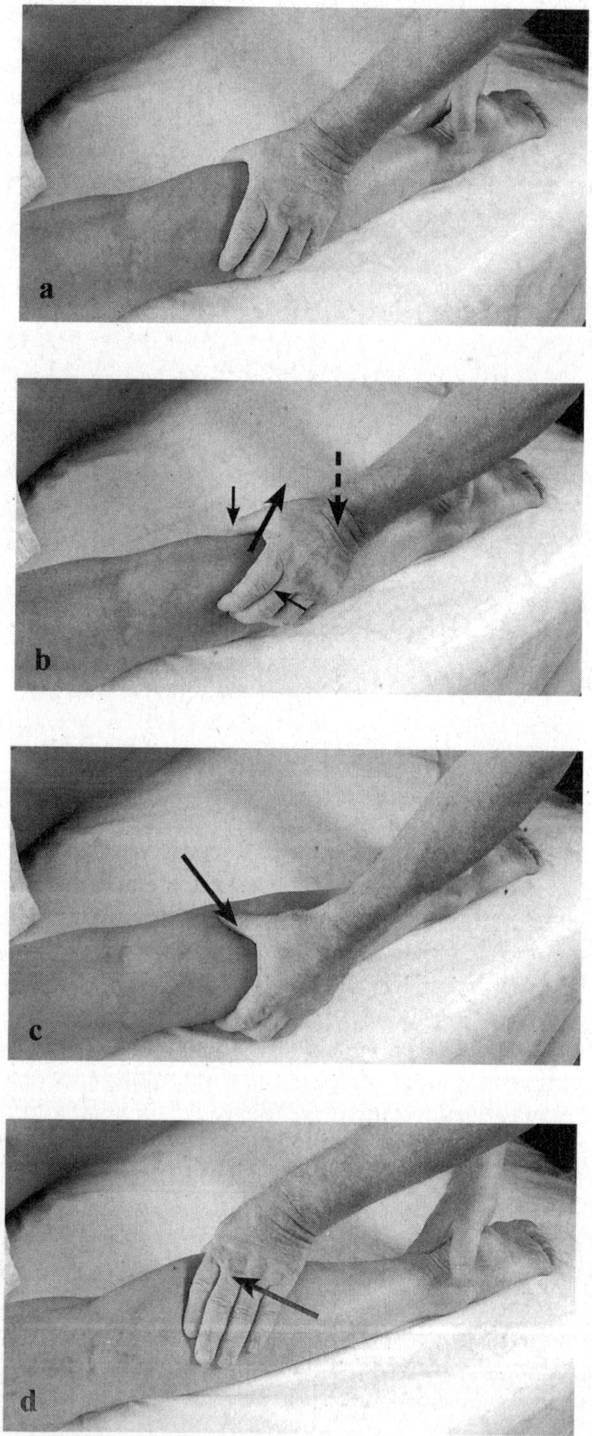

Fig. 78. Longitudinal permanent kneading

Fig. 78. Longitudinal permanent kneading
a - starting position of the hand
b - compression and lifting
c - stretching of the muscle by pushing it laterally to the direction of the thumb
d - stretching of the muscle by pushing it medially to the direction of the 2nd-5th fingers
Long solid arrow - direction of lifting **Small solid arrows** - compression from the both sides
Dashed arrow - direction of counterpressure by the base of the hand

2. TRANSVERSE PERMANENT KNEADING

To execute technique correctly place both hands perpendicularly to the axis of extremity, or to the anatomical direction of the targeted muscles. Place the maximally abducted thumbs on one side, and the rest of the fingers on the other. The tips of the thumbs should almost touch each other.

With both hands simultaneously grasp, compress and then lift the muscles (see Fig. 79 'a'). For the next step the practitioner pulls one hand toward himself and simultaneously pushes the other in the opposite direction while continue to lift tissues (see Fig. 79 'b' and 'c'). It is easier to do such opposite pull-push by rotating upper body while holding hands still. It will decrease strain on the hands and provide necessary fluidity of the strokes. Repeat these strokes 2-3 times in each area.

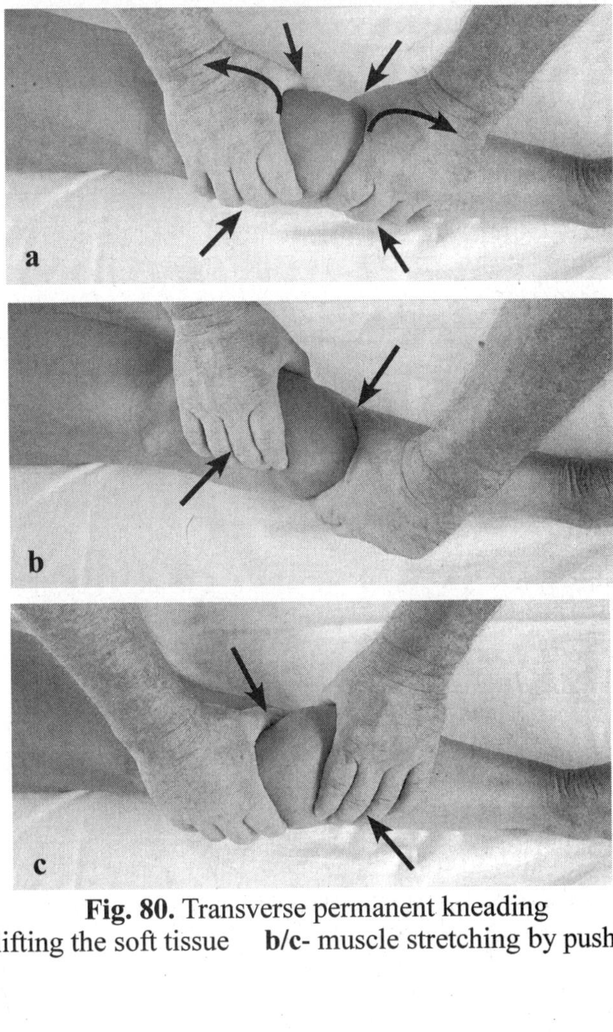

Fig. 80. Transverse permanent kneading
a - compressing and lifting the soft tissue **b/c**- muscle stretching by pushing in opposite directions

This technique can be also combined with simultaneous digital kneading (see Fig. 81). Transverse permanent kneading should be used in places of muscle belly, i.e., in the middle of the massaged muscles.

3. LONGITUDINAL AND TRANSVERSE INTERRUPTIVE KNEADING

The massage therapist may use two of the techniques we just discussed above in an interruptive mode. In such cases, the practitioner completely releases the hands after the end of each stroke and then reapplies them to the same area and repeats the entire cycle of grasping, lifting, and stretching which are a part of longitudinal and transverse kneading.

In the interruptive mode these techniques have a more stimulating impact. Permanent mode should be used during a therapeutic massage session to reduce stress and tension or during a medical massage session as a preparation for Trigger Point Therapy, for example. The same techniques in the interruptive mode should be used as part of the therapeutic massage session when the therapist wishes to make the client more alert at the end of the massage session. (e.g. client goes back to work) or during a rehabilitative sports massage session.

4. SIMPLE KNEADING

Despite its name, simple kneading is a challenging technique which requires several steps in its execution. For simple kneading, one hand is most commonly used but a two-handed variant also exists. To execute the technique correctly, maximally grasp the muscle and soft tissue between the thumb and the rest of the fingers as it is shown in Fig. 80'a'. The hand must be placed perpendicularly to the axis of extremity, or to the anatomical direction of the muscle. Compress the muscle tissue and maximally lift it (see Fig. 80 'a'). The hand must be placed perpendicularly to the axis of extremity, or to the anatomical direction of the massaged muscle. Compress the muscle and maximally lift it (see Fig. 80 'a').

Now the whole hand turns toward the operator with the tip of the thumb as a center of rotation (see Fig. 80 'b'). For the next part of the technique, the hand turns in the opposite direction but continues to hold the soft tissue firmly to prevent their sliding from the hand (see Fig. 80 'c'). Without releasing pressure bring the hand to a neutral position and now push the soft tissue forward using the thumb and thenar (see Fig. 80 'd'). At the end, bring the muscle to the starting position and without releasing the pressure reapply the technique.

This technique should be applied in areas of transition of muscles into the tendon or insertion of muscles into the bone structures as well as on the muscle belly if muscle is small.

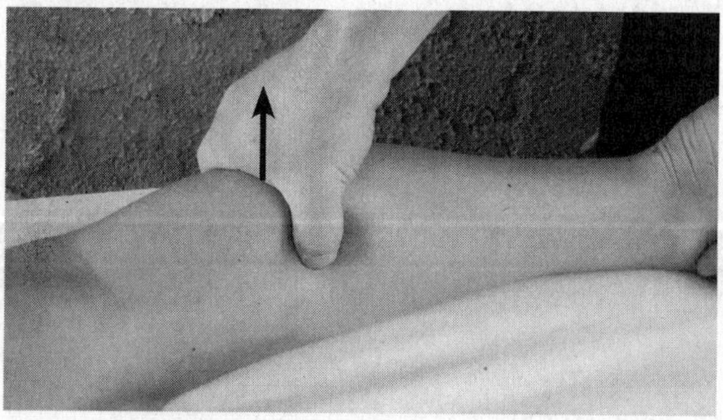

a - compression and lifting of soft tissue

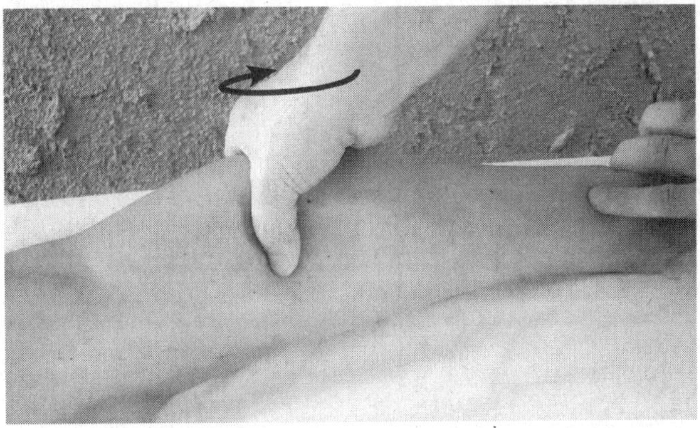

b - lateral rotation around the tip of the thumb

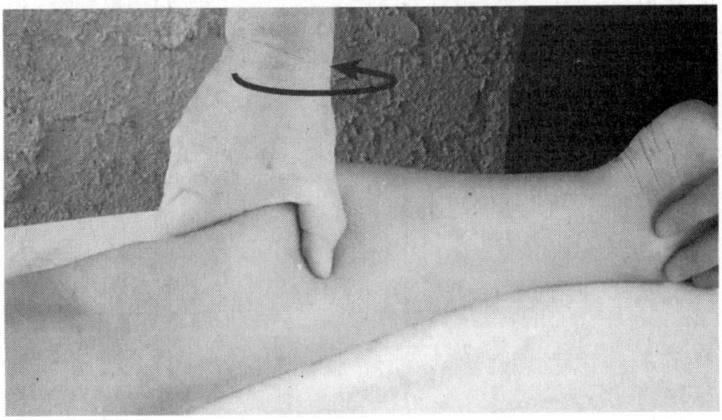

c - medial rotation around the tip of the thumb

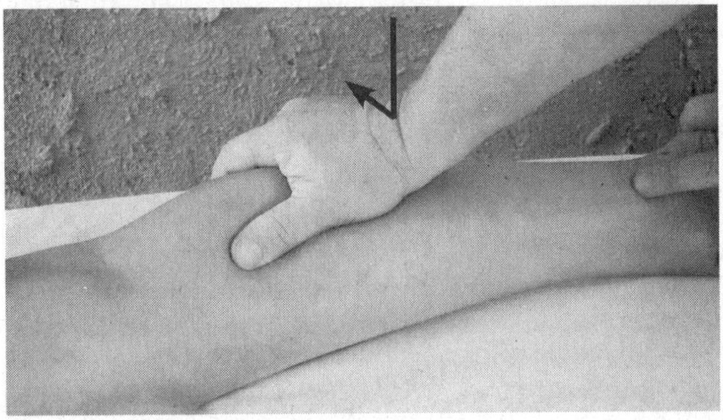

d - compressing and pushing tissues laterally using thumb-thenar area

Fig. 80. Simple kneading technique

5. DIGITAL KNEADING

The digital kneading requires some practice. For this technique, the main contact areas are the palmar surface of the hand, the thumb, and the fingertips of the 2nd-5th fingers.

The base of the hand is a main support area, the thumb provides a counterpressure, and the fingertips of the 2nd through 5th fingers are the main therapeutic tools of this technique. The actual strokes of digital kneading are similar to a piano playing. Fig. 81 illustrates the application of digital kneading on the quadriceps muscle.

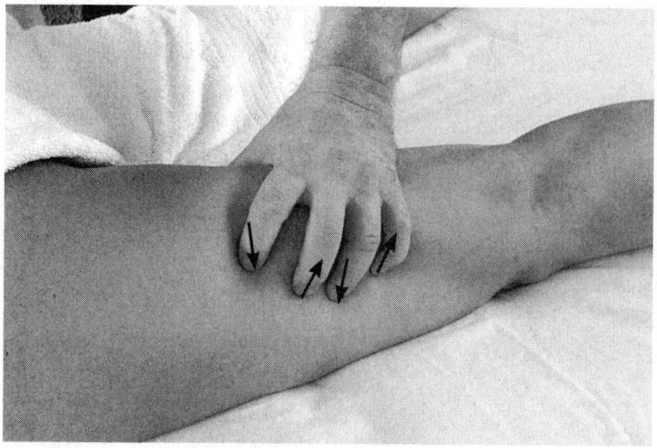

Fig. 81. The digital kneading of quadriceps muscle
Arrows indicate the different level of each finger's submergence in the soft tissue.

Place the base of the hand on the massaged area and the thumb in full opposition to the spread 2nd-5th fingers. Start to knead the soft tissue against the femur by dipping the fingertips of the 2nd-5th fingers into the soft tissue in a vertical direction. Use the base of the hand and the thumb as a counterpressure. The practitioner should press the fingertips into the tissue and alternate them with each other exactly as a piano player would.

Digital kneading is a special technique. It can be combined with other types of kneading to increase their effectiveness. With proper execution digital kneading alone feels very pleasant.

6. SCROLLING KNEADING

The name of this technique comes from the analogy of rolling the scroll. This technique is used on the upper and lower extremities, upper shoulders, edge of pectorals, etc. To perform the singular scrolling technique correctly, the operator must have some practice. Also, scrolling kneading is difficult to perform if the practitioner uses the power of the hands and arms only. All segments of scrolling kneading must be performed using body weight as the major driving force. The hand(s) just grasp and hold the tissue.

The hand is placed perpendicularly with the thumb in the maximal abduction. Push the muscle using the thenar and thumb forward without actual grasping tissue yet (see Fig. 82 'a'). As soon as the maximum of medial push is reached, grasp and compress the muscle between the thumb-thenar and the 2nd-5th fingers (see Fig. 82'b'). For the next part of technique, lift the grasped muscle (see Fig. 82 'c'), then maximally pull the muscle and soft tissue toward yourself using the 2nd-5th fingers (see Fig. 82 'd'). Be sure to slightly recline back with your entire body. Now, without releasing the hand, press the muscle down against the bone using the thumb and fingers (see

Fig. 82 'e'). As soon as you feel that all fingers have tightly compressed the soft tissue against the bone, roll the hand with tissue forward and simultaneously switch the pressure from the fingers to the palm, and later to the base of the palm and thumb (see Fig. 83 'f'). Thus, the pressure is transmitted from the fingers to the whole hand gradually, and the muscle is rolled over and against the bone. Bring the hand back to the starting position and repeat this technique 3-4 times.

All parts of this technique have to flow into each other smoothly without jerking and shaking. Don't release the soft tissue during any part of the scrolling kneading technique. The therapist must hold the soft tissue tightly.

a - pushing soft tissue forward using thumb-thenar area

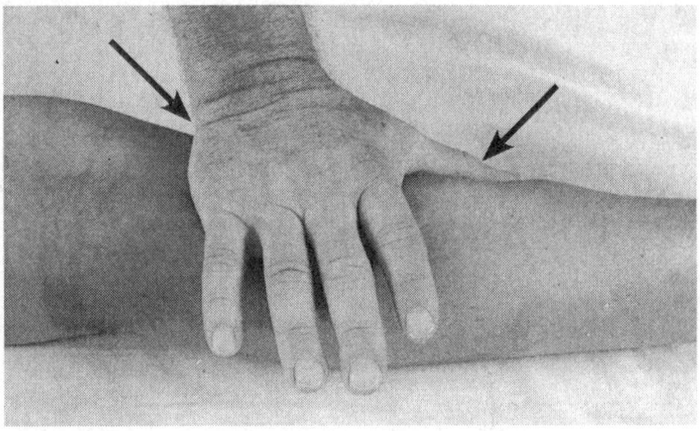

b - grasping the soft tissue

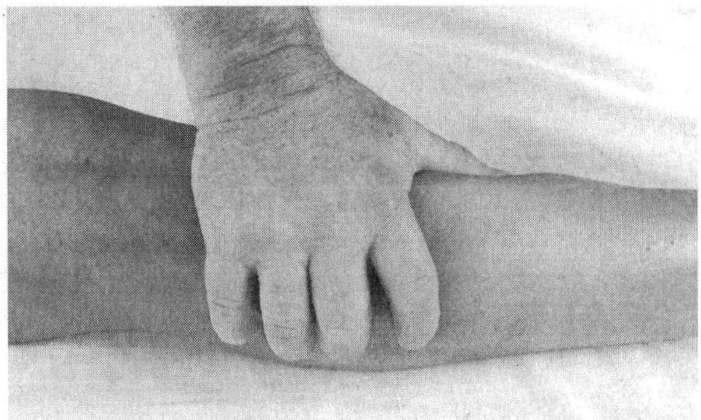

c - lifting the soft tissue

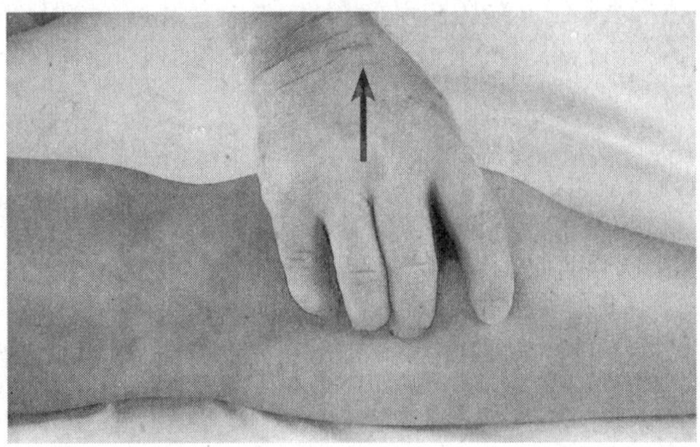

d - pushing the soft tissue toward the operator

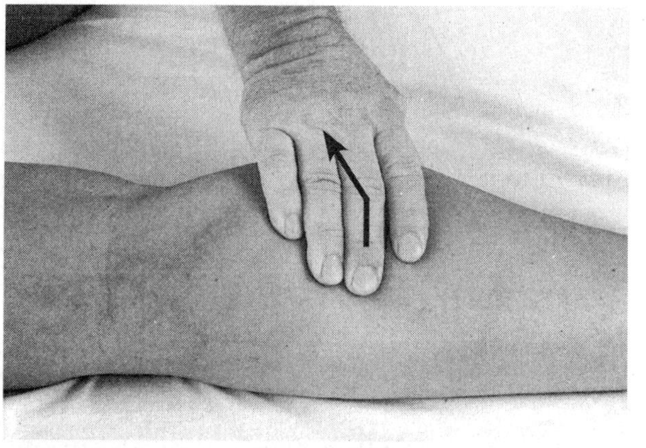

e - vertical pressure on the tissue against bone

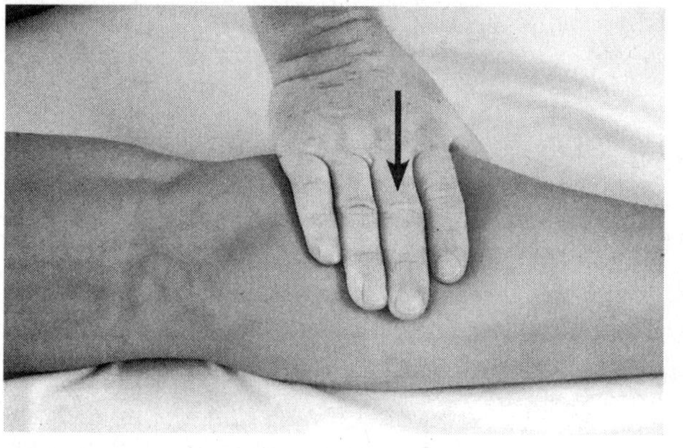

f - rolling the soft tissue forward over the bone in the sequence: fingers-palm-base of the hand

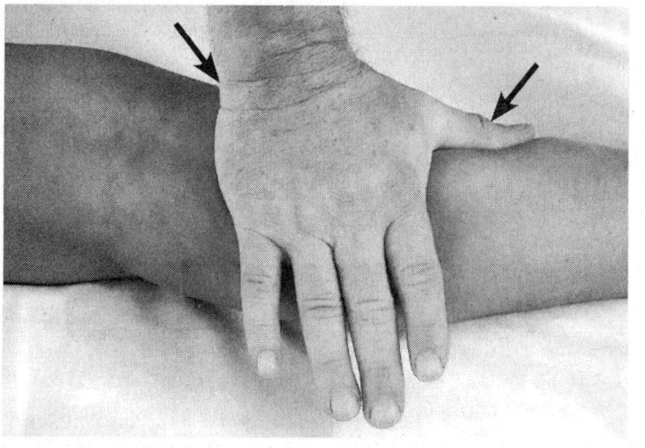

Fig. 82. Singular scrolling kneading

The scrolling kneading is a very important and effective massage technique because it targets superficial and deep muscles at the same time. Only scrolling delivers the actual kneading to deep muscles located on the large bones. First the practitioner stretches the muscles by lifting and pushing them horizontally and later roll them against the bone(s) in the contrary to simple compression, which is employed by the rest of massage techniques.

Another variant of this technique is called **bi-manual scrolling**. In the case of the bi-manual scrolling, the other (supportive) hand is placed over the fingers of the leading one. The supportive hand extends the grip of the soft tissue, 'elongating' fingers of the leading hand.

The supportive hand reinforces all strokes of the leading one and they act as one tool. This type of the kneading is especially important if the patient has large muscles which are difficult to compress and lift with one hand variant. Fig. 83 illustrates the steps of the bi-manual scrolling kneading when both hands act as one tool.

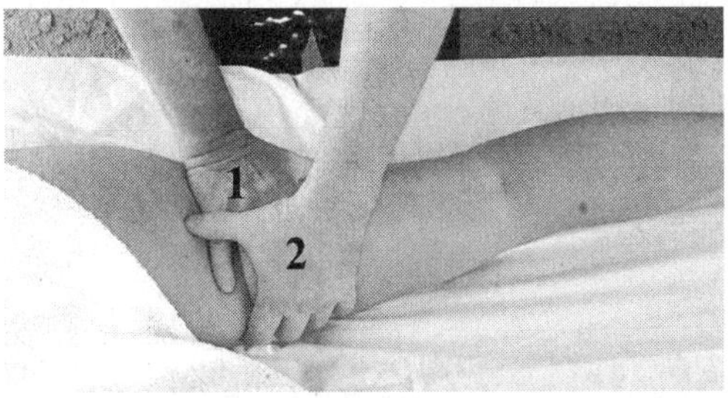

a - bi-manual grasping

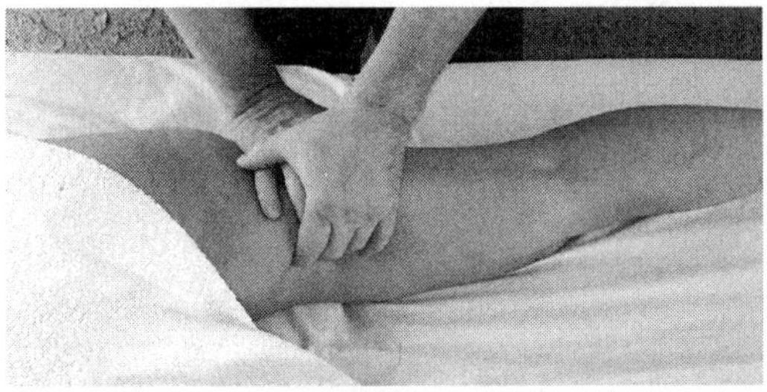

b - bi-manual lifting

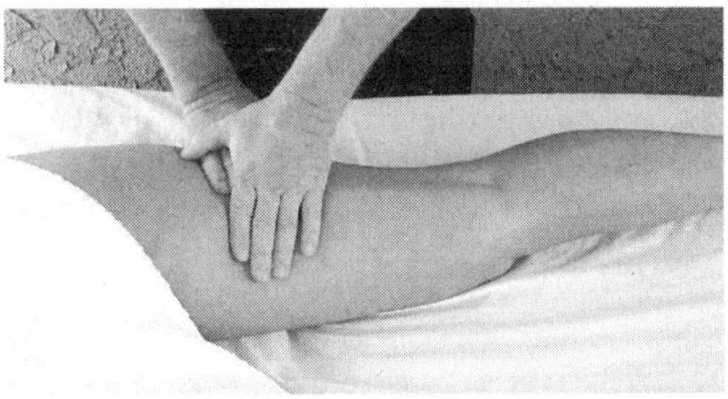

c - bi-manual pressing

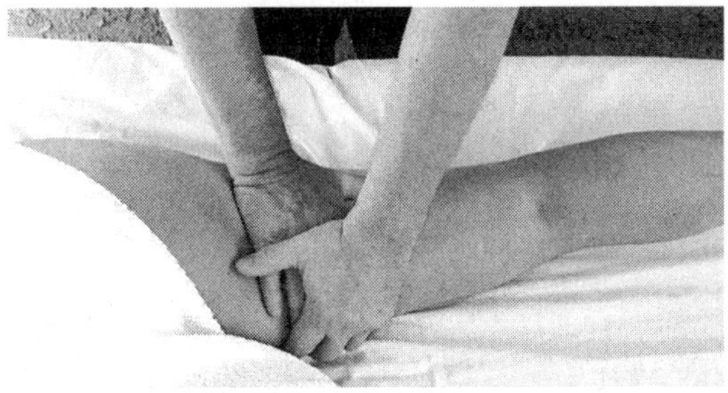

d - bi-manual rolling forward

Fig. 83. Bi-manual scrolling technique

1 - leading hand
2 - supportive hand

7. DOUBLE CIRCULAR KNEADING

Double circular kneading is used only on the extremities. Both hands are placed perpendicularly to the axis of extremity, with the thumbs on one side and the 2nd-5th fingers on the other. The main contact areas are the 1st interphalangeal spaces and both index fingers. The distance between the hands is 1-2 inches.

Grasp the muscle using both hands, compress, then slightly lift soft tissue (see Fig. 84'a'). Now, push the hands in the opposite directions (see Fig. 84 'b'). For the next step, change the direction of stretching. Change directions of stretching 3-4 times, then release the tissue to start the sequence over. The hands can be also placed with the thumbs located on the opposite sides of the extremity, with the same rules of application (see Fig. 84 'c'). With hands in this position the stretching component of the techniques is more efficient. This technique is designed to be used on the muscle belly to activate the muscle spindle receptors and slightly stimulate muscle activity and maintain healthy muscle tone.

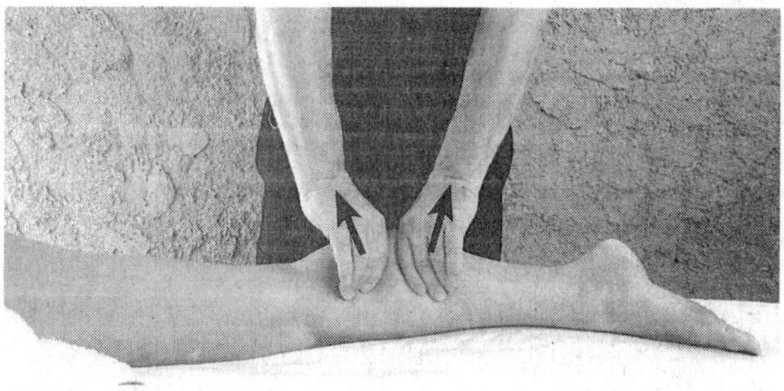

a - lifting the soft tissue

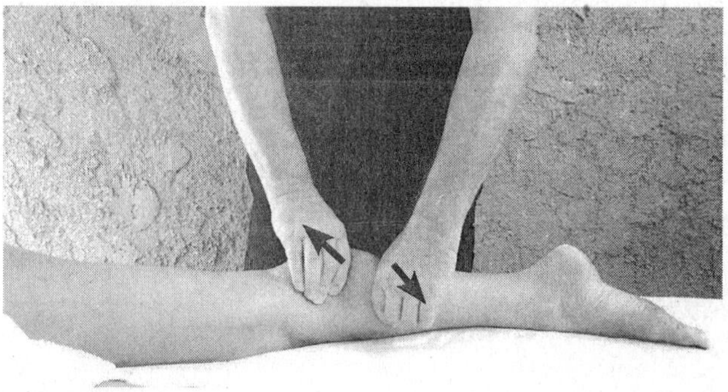

b - stretching in the opposite direction

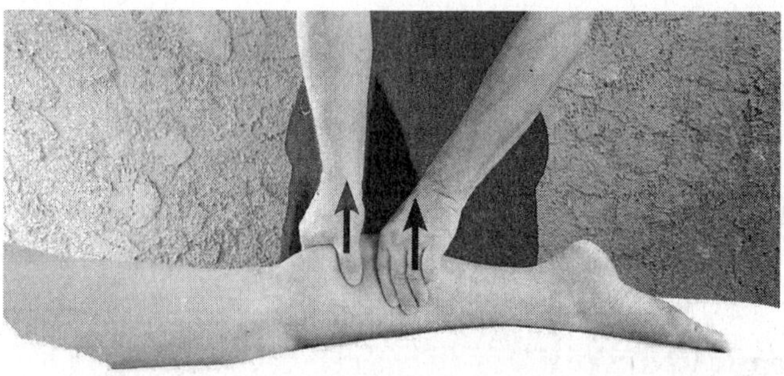

c - variant of circular kneading with thumbs on opposite sides of the extremity (starting position)

Fig. 84 Double circular kneading

8. MOBILE KNEADING

The mobile kneading is also designed for the arms and legs. Generally speaking, kneading is a local technique and mobile kneading is the only type where the therapist's hands are moving along the massaged segment while kneading is being applied. The mobile kneading is a bi-manual technique. Fig. 85 illustrates the application of mobile kneading on the posterior surface of the leg.

The 2nd-5th fingers of the leading hand are placed on the posterio-lateral surface of the leg, and the thumb is placed on the anterior surface. The supportive hand is placed similarly on the medial surface and slightly behind the leading one.

The operator starts to lift tissue up and push it down using the leading hand while slowly moving forward along the massage segment. While doing so his or her thumb simultaneously makes small circular friction strokes and 2nd-5th fingers may execute digital kneading (see Fig. 85 ‘a’). Thus, kneading combines with the deep circular friction and digital kneading. While leading hand does all that the supportive hand holds the arm or leg down to create counterpressure.

For the next part of the technique, the leading hand starts to play a supportive role and the supportive hand becomes the leading one with the same rules of application (see Fig. 85 ‘b’) until leading hand catches to the level where supportive hand is now positioned and they switch their roles again. The mobile kneading technique is used along the massaged segment from its distal to the proximal regions. The proper amount of lubricant should be used.

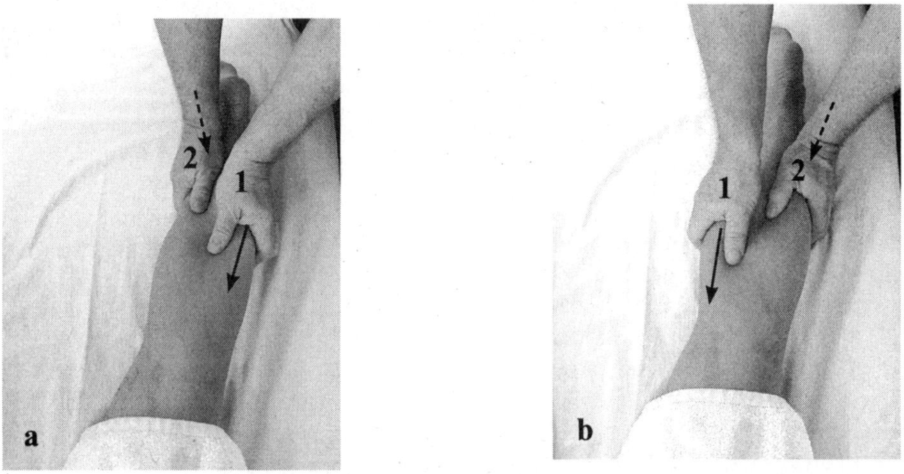

Fig. 85. Mobile kneading on the posterior leg
a - mobile kneading using right hand
b - changing hands during the same stroke
1 - leading hand
2 - supportive hand which provides the vertical counterpressure
Solid arrows - direction of the stroke by leading hand
Dashed arrows - conterpressure provided by supportive hand

9. PINCHING KNEADING

Pinching kneading is a one- or two-handed technique. The contact areas are the middle and distal phalanges of the fingers. This technique is used mostly on the small muscles of the hands or feet. The practitioner can use the thumb and the 2nd, 2nd-3rd or 2nd-5th fingers (it depends on the size of the massaged area.) The fingers are placed approximately 1 inch apart. Usually the thumb is placed on one side of the muscle, and the rest of the fingers on the other. Grasp, compress, lift and knead the soft tissue between the fingers. The effectiveness of this treatment increases if both hands are applied. Other kneading techniques (e.g. scrolling kneading) can be applied in the pinching mode. Fig. 86 illustrates the pinching kneading technique on the foot.

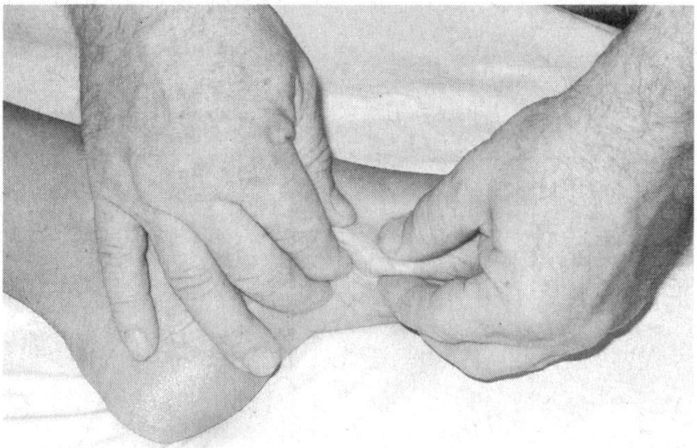

Fig. 86. Pinching kneading on the foot along medial arch

10. WAVE KNEADING

Wave kneading is a two-handed technique. This is one of the few massage techniques which can be effectively used to work on the abdominal muscles.

The supportive hand is tightly placed on the ulnar edge with slightly bent fingers at an angle of 45-50 degrees to the skin. The leading hand grasps the muscles (see Fig. 87 'a'), moves, and then compresses them against the passive hand (see Fig. 87 'b'). In another variant of this technique, the therapist compresses the soft tissue against the passive hand which makes the fist. The operator has to repetitively compress and release the tissue with a rhythm of waves coming to the shore.
The passive hand must be placed along the muscle fibers.

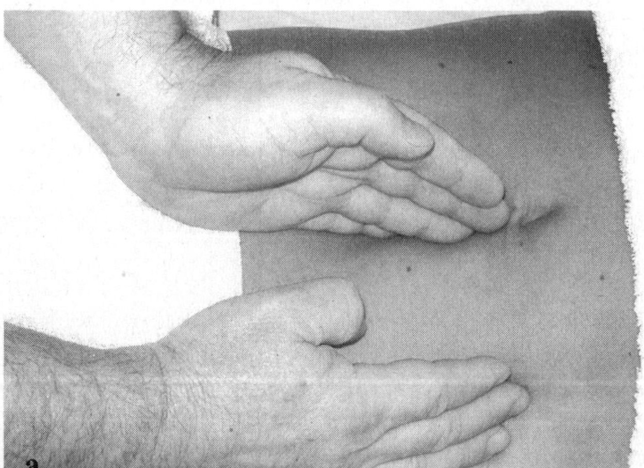

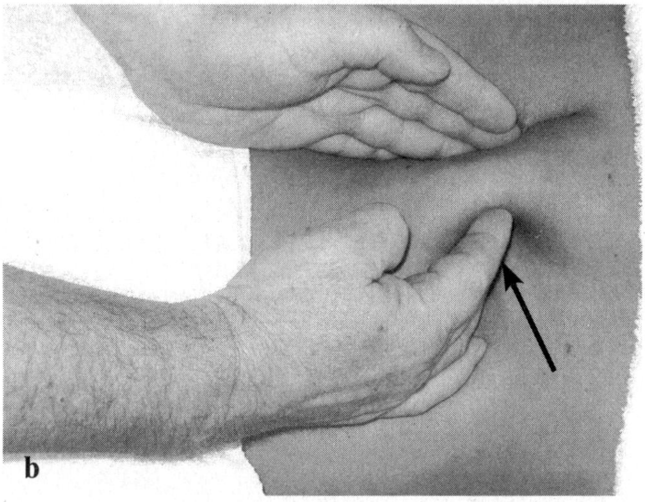

Fig. 87. Wave kneading of the right rectus abdominis muscle
a - grasping of the soft tissues
b - compressing tissues against supportive hand

As mentioned previously, the wave technique is a unique method of kneading the abdominal muscles. Also the repetitive application of this technique normalizes the motor and secretory functions of the inner organs in the abdominal cavity. The practitioner is able to stimulate the gastric and intestinal motility if he or she performs the wave kneading along the anatomical pathway of gastro-intestinal tract.

11. ROLLING KNEADING

The contact areas for rolling kneading are the palmar surfaces of both hands. This technique is used on the upper or lower extremities only. Extend and tighten both hands in the wrist joints, press the 2nd-5th fingers together, then slightly abduct the thumbs. The hands suppose to be parallel to each other, on the opposite sides of the extremity. The therapist compresses the soft tissue against the bone first, then rolls the muscles back and forth between the hands and the bone in opposite directions.

If the amplitude the of rolling is small, the rolling kneading is a gentle technique while increased amplitude and pressure have stimulating impact of the muscles. Gentle rolling is used for rehabilitation purposes after muscle overload (e.g. part of the sports massage), surgery or prolonged immobilization in the cast. Fig. 88 shows the example of rolling kneading of the arm muscles.

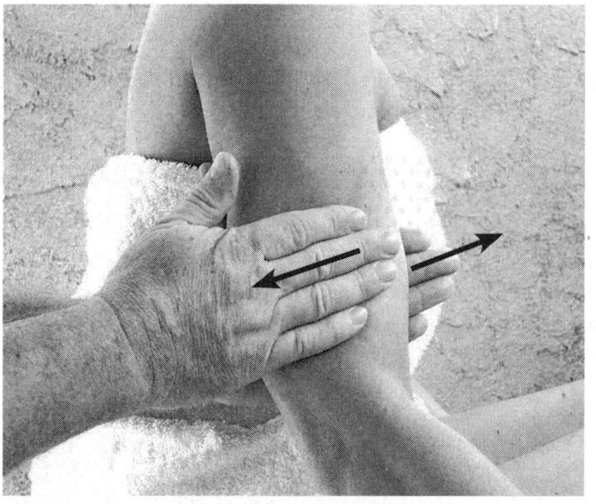

Fig. 88. The rolling kneading of the arm muscles

Rolling kneading can be also performed in the horizontal direction when both hands are placed next to each other. Figure 89 shows this variant of rolling kneading on leg muscles.

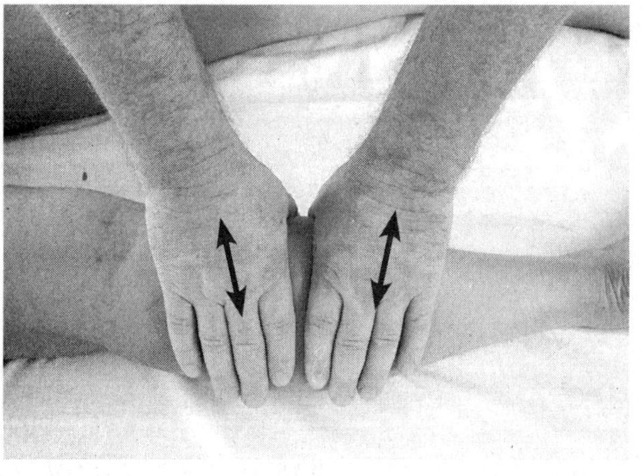

Fig. 89. Rolling kneading on the posterior leg

12. STRETCHING KNEADING

The contact areas for stretching kneading are the fingertips and palmar surface of both hands. The therapist grasps the muscles perpendicularly to direction of fibers using both hands. Be sure to have a fold of skin between the hands. Try to use direction of lines of cleavage as much as possible (see Fig. 60). For the next part, compress the soft tissue and lift them (see Fig. 90 'a'). As soon as therapist reaches maximum lift he or she should slowly stretch the muscles by rolling both hands in opposite direction (see Fig. 90 'b'). The practitioner must use ulnar edges of both hands as major stabilization points. Release the muscles and repeat the sequence 2-3 times before moving to the neighboring area.

For the best performance of this technique, do not use any lubricant. Stretching kneading is even more effective when combined with digital kneading (see Fig. 81).

If technique is applied on the distal or proximal end of the muscle, the therapist alternates the stimulation of the muscle spindle and the Golgi tendon organ receptors during the same stroke.

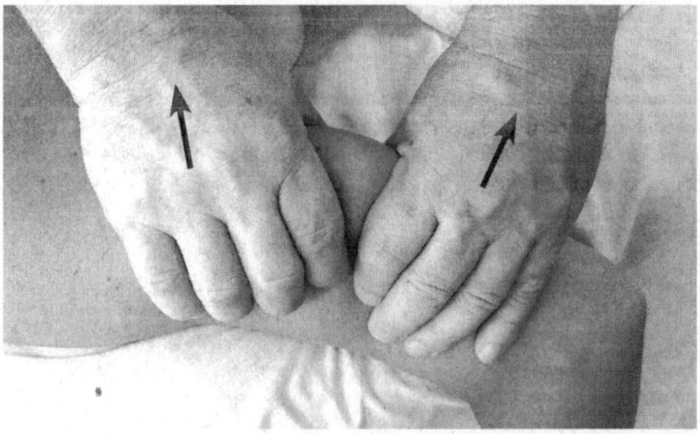

a - lifting of soft tissue (notice the fold of skin between the operator's hands)

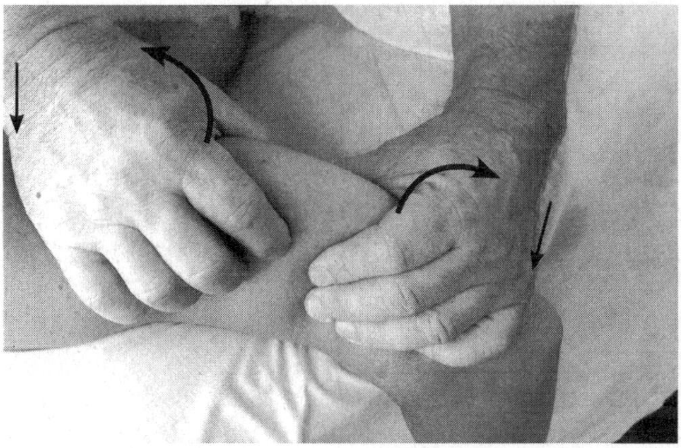

b - stretching kneading (small, vertical arrows show the direction of counterpressure on the ulnar edge of the hands)

Fig. 90. Stretching kneading on left triceps brachii muscle

13. TISSUE DISPLACEMENT KNEADING

The main contact area for this technique is the thenar-hypothenar area. The best place to perform this technique is the erector spinae muscles. Place the leading hand perpendicular to the anatomical direction of the muscles, and put the supportive hand over the leading one (see Fig. 91).

The supportive hand increases the pressure and, additionally, controls the leading hand. The contact area of the hand has to be placed on the medial edge of the erector spinae muscles. Be sure to have a fold of skin behind the hand because it will additionally help to stretch muscles. Press the contact area of the hand into the soft tissue in front of medial edge of lumbar erectors and push the muscle forward. To do this, the operator must apply significant pressure in the horizontal direction and it is the beset to engage body weight into each stroke. Vertical pressure is used only to tightly press the leading hand against the massaged area.

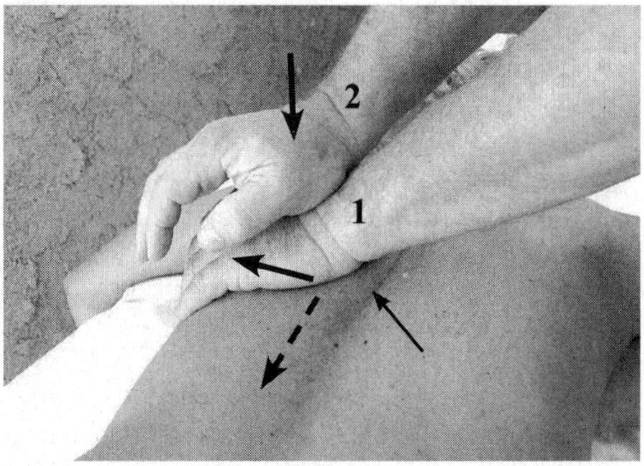

Fig. 91. Tissue displacement of erector spinae muscles; starting position of the hands
Vertical solid arrow - vertical pressure at contact area
Horizontal solid arrow - pressure to stretch the erector spinae muscles
Dashed arrow - direction of the stroke
Thin solid arrow - indicates fold of skin behind the leading hand to effectively stretch muscles during the stroke
1 - leading hand
2 - supportive hand

In another variant of this technique, the main contact areas are the thumb and thenar. The practitioner has to push the muscles in the direction of the 2nd-5th fingers (see Fig 92), lift it up and push it down again while compressing and knead the soft tissue between the thumb-thenar area and the 2nd-5th fingers. The digital kneading can be added (see Fig. 81).

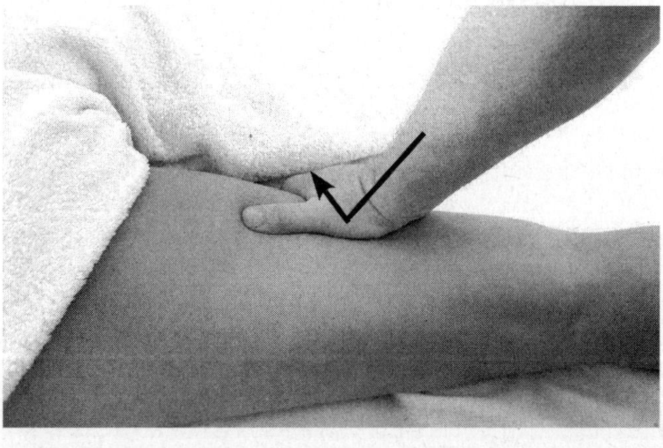

Fig. 92. Tissue displacement kneading using the thumb-thenar on the hamstring muscles

Both of these types of tissue displacement kneading are effective on the long muscles. The practitioner stretches the massaged muscle between its points of origin and insertion.

VIBRATION

A. GENERAL CHARACTERISTICS

Vibration was considered a therapeutic agent centuries ago. In 2nd century A.D. the Roman physician Galen was the first to incorporate a vibration technique in massage therapy. At the beginning of our century, vibration, especially electric vibration, was one of the most frequently used methods of physiotherapy. Professor A. Sherbak, MD (1903), of Russia and Dr. M. Snow, MD (1917) of the US spent a lot of effort studying the effects of vibration on the human body. Later, vibration massage was forced out by newer, more powerful methods of medical massage and physiotherapy. After World War II, interest in the therapeutic benefits of vibration was renewed in many countries, especially in cases of pathology of the central and peripheral nervous systems.

Vibration is a powerful stimulus for all living objects. It surrounds us in everyday life and is produced by different sources. The human body itself is a complex vibro-mechanical system. Each inner organ and system is affected by vibration during every body movement. The heartbeat and the pulsation of large vessels are sources of permanent inner vibration. Any outside source of vibration provides additional energy, which evokes a variety of physiological responses. Humans can detect vibration in the range of l2-8.000 Hertz (Hz).

Pacinian corpuscles are the primary receptors that analyze and encode vibration (Intyre, 1966; Vega et al., 2009). They are located in the dermis layer of the skin and in the subcutaneous tissue, in the ligaments and other connective tissue structures and they do not spread equally through the body. This is why we feel vibration in different parts of the body, and to various degrees. The structure of a Pacinian corpuscle is shown in Fig. 93.

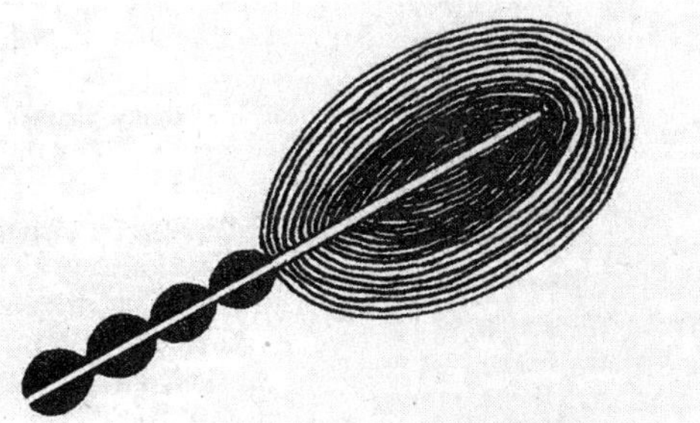

Fig. 93. Pacinian corpuscle

Pacinian corpuscles react to a vibration between 50 and 500 Hz. These receptors are activated as a result of their mechanical deformation. They are very rapidly adapting receptors. To constantly stimulate Pacinian corpuscles, vibratory stimuli have to be removed and reapplied each time. It is very important to apply the vibratory techniques correctly.

In addition to Pacinian corpuscles, deep receptors in the ligaments, tendons and periosteum are also activated as a result of exposure to a vibration stimuli. However these receptors are activated later, after the vibration has been applied to the same area reaches the posterior horns of the spinal cord. Vibration, together with pain and temperature sensation, are transferred to the brain trough dorsal columns of the spinal cord. Scientists consider the center of vibratory sensibility to be located in the temporal lobes of the brain (Kreimer, 1989).

Total body water comprises about 60% of the body weight in young males. It is distributed as follows: muscles - 50%, skin and connective tissue - 20%, inner organs - 20%, and blood ~ 10%. Therefore, vibratory oscillations transmitted from tissue to tissue similarly to waves spreading through the water surface. Thus, even application of local vibration eventually affects distant parts of the body. Vibration has many therapeutic effects on the human body. By referring to the results of Professor Kreimer's (1989) experimental and clinical study, I will enumerate the main therapeutic outcomes of vibration:

1. ANALGESIC EFFECT

Low-frequency vibration raises the threshold of the activation of peripheral receptors and decreases the amount of noxious stimuli which flow to the spinal cord and brain. The central nervous system reacts by closing the "gates," and suppresses the central sensory-analyzing centers and pathways. As a result, the cortex is inhibited as well and pain is suppressed.

2. VASOMOTOR EFFECT

Low-frequency vibration first causes initial vasospasm, but after 1-2 minutes of exposure to the same vibratory stimuli the vasodilation is triggered and the peripheral arterial resistance drops causing the decrease in blood pressure. In the contrary the high-frequency vibration produces vasospasm and an increase in blood pressure.

3. EFFECT ON THE NEURO-MUSCULAR STRUCTURES

Strong, interruptive vibration with a frequency of more than 120 Hz stimulates the nervous system and increases the resting muscle tone. Strong, sustained vibration with a frequency of around 60-100 Hz has the opposite effect on neuro-muscular structures. This dual effect of vibratory stimuli has to be remembered when vibration techniques are applied on the muscles with any kind of the hypertonic pathology.

4. EFFECT ON THE ENDOCRINE SYSTEM

Vibration stimulates the functions of the adrenal and pituitary glands. At the same time, the thyroid gland shows signs of hypofunction.

In cases of medical massage, the main indications for vibration are pain suppression and treatment of abnormalities of the central and peripheral nervous systems. Vibration plays an important role in the rehabilitation of patients after a stroke. Gentle vibration on the affected extremities is an important part of the rehabilitation program for these patients. It supports the process of the formation of new motor pathways in the brain, around the damaged area. Thus, affected motor functions are improved.

Vibration can be conducted both manually and with the aid of electrical vibration devices. Professor Kreimer recommends electrical vibration. At the same time, many authors recommend manual vibration, especially for the treatment of patients with cerebral palsy (Bortfeild, 1979).

Vibration using electrical devices does not warrant any special discussion because it is a common and easy procedure. Besides this, information about any particular vibrator can be found in its user manual. Remember that the massager has to be moved very slowly over the massaged area.

Manual vibration is the most physically challenging massage technique. The overall success of the treatment and the conservation of the operator's energy depend on the proper technical application of vibration.

A simple test can help to determine whether if manual vibration is being conducted properly. Put a glass full of water in the middle of a small table and create the vibration using entire hand placed flat. With the proper application of the vibration, the waves will spread over the water surface but the water will not spill out of the glass.

B. TECHNICAL DISTINCTIONS

1. CONTACT AREAS

The fingertips are the main contact areas for direct vibration. Another contact area for the supportive technique of vibration is the palmar surface of hand.

2. DIRECTION OF STROKES

Direct vibration can be either mobile or fixed. In the case of mobile vibration, the operating hand moves through the massage segment. The direction of mobile vibration can be longitudinal, perpendicular, spiral or Z-shaped to the axis of the massaged segment.

3. SPEED AND PRESSURE

The effectiveness of vibration depends directly on the speed of the oscillations. Thus, the speed of direct vibration fluctuates between 100 and 350 oscillations per minute. In the case of supportive vibration, the speed is lower and approximately equals 80-100 oscillations per minute.

Kunichev, (1985) recommends to start the vibration massage at an oscillation range of about 100 per minute. Then, slowly increase the frequency to 200 oscillations per minute and finally, at the end of treatment, decrease it again to 100. However other authors recommended a higher speed (Birach, 1985; Kreimer, 1989). Our personal clinical experience also shows that the therapeutic effect of manual vibration with higher frequency of oscillation (around 300-350 oscillations per minute) has more expressive therapeutic potential.

Applied pressure is another important parameter. The amount of pressure during vibration depends on the final goal of the therapy. If the practitioner works with the skin or fascia, the pressure is superficial. It significantly increases if vibration is delivered to the deeper structures (e.g., muscles, periosteum). Permanent vibration has an inhibitory effect and interruptive vibration has a stimulating effect. Vibration must be always alternate with effleurage in the direction of drainage.

Vibration is the most physically challenging technique for the practitioner. It has to be done in the proper manner in order to reduce both muscle strain and fatigue. Let's discuss the application of vibration from this point of view. First of all, the client's muscles in the massaged area have to be completely relaxed as much as possible. As soon as the right protocol of vibration is selected, have a hand or a part of the hand act as a transmitter of vibration waves which should come from the shoulder, down to the forearm and, finally, to the hand. Try to relax the muscles as much as possible during vibration strokes. Have a clock nearby to control the frequency of oscillations.

C. TYPES OF VIBRATION

Manual vibration can be direct or supportive. In the case of direct vibration, the therapeutic impact is delivered to one (usually small) area of the body (Birach, 1985). In cases of supportive vibration, the treatment applies to a whole anatomical structure (e.g. larynx) or entire segment or part of the body (e.g. abdomen, thorax). Fig. 94 graphically represents the classification of direct and supportive techniques of the manual vibration.

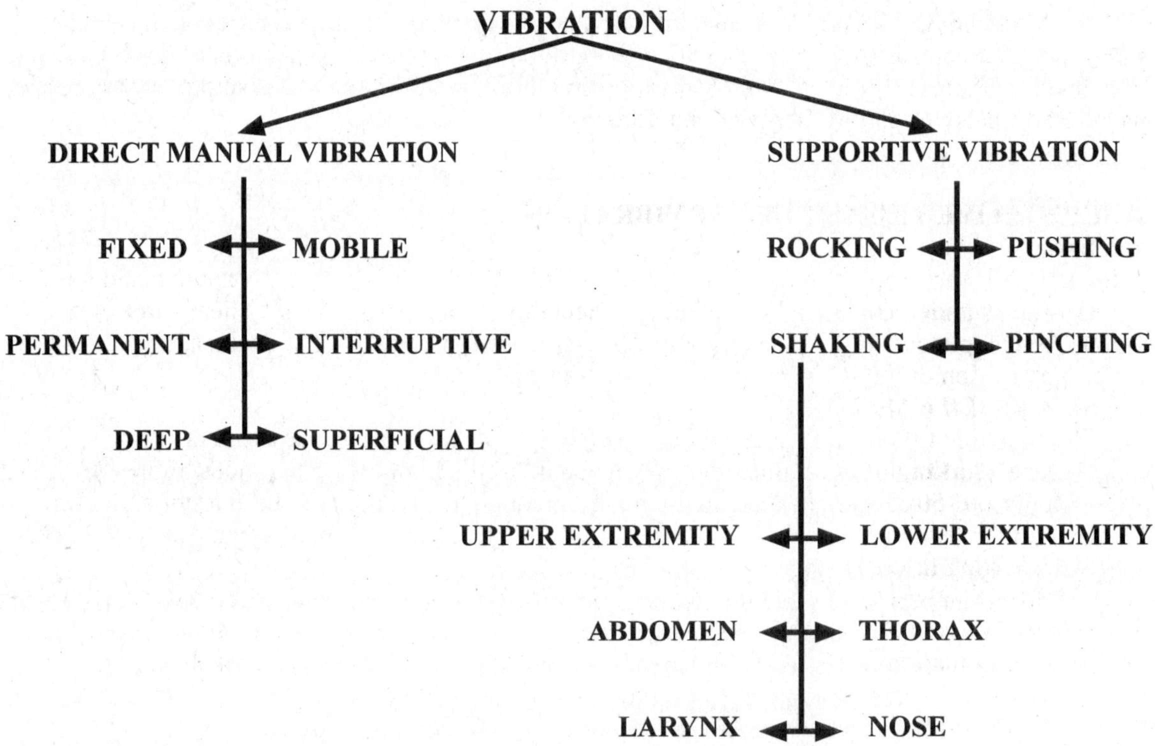

Fig. 94. Classification of vibration techniques

1. DIRECT MANUAL VIBRATION

a. Fixed Vibration

During fixed vibration, the therapist places the hand or fingers on the massaged area and creates vibratory oscillations. The hand itself does not move throughout the massaged segment.

b. Mobile Vibration

During mobile vibration, the therapist places the hand or fingers on the massaged area, starts the vibration while moving the hand through the massaged segment. Lubricant must be used.

c. Permanent Vibration

During permanent vibration, the therapist creates vibration in the part of the body for a determined period of time, usually 2-3 minutes. This technique is considered an inhibitory treatment.

d. Interruptive Vibration

During interruptive vibration, the therapist creates vibration and applies and withdraws pressure during the application. Every time the hand touches the skin's surface, Pacinian corpuscles are activated and action potentials are generated. Thus, interruptive vibration is a stimulating therapy.

e. Deep Vibration

This type of direct vibration affects the deep layer of soft tissues. The closer the practitioner's hand is to a 90 degree angle to the body surface, the deeper the vibration is achieved. This technique is a good tool for stimulating deep receptors in the periosteum, ligaments and tendons.

f. Superficial Vibration

Superficial vibration is created using the fingertips as well as whole hand. Superficial vibration activates receptors which are mostly located in the skin, ligaments and fascia.

All techniques of direct manual vibration can be combined in any order, even during the same session, to create an optimal regime of therapy. However, use a combination of both fixed and permanent vibration only in the case of massage in inhibitory regime as, for example, with cerebral palsy, Bell's palsy or part of Trigger Point Therapy.

2. SUPPORTIVE TECHNIQUES OF VIBRATION

a. Shaking

Shaking is a very important technique which is, unfortunately, not frequently applied and its real value is underestimated. For the proper execution of this technique, the client's muscles must be completely relaxed. This is why shaking is used as a final part of a massage treatment. The application of this technique varies with different parts of the body.

Shaking of the Abdomen

The shaking of the abdomen mostly affects the inner organs. It can be general or local.

General shaking of the abdomen is conducted with two hands placed on sides of the abdomen, with the 2nd-5th fingers located on the back and the thumbs placed on the anterior abdominal wall on the level of the navel. Gently compress both hands against each other. Apply and alternate shaking in vertical and horizontal directions (see Fig 95). If the client is not heavy, the operator can also slightly lift the middle section during shaking. The speed of shaking is about 100 oscillations per minute. The general shaking of the abdomen stimulates arterial and venous circulation, increases lymph drainage, and stimulates gastric and intestinal motility.

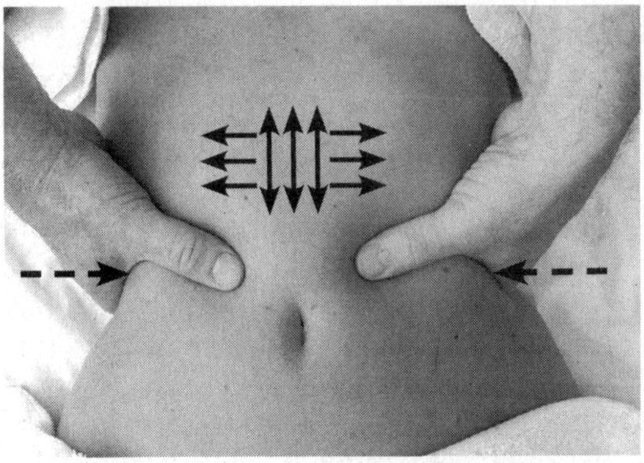

Fig. 95. General shaking of the abdomen

Dashed arrows - side compression
Solid arrows - direction of shaking

Local shaking of the abdomen is applied to the area of the targeted inner organ. It can be performed with one or two hands placed next to each other with slightly bent fingers. Be sure to have a fold of skin between the hands. Decision whether to use one or two hands has to be based on the size of the abdomen. Put a hand on the chosen area (e.g. stomach), slightly press hand into abdomen, then apply shaking permanently changing its direction. If a two-handed variant is chosen, draw the hands close and away from each other during the application. This technique is effective if the client has intestinal atonia, constipation, chronic gastritis with low acidity, or atonia of stomach and gall bladder. Local shaking also increases blood circulation, lymph drainage and gastric, pancreatic and biliary secretion (Belaya, 1974). Fig. 96 illustrates local shaking of the stomach with one hand.

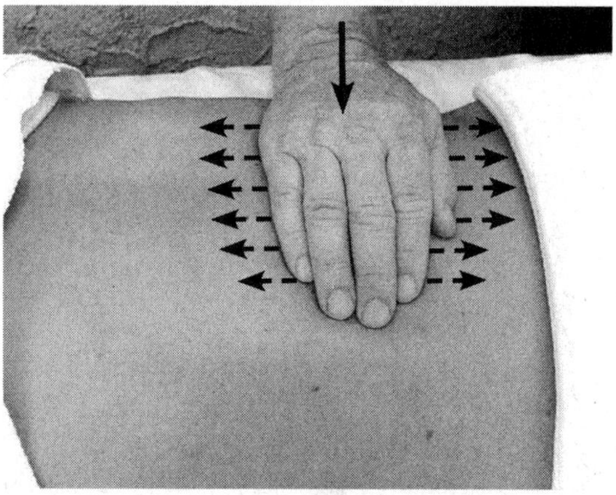

Fig. 96. Local shaking of the stomach using right hand
Solid arrow - vertical pressure
Dashed arrows - shaking of the abdomen

Shaking of the Thorax

Shaking of the thorax is conducted in exactly the same manner as general shaking of the abdomen (see Fig. 96), with the only two differences. First of all, the thorax must be compressed harder during shaking. The practitioner must apply thorax compression and shaking only during the client's exhalation. Therefore, ask the client to adopt a long, slow pattern of breathing. This will prevent the hyperventilation.

Another difference between shaking the thorax and the abdomen is that during general shaking of the abdomen the operator's hands stay still. In the case of shaking of thorax, the operator starts the application of the shaking from the lower parts of the thoracic cage and moves to the upper segments, each time releasing and reapplying hands to the next area.

Shaking of the thorax is effective in cases of pulmonary disorders which produce sputum: chronic pneumonia, bronchitis and bronchiectasis. The therapeutic impact of shaking increases if the client is positioned on the stomach, with the lower part of the body elevated. This accelerates the drainage of sputum and helps to clean the bronchial tree.

Shaking of the Larynx

Shaking of larynx is a very gentle and helpful procedure which is performed using the thumb and the 2nd-3rd fingers of one hand. The client has to be on the back, with the head slightly bent backward. Put the ulnar edge of the hand on the upper part of the sternum for stability and very gently hold the larynx with the thumb on one side and the 2nd-3rd fingers on the other. First carefully move the larynx from left to right to test its mobility. After this very gently start to shake the larynx with a small amplitude. This treatment has to be done separately with the client's mouth both opened and closed. Apply shaking no more than 1-2 minutes. This technique can be unpleasant if client wasn't prepared. Thus, the practitioner must explain every detail before the treatment is started.

The shaking of the larynx has to be applied if a client has laryngitis, laryngeal tension, tracheitis or vocal cord paralysis. It reduces the spasm of the smooth muscles inside the airways, stimulates the passage of sputum, reduces the dosage of broncholitic drugs needed, and balances the respiratory cycle. Fig. 97 illustrates the shaking the larynx.

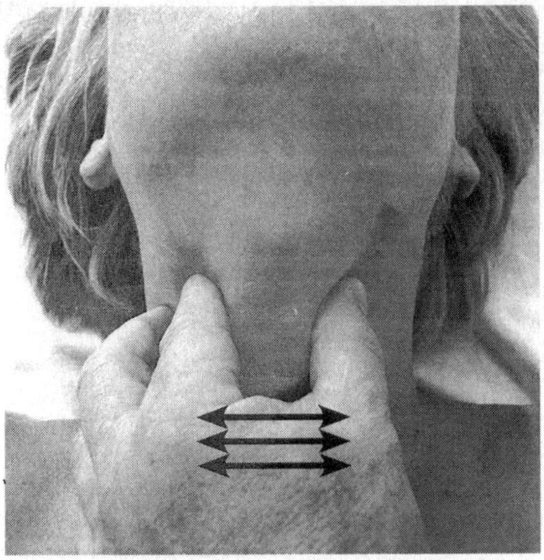

Fig. 97. Shaking the larynx with mouth closed

Shaking of the Nose

Shaking of the nose may look and feel weird, but in many cases it is very helpful. The practitioner should use the thumb and index finger of one hand. Gently hold the cartilaginous part of the client's nose and shake it from side to side. Do not compress nose hard, and release fingers frequently.

Start from the tip of the nose, then move the fingers up to the connection of the cartilaginous part of the nose with its bony part. This procedure usually should take about 2-3 minutes. The shaking of the nose has to be the final part of the treatment of clients who suffer from sinusitis. It reduces pressure in the sinuses and increases their drainage. Fig. 98 illustrates the shaking the nose technique.

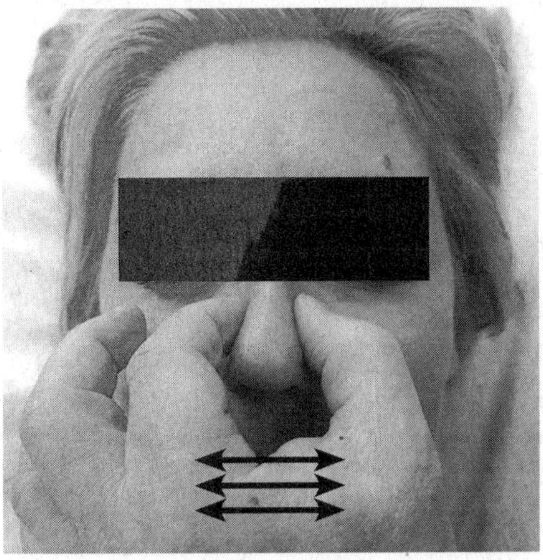

Fig. 98. Shaking the nose

Shaking of the Extremities

The shaking is a final part of massage of upper or lower extremities. The operator can apply shaking to the whole extremity or to its segment. This depends on what part of the extremity the practitioner holds during the shaking. For shaking the whole limb, the operator must grasp the most distal part (i.e., fingers or toes) of the extremity.

Shake the entire limb rhythmically at a medium speed, about 90-100 oscillations per minute. In this case, shaking has a relaxing effect. The quick shaking with a different rhythm has a stimulating impact on the muscles. Therefore, this type of shacking is an important part of sports massage which should be performed just prior to the competition. Slow, rhythmical shaking has a deep relaxing effect on muscles, and is used during the breaks of competition or after the event.

b. Rocking

Rocking is a variant of slow shaking. It is usually applied to the whole body, or to the extremity. Put both hands on the part of the body which undergoes treatment and push it from side to side. Don't change the hands' position during the rocking. Release and relocate hands if you need to apply rocking on another area.

Rocking has to be slow and rhythmical. It can be compared to the rocking of a baby. This technique has a sedating effect on the patient's central nervous system, and can be used at the beginning of the every session especially during the first treatment to calm the client down and create bond of trust between the client and practitioner. Fig. 99 illustrates rocking of the body.

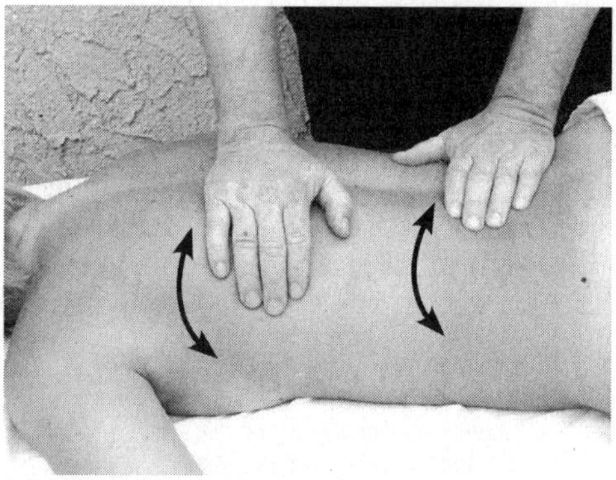

Fig. 99. Rocking the body

c. Pushing

Pushing is a technique which is applied on the abdomen and it targets the inner organs of the abdominal cavity. Despite the fact that this technique looks similar to wave kneading, they are significantly different. During wave kneading, the therapist works with the abdominal muscles, but pushing targets a particular inner organ. Therefore, in the case of pushing the target is not soft tissue but abdominal organ and it is performed at a quicker rate.

Like wave kneading, pushing is also two-handed technique. The operator gently presses the supportive hand into the abdomen in the area of targeted inner organ. The main contact areas are the hypothenar and ulnar edge of the hand. The leading hand is placed next to the supportive one. The operator presses the leading hand down and rhythmically pushes it in the direction of the passive hand.

Compare Fig. 87 and Fig. 100 and notice that there is no actual tissue compression between the leading and supportive hands in the case of the pushing technique. The pushing stimulates gastric and intestinal motility, and also increases biliary, gastric or pancreatic secretion.

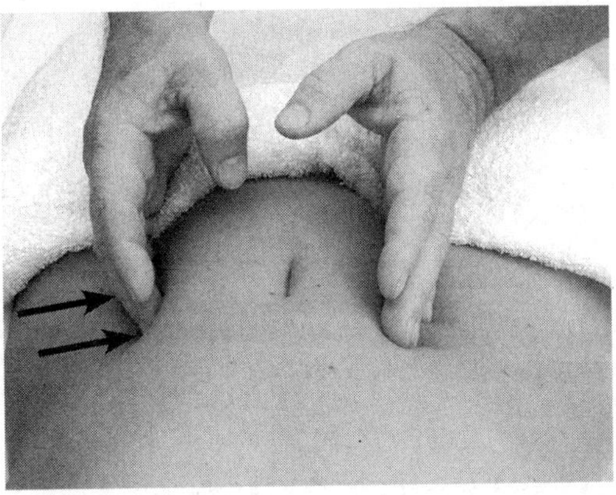

Fig. 100. Pushing in the area of the stomach

Gentle repetitive pushing is used in Lymph-Drainage Massage to stimulate drainage and in these cases it is called **pumping**.

d. Pinching

The pinching technique is designed to affect the major nerves in the areas of their closest anatomical location to the skin. This technique is performed with the thumb and index fingers, or the thumb and the 2nd-3rd fingers. The practitioner quickly grasps the skin between the fingers, compresses, lifts, then releases it.

Pinching strokes have to be quickly reapplied with a speed of approximately 130-150 per minute. During the first 10-15 pinches, the operator has to pull the skin distally (see Fig. 101 'a'). After this, gently press the soft tissue using the index finger for 10-15 seconds (see Fig. 101 'b') or use light, permanent vibration. The next step is another series of 10-15 pinches, but this time the skin should be pulled in the proximal direction (see Fig. 101 'c'). Again, compress the soft tissue for 10-15 seconds. Repeat whole protocol 3-4 times. Fig. 101 illustrates the pinching in the area of common peroneal nerve on the lateral surface of the upper leg

This technique is mostly applied in cases of medical massage when client have peripheral neurological disorders: neuritis, neuralgia, causalgia, etc. The pinching technique must be used only after the acute symptoms are gone and the cleint is ready for a rehabilitation program.

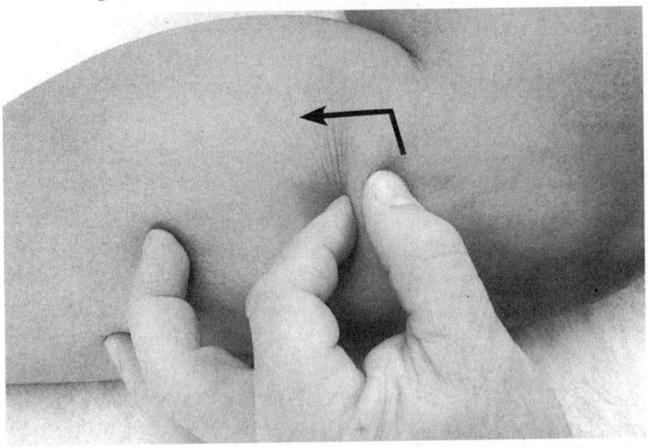

a - pulling and pinching fold of skin distally

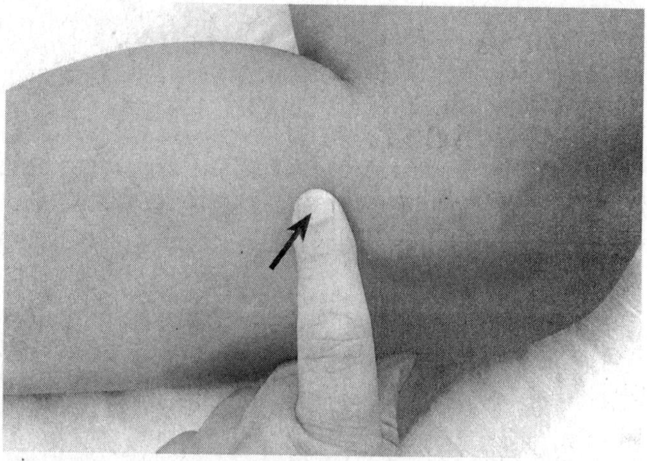

b - vertical compression

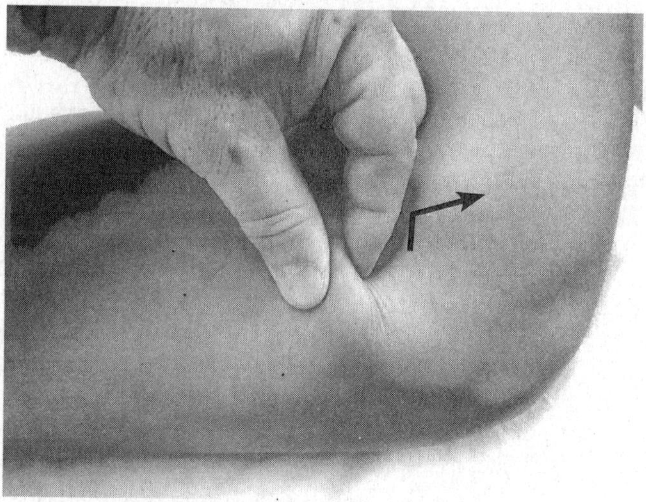

c - pulling and pinching fold of skin proximally

Fig. 101. Pinching in the area of the common peroneal nerve

PERCUSSION

A. GENERAL CHARACTERISTICS

Percussion can be considered a variant of vibration. However, to be academically accurate, percussion should be discussed as a separate technique. The physiological effect of percussion is a result of a combination of vibration and rhythmic compression. Its therapeutic impact mostly depends on the speed of applied strokes.

During percussion, the practitioner rapidly strikes the massaged area using different parts of the hand. To successfully perform percussion, the operator must immediately withdraw the hand after it makes contact with the massaged area. It seems, that the hand bounces back like a rubber ball from a wall. This is called **elastic percussion**. It demands some practice, but elastic percussion prevents the client's tissue from excessive damage during application of this intense technique.

The sweep of the stroke and the force of percussion are other important elements. Percussion delivers shock waves through the massaged area and the entire body. This impact elicits different physiological responses from the systems and organs of the client's body.

Rhythmic percussion causes a reflex contraction of the skeletal muscles and, consequently, their stimulation, plus an increase in muscle tone. These effects of percussion are helpful in cases of muscle weakness caused by neurological disorders, or long immobilization in fixing casts. It is also very useful to apply percussion strokes as a part of sports massage directly before competition. The stimulating effects of percussion are especially noticeable if this technique is applied to the motor points or on the tendons.

1. PERCUSSION OVER THE MOTOR POINTS

The motor point is the area where the motor nerve that provides the innervation of the skeletal muscle enters it. The motor point cannot be found by palpation or any other type of examination. Electromyographically, the motor point is the area where the externally applied electrical current with lowest magnitude is able to produce a full scale muscle contraction. The percussion strokes over the area of the motor point have the great stimulating effect on the muscle.

The area of the motor point is easy to find because it is in the **middle of the muscle belly**. However, this simple recommendation has one important element which is frequently missed. The middle of the muscle belly does not always match the middle of the massaged muscle.

For example, percussion in the middle of the anterior thigh will target the motor point in the rectus femoris muscle because middle of massaged segment (anterior thigh) coincides with the middle of muscle belly of the quadriceps muscle (see Fig. 102 'a') At the same time, to perform percussion on the motor point of the extensor digitorum muscle the operator has to apply this technique proximally to the middle line of the forearm because the middle of the extensor digitorum muscle's belly does not coincides with the middle of the forearm (see Fig. 102 'b'). This happens because the extensor digitorum muscle has a long tendinous part. Thus, to perform the percussion over the motor points correctly, the practitioner has to keep in mind the muscle anatomy of the massaged area. Fig. 102 illustrates the percussion over the motor points in both discussed cases.

2. PERCUSSION ON THE TENDON

Percussion on the tendon is another great way to stimulate the skeletal muscles. It activates the muscle spindle receptors, which increase the muscle tone and prepare the muscle for optimal performance. The more widely known example of percussion on the tendon is the **knee-jerk reflex**.

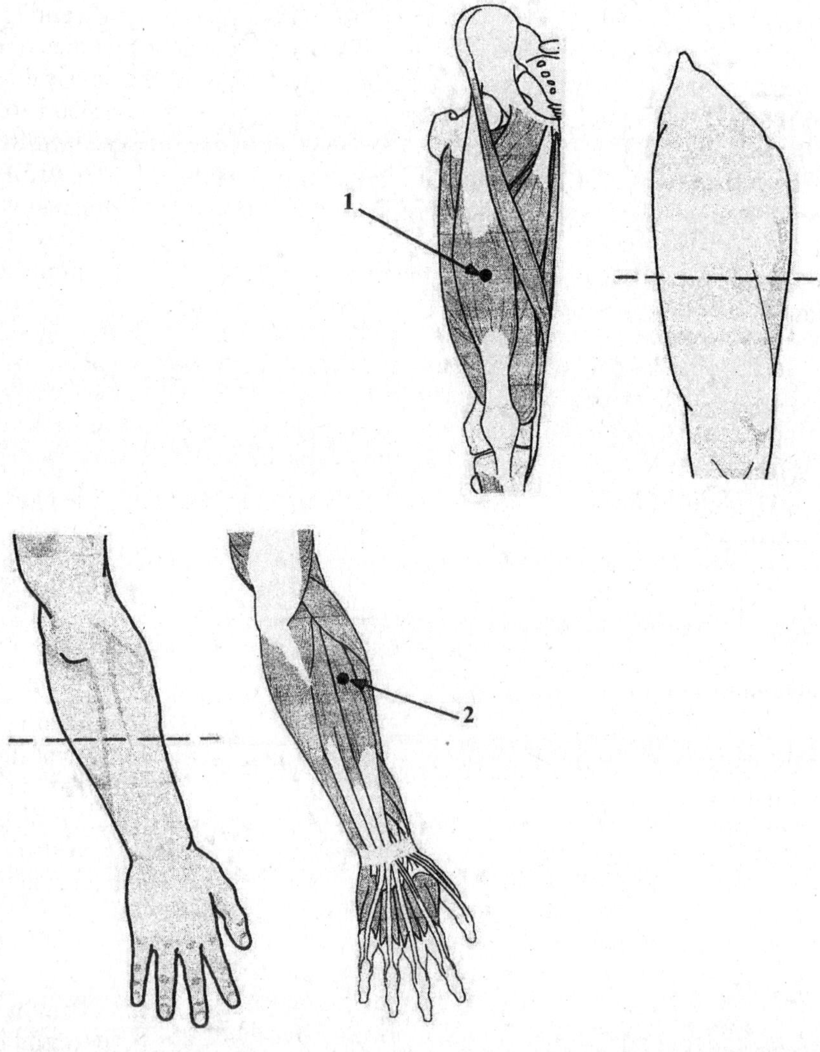

Fig. 102. Location of the motor points in the rectus femoris and extensor digitorum muscles
1 - motor point in the rectus femoris muscle
2 - motor point in the extensor digitorum muscle
Dashed line - middle of the segment

Despite the initial stimulating effect of percussion, the light prolonged application of this technique on normal muscles produces their relaxation. This paradoxical phenomenon never happens with muscles that have any type of hypertonic pathology: hypertonus, trigger point or myogelosis. This is why any percussion technique in these areas is always contraindicated.

During percussion, the practitioner compresses the walls of the arterial and venous vessels. As a result of rapid interruptive compression, the vessels respond with vasodilation and increased local circulation. The stimulation of local blood circulation is achieved more quickly after percussion than after any other massage technique; however, its effect is not as long lasting compared to kneading, for example.

Percussion has profound effects on the client's body because of its shock-delivering impact. As a result of percussion, the sympathetic division of the autonomic nervous system is stimulated and this is why percussion frequently used as a treatment tool for the abnormalities of inner organs. Like vibration, percussion waves spread throughout the body. However, the physical impact of percussion stronger than vibration, and its waves spread further. Thus, the percussion is only technique which delivers the great amount of mechanical oscillations to the inner organs even from a distance.

In the significant body of articles, the benefits of thorax percussion for patients with chronic pulmonary disorders is discussed (see Chapter I, section 'F'). The common conclusion is that percussion stimulates sputum drainage and cleaning of the bronchial tree, enhances the breathing, increases blood oxygenation, reduces tension in the respiratory muscles, and diminishes the amount of bronchodilating drugs taken by the patients.

B. TECHNICAL DISTINCTIONS

1. CONTACT AREAS

During percussion, the therapist may use different parts of the hand. The chosen contact area, or even the shape of the operator's hand, play a more important role for the percussion than in any other massage technique. The main contact areas are: the entire palm, the fingertips, the thenar-hypothenar area, the ulnar edge of the hand, the dorsal surfaces of the 2nd-5th fingers, and the ulnar and palmar surfaces of the fist(s).

2. DIRECTION OF STROKES

During percussion, the actual contact between the practitioner's hand and the massaged area is brief. Thus, the strokes can be directed along the drainage as well as against it. However the direction of the final series of strokes should follow the direction venous drainage. The best way to perform percussion is to apply strokes along the segment, constantly change their direction.

There is another important matter relating to the direction of percussion strokes in the case of medical massage treatment. Light to moderate percussion plays an important role in the treatment of peripheral neurological abnormalities (e.g. various neuralgias, casualgia, etc.). In such cases, percussion should be applied along the pathway of the affected nerve. However, the choice of the correct direction for percussion strokes completely depends on the clinical picture.

If the motor part of the peripheral nerve is mostly affected; i.e., the patient has muscle weakness, quick muscle fatigue or hypertonic abnormalities; light percussion should be performed from the proximal to distal parts; i.e., along the efferent or descending pathway of motor impulses from the central nervous system. In cases when peripheral nerve disorders are seen mostly as sensory abnormalities; i.e., numbness, paraesthesia, etc. light percussion should be applied along the nervous pathway from the distal to the proximal areas. In this case percussion strokes follow the ascending or afferent flow of sensory impulses from peripheral receptors to the CNS.

3. SPEED AND PRESSURE

As mentioned above, the therapeutic impact of percussion depends on the speed of the strokes. It has to be significant, around 200-250 strokes per minute.

The correctly used pressure is another important factor. Because the speed of the strokes is high, the pressure cannot be significant. The amount of applied pressure depends on the actual energy of the blow and its angle. The more vertical direction, the more the strokes compress the soft tissue. Thus, in the case of percussion technique, the speed and pressure have a strong inverse correlation: a higher speed of strokes demands lower pressure and *vice versa*.

The rhythm of the percussion strokes is important issue. With stable rhythm, longer percussion has a less stimulating impact, compared to the same strokes which are delivered with a constantly changing rhythm. Thus, the operator can use a changing rhythm of strokes as an additional therapeutic tool. The percussion should be used during the client's exhalation.

C. TYPES OF PERCUSSION

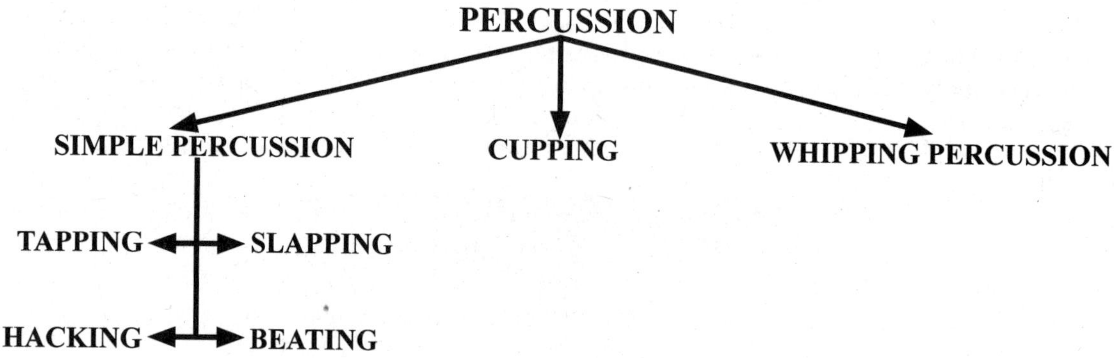

Fig. 103. Classification of percussion techniques

1. SIMPLE PERCUSSION

For simple percussion, the operator must lift the hand(s) and strike the massaged area from a height of about 2-4 inches. Simple precussion includes tapping, slapping, hacking and beating.

a. Tapping

Simple percussion with the fingertips is called tapping. It is more effective when both hands are used. Slightly bend the phalanges, spread the fingers, and gently hit the massaged area using the pads of the fingertips. The fingers should alternate with each other when they hit the massaged area as, for example, during typing. The more vertical position the fingers have, the harder impact is. Fig. 104 illustrates the tapping on the face. Notice that the tapping is conducted by the flexion-extension in the metacarpophalangeal joints with wrist joints tightened.

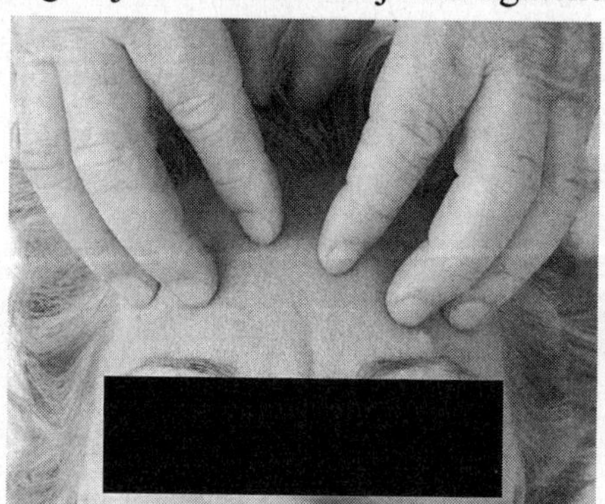

Fig. 104. Tapping on the face

Another variant of tapping is applied in cases of pseudoarthrosis or the delayed union of fractures. This type of tapping is more vigorous and demands more energy. The practitioner can use tapping which is illustrated in Fig. 105. However, it is better in these case to use tapping where the fingers don't alternate with each other, but instead hit the massaged area simultaneously. In this case, the tapping has a stronger therapeutic impact to stimulate callus formation. Usage of small wooden hummer is another alternative.

Bend the phalanges, place the fingers strictly vertically, and tighten the metacarpophalangeal joints. This treatment is effective only in areas where the bone is covered by skin only, e. g., anterior surface of the tibia or ulna. The speed of percussion is about 120-150 per minute and the operator must apply this kind of stroke for at least 3 minutes. Fig. 105 illustrates application of tapping on the anterior surface of the tibia. Notice that the tapping is conducted by flexion-extension in the wrist joints while the metacarpophalangeal joints tightened, in difference with tapping illustrated in Fig. 104.

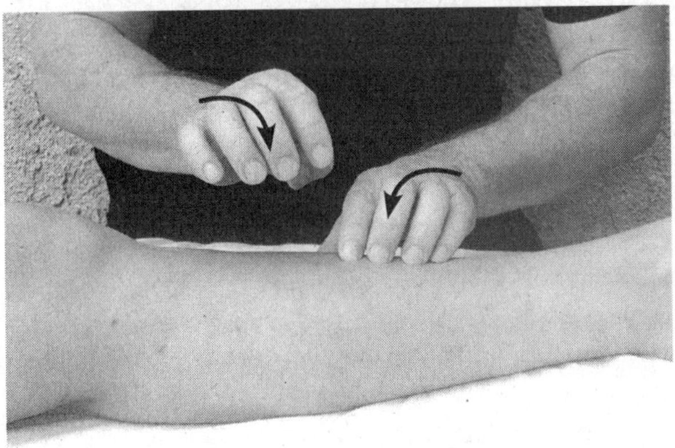

Fig. 105. Tapping on the anterior surface of the tibia

b. Slapping

Simple percussion using the palms is called slapping. It can be a one- or two-handed technique. To perform slapping, tighten all hands and wrist joints, slightly abduct the thumbs, and then rhythmically hit the massaged area with both or alternating hands. In another variant, slapping can be done by relaxing wrist and hand joints. Fig. 106 illustrates slapping on the back with all joints tightened.

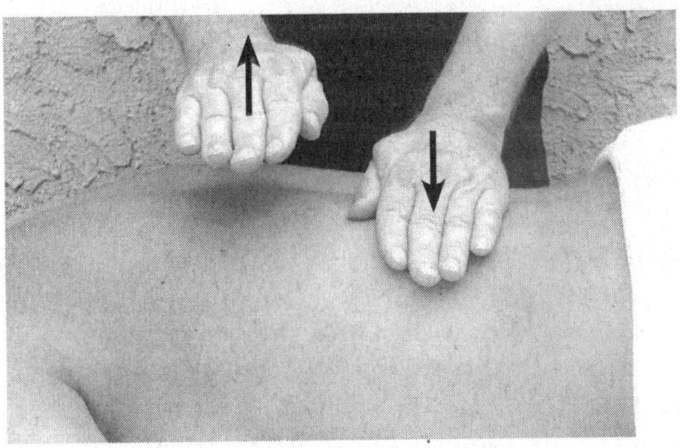

Fig. 106. Slapping on the back

c. Hacking

Hacking is percussion delivered by the ulnar edge of one or, more frequently both hands. The practitioner has to place hands on the ulnar edges at a distance of about 1 inch apart and strike the massaged area by the alternating hands or by both hands at the same time. The hands are always placed perpendicularly to the direction of the muscle fibers in massaged area.

An important element in hacking is the degree of tightness in the wrist and interphalangeal joints of the operator's hands. If hacking is performed with relaxed hands, the applied strokes are moderate (see Fig. 107 'a'). If the operator presses his or her fingers together and tightens the wrist joint, the force of the strokes increases dramatically (see Fig. 107 'b'). In this case, the practitioner has to be very careful to not damage the soft tissue against the underlying bone structures.

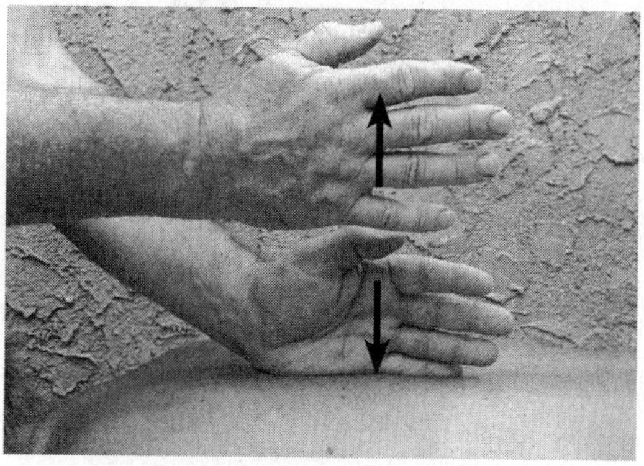

a - hacking with a relaxed hand

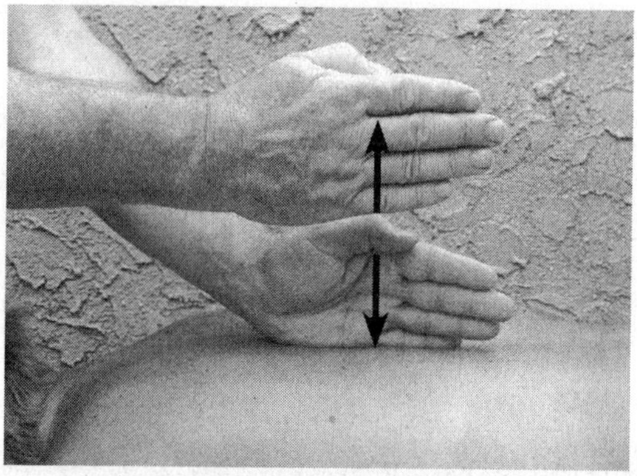

b - hacking with a tightened hand

Fig. 107. Hacking technique

Hacking stimulates the functions of the inner organs. In the abdominal area, this technique must be performed lightly and only with relaxed hands. On the thoracic cage, hacking can be done with a tightened hand and the fingers pressed together to increase the therapeutic impact.

It is helpful to apply hacking along intercostal spaces on patients with chronic pulmonary disorders, using a one-hand variant of hacking. In such a case, the ulnar edge of the hand or the 5th finger has to strike exactly between the two neighboring ribs into intercostal space (see Fig. 108). It is also helpful to completely abduct the client's upper extremity in the shoulder joint to additionally "open" the intercostal spaces.

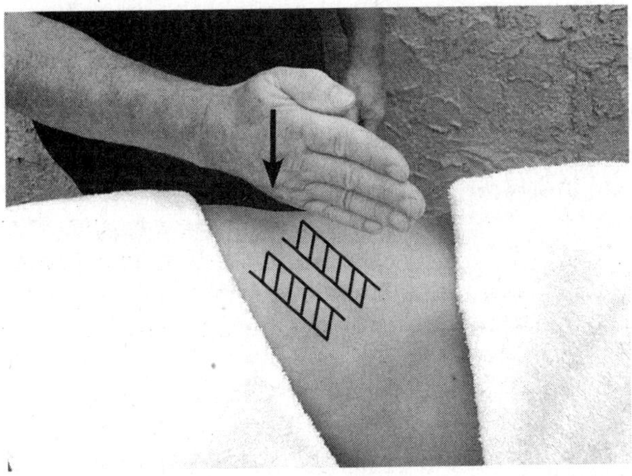

Fig. 108. Hacking along intercostal space

Dashed stripes indicate two neighboring ribs
Space between two dashed strips is the intercostal space
The client is positioned on the right side with left upper extremity completely abducted and placed over the head

d. Beating

Beating is a type of simple percussion in which the operator uses one or both fists. The massage practitioner can use two contact areas for this percussion technique: the ulnar edge of the fists or the palmar surface of the fists.

Beating using the ulnar edges is usually more vigorous than in the case of using the palmar fists. The practitioner may alternate fists or strike the massage area with both fists at the same time. Beating is contraindicated over the abdomen and on the anterior surface of the thoracic cage in the area of the heart. Always correlate the intensity of the technique with your client's level of comfort. Fig. 109 illustrates both variants of the beating.

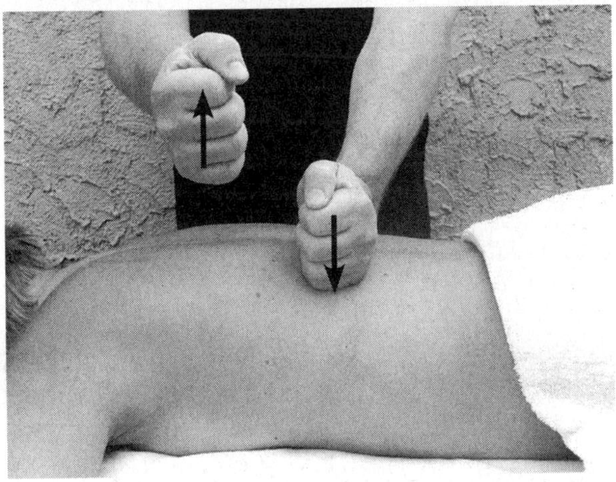

a - beating using the ulnar edge of the fists

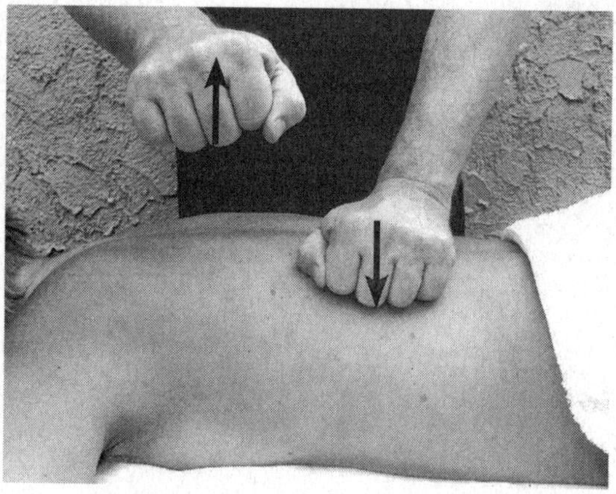

b - beating using the palmar surface of the fists

Fig. 109. Beating technique

2. CUPPING

Cupping is a unique technique because it combines several factors to produce a therapeutic impact. Besides rhythmic compression and vibration, cupping also employs the impact of air compression. This technique can be performed with one or two hands. The main contact areas are thenar-hypothenar, the thumb, the 5th finger and the fingertips of the 2nd-4th fingers. Thus, the hand has a cup-like shape. All fingers have to be tightly compressed against each other. The goal of this hand position is to generate the maximum therapeutic impact from the air compression during the stroke. With the correct execution of cupping, air comes out only between the hand and the massaged surface, but not between the fingers.

Lift the hand(s) and hit the massaged area. With proper execution, a loud, shooting noise is produced by air blowing against the massaged area. The more flatly positioned the hand is, the less intense the noise is and the less air compression is involved in the treatment. In such case cupping becomes simple slapping technique we discussed above (see Fig. 106). Fig. 110 shows the starting and final positions of the hand during cupping.

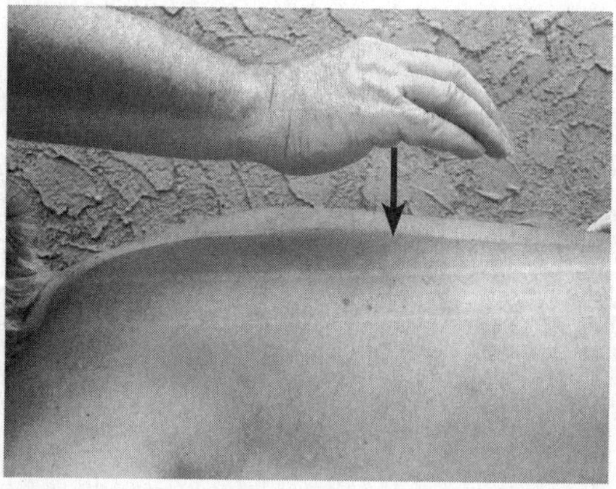

a - starting position of the hand; the solid arrow is direction of the stroke

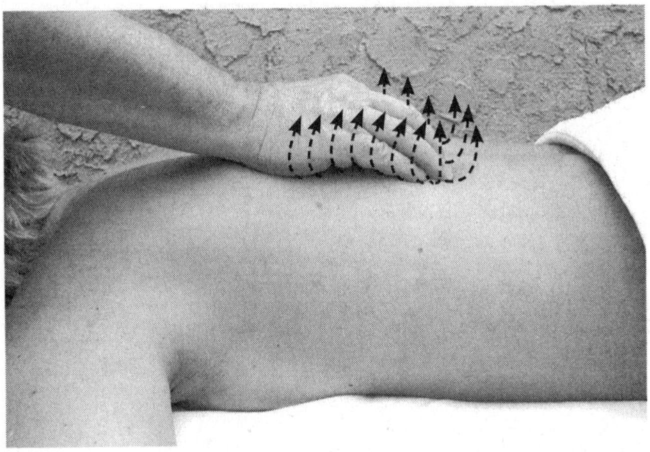

b - final position of the hand; the dashed arrows indicate the air compression

Fig. 110. Cupping technique

Slow, gentle cupping with several strokes in the same area produces local vasoconstriction. It also causes bradycardia. Fast, energetic strokes over the same area produce local vasodilation and have a strong analgesic effect. Energetic cupping is an extremely effective method of treating patients with degenerative joint disease (i.e., osteoarthritis), especially in the knee joints. Cupping reduces pain and, more importantly, the regular application of this technique slows down the progression of degenerative changes in the affected joint.

3. WHIPPING PERCUSSION

During whipping percussion, the operator strikes the massaged area with a hand(s) placed at a sharp angle to the body surface. The contact areas are the palmar surface of the 2nd-5th fingers only, the whole palm, or the dorsal surfaces of the 2nd-5th fingers. It works best to use both hands, but one hand can be used as well. The hands can have the same (i.e., follow each other) or opposite (i.e., alternate with each other) direction of stroke.

During this type of percussion, the operator uses the hand(s) as a whip. The actual area of therapy is restricted to the size of the practitioner's hand(s) because there are not any strokes along the massaged segment. If the operator wants to apply whipping percussion to a neighboring area, he or she must relocate the site of actual contact between the hand and massaged surface.

Tighten all joints in the hand and wrist, compress fingers together and slightly abduct the thumb. Start the stroke up in the air (see Fig. 111 'a'). The hand has to "fly" down, with a gradually decreasing height, until it hits the body surface (see Fig. 111 'b'). As soon as the hand makes contact with the massaged area, lift it up in the air again (see Fig. 111 'c'). The second hand immediately follows from the same side or from the opposite side and hits exactly the same area.

The higher the operator's hand is positioned at the beginning of the stroke, the less frequently the operator makes contact with the massaged area. A lower height allows the operator to significantly increase the speed of the strokes and stimulating impact of whipping percussion dramatically increases.

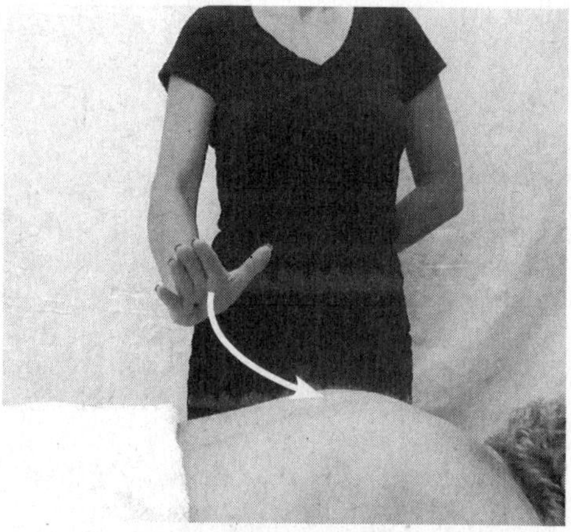

a - starting position of the hand

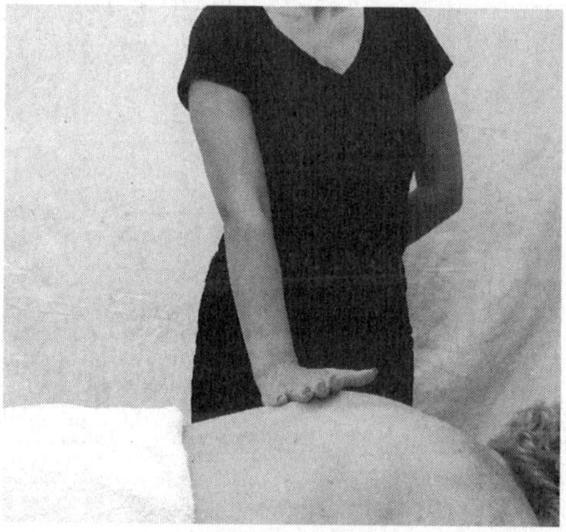

b - contact between hand and massaged area

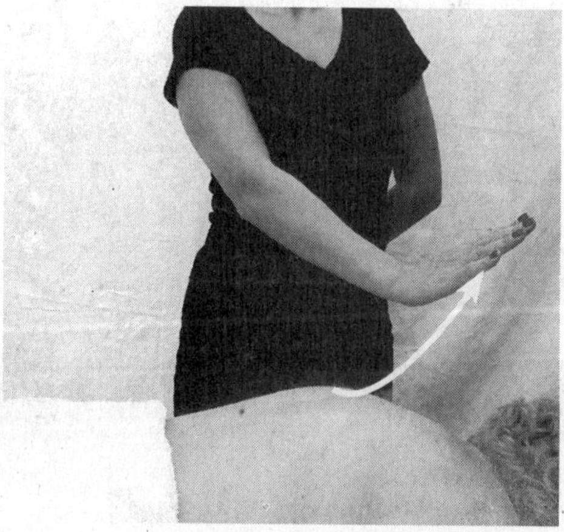

c - final position of the hand

Fig. 111. Whipping percussion

If strokes are performed in the opposite direction, the hands can alternate and touch the massaged area at different times, or they can make contact with the same area simultaneously. In the latter case the operator also uses the element of stretching. Stretching can be effective only under one condition: both hands have to make contact with the massaged area at exactly the same moment. Fig. 112 illustrates this variant of whipping percussion.

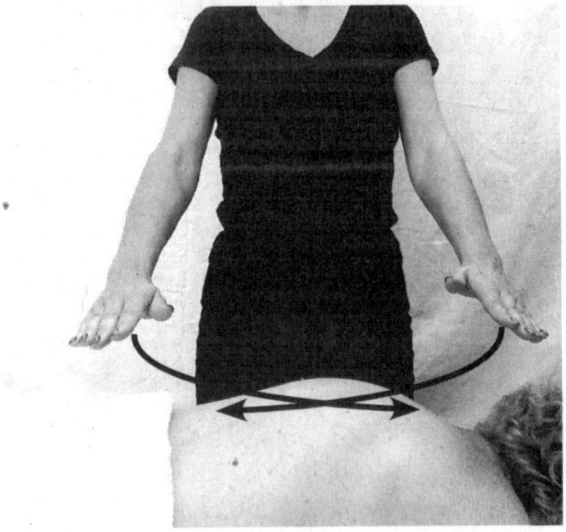

a - starting position of both hands and direction of strokes

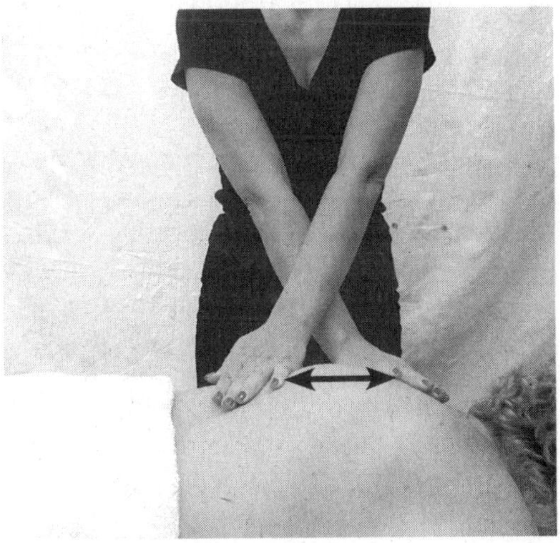

b - position of the hands during actual contact with massaged surface

Fig. 112. Whipping percussion with oppositely directed hands
Solid arrow - element of stretching between both hands
Dashed arrows - positions of both hands at the end of the stroke

The whipping percussion is a powerful method of stimulating the nervous system and skeletal muscles, and producing local hyperemia. Whipping percussion is also helpful on areas of scar tissue and in cases of massage treatment for obesity.

COMPRESSION

A. GENERAL CHARACTERISTICS

The compression technique delivers a certain amount of pressure to the massaged area. Even Hippocrates (450-3 80 BC) emphasized the importance of the right amount of applied pressure. His famous statement, “Hard pressure binds and soft pressure loosens,” which was written almost 2.500 years ago, still applies today and can be found in every modern book of manual medicine.

The pressure is a force per unit area. Therefore, compression over a small area has a greater impact than the same compression over a large area. This is one of the fundamental principles of treatment by the compression techniques.

Compression is a technically simple manipulation, but has several important considerations. First of all, one has to know the exact purpose of the compression, because the regional compression and ischemic compression have completely different indications and approaches.

Before applying any pressure, especially in sensitive areas, the massage practitioner has to determine the client’s personal pain threshold there. Thus, the therapist must have a clear idea if he or she will or will not activate the pain analyzing system during compression. In any case, the pressure has to be applied carefully and increased slowly.

We previously discussed the local effects of compression in Chapter 3. This technique has another important benefit. As it was reported by Kukulka, et al. (1985 and 1986), permanent and intermittent compression of the tendon causes immediate reduction of muscle tone and triggers muscle relaxation. In both studies, the excitability of alpha-motoneurons in the spinal cord was estimated by measuring the changes in H-reflex amplitude.

The authors detected a maximum depression of the H-reflex (45% compared to the control group) after intermittent tendon compression within 30 seconds of application. Despite the fact that this effect was short-lived and disappeared after the cessation of compression, it is very useful to apply intermittent compression to the tendons of muscles just before stretching. This simple procedure will better prepare muscles for stretching and reduce the risk of complications.

Another important benefit of a tendon’s compression is its effect on muscles with hypertonic abnormalities. This technique reduces protective muscle tension and prepares muscles for the Trigger Point Therapy or for Postisometric Muscular Relaxation (PIR).

B. TECHNICAL DISTINCTIONS

1. CONTACT AREAS

Basically every part of the hand can be used for the compression. In cases of deep pressure, the operator must be aware of possible injury to the hand or fingers. To avoid that try to support the operating hand with the other hand.

The operator can use an elbow on patients with a large muscle layer. The main disadvantage of compression by elbow is the difficulty in controlling the degree of applied pressure, as well as its direction, which is extremely important during the trigger point treatment. Besides this the elbow has a larger contact area (compared to the thumb, for example) and, as mentioned above the pressure is a force per unit area.

All these negative characteristics make the benefits of compression using the elbow very questionable especially during its application in cases of hypertonus, trigger point even risky. As mentioned above, the many of authors agreed that uncontrolled application of excessive pressure is responsible for the progression of hypertonic muscle pathologies on the long run, despite visible pain relief immediately after the treatment.

2. DIRECTION OF STROKES

Compression is a local technique, without actual advance through the massaged area. However, it can be applied as a series of compressions along the massaged segment. In this case, compressions should be applied along venous and lymphatic drainage. Soft tissue can be compressed between the operator's hands, or between the hand and underlying bones.

3. SPEED AND PRESSURE

The maximum amount of applied pressure should be on the level of client's pain threshold or exceed it slightly. Any further increase in pressure is useless. As a response to excessive pain the client will generate a protective tension, and additional pressure will only damage soft tissue. This is especially important in cases of treatment of hypertonic muscle abnormalities.

Deep pressure beyond the client's threshold of pain is part of ischemic compression treatment. However, it has to be done the correct way. We will discuss this special procedure in detail later.

The depth of compression directly depends on the direction of applied pressure. The closer the operating hand comes to an angle of 90 degrees to the surface of the body, the more pressure is achieved with the same amount of applied pressure. During compression, the applied pressure can be constant, slowly increased or intermittent. In the latter case the operator rhythmically compresses the soft tissue in the massaged area by applying and releasing the hand. In the another variant, the operator maintains some basic level of compression and rhythmically increases the pressure from this level without actually releasing the hand.

C. TYPES OF COMPRESSION

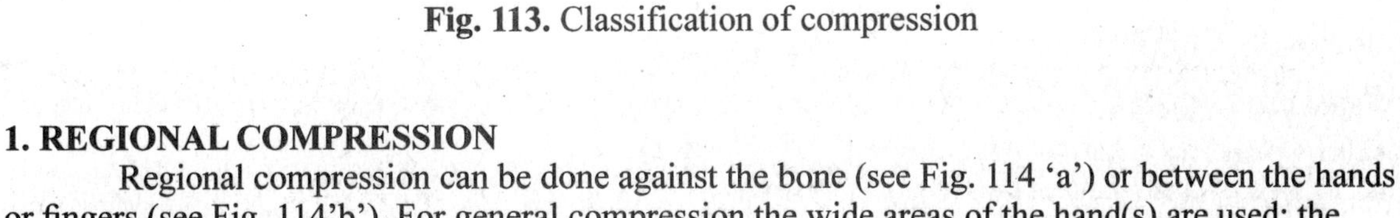

Fig. 113. Classification of compression

1. REGIONAL COMPRESSION

Regional compression can be done against the bone (see Fig. 114 'a') or between the hands or fingers (see Fig. 114'b'). For general compression the wide areas of the hand(s) are used: the palm, the thenar-hypothenar, the palmar surface of fingers or the dorsal surface of middle phalanges.

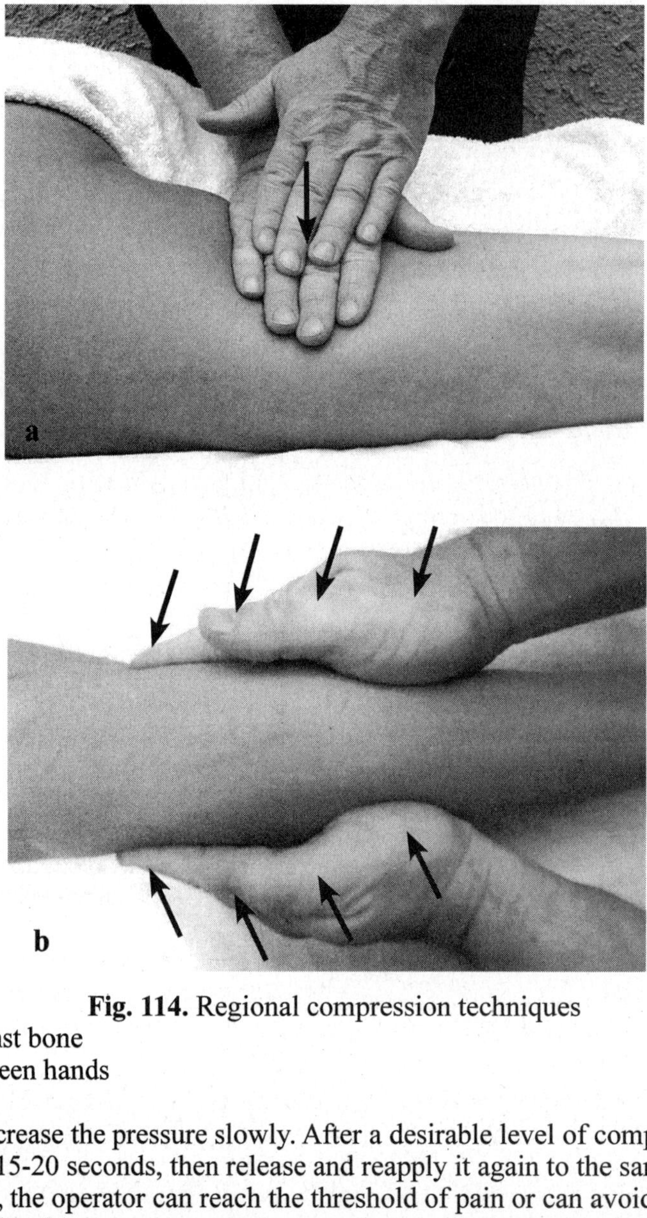

Fig. 114. Regional compression techniques

a - compression against bone
b - compression between hands

Apply and increase the pressure slowly. After a desirable level of compression is reached, hold the pressure for 15-20 seconds, then release and reapply it again to the same area. During regional compression, the operator can reach the threshold of pain or can avoid it.

If the threshold of pain is not reached, general compression has a relaxing effect on the skeletal muscles. If the pain analyzing system is activated, general compression stimulates the muscles and central nervous system. These make the patient alert. Watch the client's reaction closely!

2. PUMPING

Compression in an interruptive regime, also called pumping. For the correct execution of pumping, pressure has to be applied and released completely from the massaged area. Pumping is one of the key techniques of Lymph Drainage Massage. It is usually applied in the area of lymphatic nodes to drain pack of lymph nodes and accelerate lymph passage through the massaged segment. Fig. 115 illustrates pumping in the area of inguinal lymph nodes.

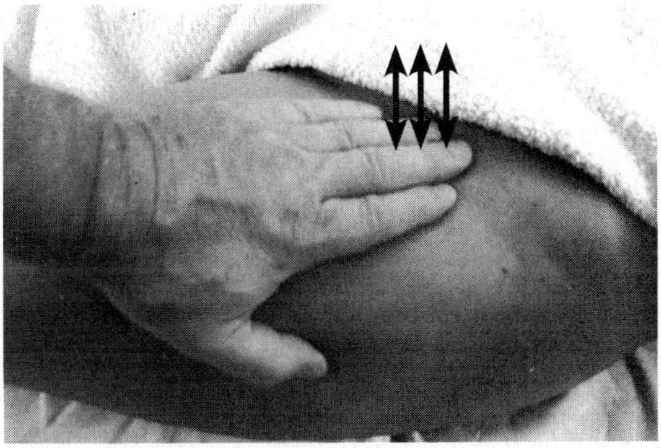

Fig. 115. Pumping in the area of inguinal lymph nodes

In another variant of interruptive compression, the operator applies a basic amount of pressure and maintains it during the stroke while rhythmic compression is delivered from this basic level. Thus, after every compression, the operator does not release the hand but returns the level of basic pressure.

3. ISCHEMIC COMPRESSION

Ischemic compression is a powerful method of treatment of hypertonic muscle abnormalities - i.e., hypertonus, trigger point, and myogelosis - as well as cutaneous and periosteal trigger points. When it is applied correctly, ischemic compression plays a critical role in the successful treatment of these of muscular abnormalities.

The massage therapist may apply ischemic compression using the thumb or 2nd or 3rd fingers. It is best to use the thumb adducted to the hand which makes the first (see Fig. 28 'a'). During ischemic compression, the operator has to reach the client's pain threshold and go beyond it without provoking protective muscle tension. Therefore, pressure has to be increased slowly and gradually using 'stop and go' approach.

Let's discuss ischemic compression in the area of the trigger point in the skeletal muscles. After the operator reaches the threshold of pain, he or she should stop and maintain the same pressure to let the client to adapt to this new sensation. Use all four mechanisms of pain control as discussed above (see pp 75-79).

As soon as the client is comfortable with the degree of applied pressure, the operator once more increases it and stops again as soon as client reports increase of pain generated by new level of compression. After the desirable submergence into the tissue of the trigger point is reached, the practitioner quickly releases the hand. This will help to increase reflex vasodilation at the site of compression.

If the practitioner repeats the gradual steps of ischemic compression, he or she can reach the maximum submergence into the trigger point without evoking protective muscle tension. The application of soft tissue compression when a client exhibits protective muscle tension is a common mistake a lot of massage practitioners do.

Why is control over protective muscle tension such an important matter? I think this subject deserves a separate discussion. The modern view on the mechanism of trigger point formation views the vasospasm as its fundamental cause (Fassbender and Wegner, 1973; Popelnasky, et al., 1976; Travell and Simmons, 1983; Yumashev and Furman, 1984; Asdonik, 1985; Kimura et al. 2009). This vasospasm can be triggered by different factors: injury, infections and intoxication, referred visceral or somatic sensory impulses, etc. In any case, the vasospasm combines with increased muscle tension, and painful hypertonus and trigger points are formed. The pain stimuli from the affected area flow to the central nervous system and additional tension in the hypertonically changed area is triggered. As a result, the already constricted vessels are additionally compressed between tensed muscle fibers in the areas of the hypertonus and trigger point. This increases local ischemia. Thus, blood circulation is compromised in the area of the hypertonus with the peak of this decrease in the area of the trigger point. All these events happen not only during muscle contractions, but also when a client's muscles are relaxed.

Now let's see what happens if the operator does not pay attention to the protective muscle tension during the application of ischemic compression. The goal of ischemic compression, as discussed above, is reflex vasodilation after pressure is released. However, the operator is interested in the normal blood circulation in the tissues around the compressed area. In this case, at the moment of releasing the pressure, the maximum amount of blood rushes into hypertonically changed muscle tissue and restores normal oxygenation. If the client exhibits and maintain protective muscle tension during the ischemic compression, the blood circulation in the entire segment is significantly reduced because of increased peripheral vascular resistance caused by protective muscle tension. In such a case, at the moment of pressure release and reflex vasodilation, a lesser amount of blood comes into the hypertonically changed area because the afferent blood vessels are compressed between muscle fibers and, consequently, contain a lesser volume of oxygenated blood. Thus, the therapeutic result of ischemic compression is lowered, and in the best variant it puts the trigger point into a "sleeping" state instead of eliminating it completely.

If the operator decides to use the method of ischemic compression he should not try to reach the maximum submergence in one or two sessions. To completely eliminate the trigger point, several sessions are needed. The same rules apply to the periostal and cutaneous trigger points. Fig. 116 shows an example of ischemic compression on the periostal trigger point located on the anterior surface of the tibia.

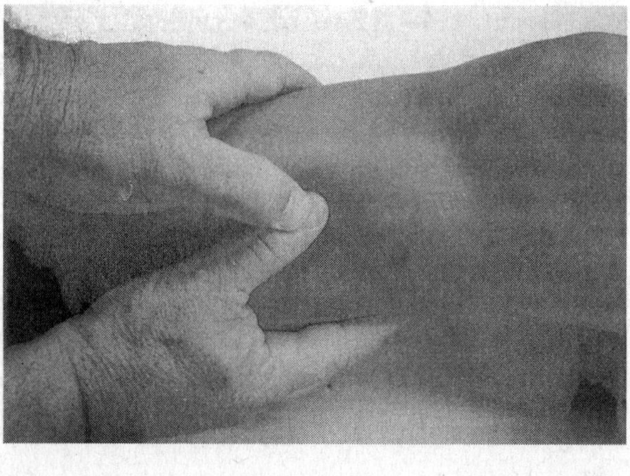

Fig. 116. Ischemic compression in the periosteum of tibia

Ischemic compression in the areas of cutaneous trigger points is best applied using the compression of a skin fold between the thumb and index finger or the thumb and the 2nd-3rd fingers (see Fig. 117 "a"). Another variant is strong stretching of the area of cutaneous trigger points between two fingers; e.g., thumbs (see Fig. 117 "b").

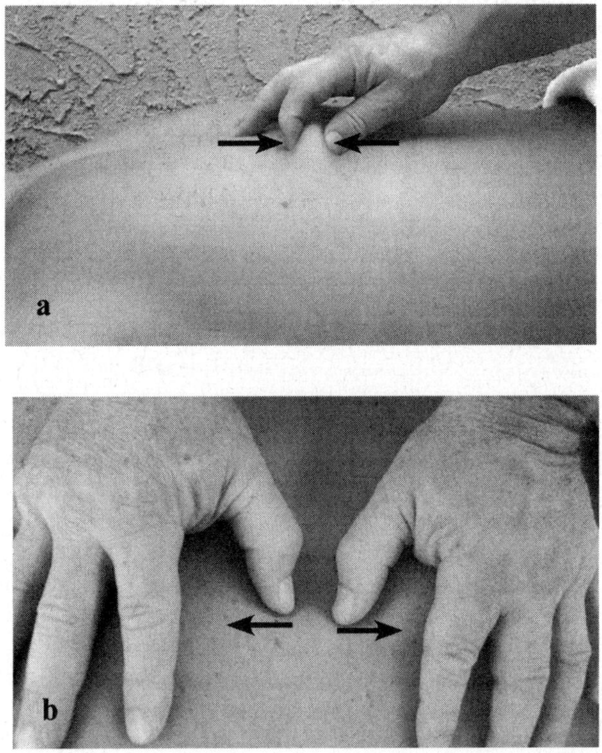

Fig. 117. Ischemic compression in the area of cutaneous trigger points.
a - compression of a fold of skin
b - strong local stretching

For the correct application of ischemic compression, the operator has to be absolutely positive about the exact direction of applied pressure. If the pressure affects only the tissue which surround the trigger point, the efficiency of the treatment significantly decreases. If the trigger point chosen for the therapy is highly painful, the practitioner should begin the treatment on surrounding tissue while gradually moving to the trigger point's epicenter.

Ischemic compression produces temporary local hypoxia in the trigger point. After the pressure is released, reflex vasomotor reactions are triggered and the local vascular spasm is substituted by vasodilation. As a result of vasodilation, microcirculation in the trigger point is restored and increased. Furthermore, partial damage of the capillaries leads to microhemorrhage into the muscle tissue and controlled inflammation. This hemorrhage stimulates the local metabolism. All these processes eliminate trigger points, though this may take several sessions.

PASSIVE STRETCHING

A. GENERAL CHARACTERISTICS

There are several types of stretching that can be used for different purposes: passive, active, passive-active, and stretching as a part of muscle energy techniques. We will discuss here only passive stretching because this technique is the integrative part of therapeutic massage session.

During passive stretching, the therapist stretches a part or segment of the body with the client's muscles completely relaxed. This technique is usually applied at the end of the treatment. The main therapeutic effects of stretching are: additional muscle relaxation through the activation of the Golgi tendon organ receptors, straightening the tendons and ligaments around the joints, restoration of soft tissue tensility and flexibility, the stimulation of blood circulation in the muscles, and the inactivation of some trigger points in the muscles, especially if they were recently formed.

Any mechanical stimuli, especially stretching, stimulates the myogenic tone of the vascular walls; i.e., causes vasoconstriction with following vasodilation after the release of pressure (Laher and Bevan, 1983). Lakin, (1990) examined the effect of stretching on blood circulation in the muscles. The author registered an increase in blood circulation of up to 30% after the passive stretching of muscle on 0.5 cm.

There are numerous results of the effect of stretching on new capillary formation (i.e., proliferation of the endothelial cells) in the muscles. Hudlicka and Brown, (1983) concluded that:

> "Repeated stretch and relaxation could be an important factor in addition to increased capillary wall tension and increased shear stress, in the remark able degree of capillary proliferation in stimulated muscles."

Stretching is a simple technique, but the client can be easily hurt by its inappropriate application. As a result of overstretching, muscles, tendons and ligaments can be over stretched and strained. To avoid these problems, the client's muscles have to be completely relaxed, and the therapist has to carefully estimate the amount of stretching to be applied.

Finally, for passive stretching to be effective, it must be conducted during a client's prolonged exhalation because during a physiological inhalation, all the skeletal muscles slightly increase their tone.

B. TECHNICAL DISTINCTIONS

1. CONTACT AREAS

For the correct application of stretching, the therapist must tightly grasp the distal part of the stretched segment. Thus, the main contact areas are the whole palms and the 1st-3rd (or all) fingers.

2. DIRECTION OF STROKES

Stretching can be applied in longitudinal, diagonal and perpendicular directions to the axis of the extremity, or in the direction of muscle fibers.

3. SPEED AND PRESSURE

Before stretching the therapist must detect the level of individual elasticity in the client's soft tissue. This characteristic varies from person to person. A simple test will allow the practitioner to estimate individual elasticity of soft tissues: Ask the client to passively adduct the thumb to the forearm using the other hand. Fig. 118 shows examples of this test in cases of low and high elasticity of the soft tissue.

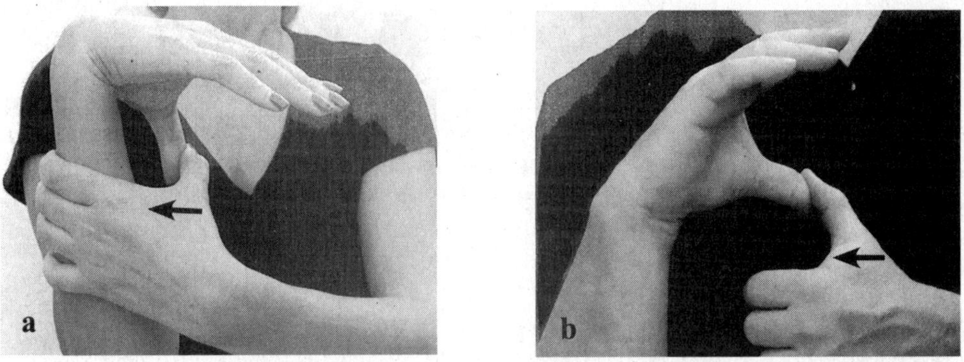

Fig. 118. The detection of individual tensility of the soft tissues
a - high tensility of soft tissues **b** - low tensility of soft tissues

The practitioner can use the movements in the joint as a tool to stretch the soft tissue. In this case, before stretching, the practitioner must detect the physiological range of movements in the joint. This allows to avoid unexpected complications.

The applied pressure has to be strong enough to grasp and securely hold the stretched part of the body. It is best to remove any lubricant before the application of stretching, or to use, for example, a towel to prevent the operator's hand from slipping off the stretched part.

C. TYPES OF PASSIVE STRETCHING

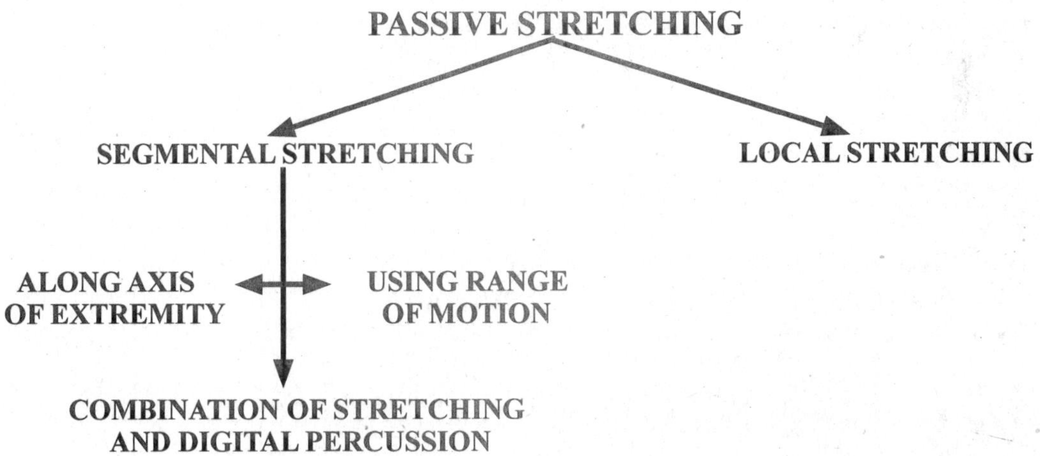

Fig. 119. Classification of passive stretching techniques

1. SEGMENTAL STRETCHING

During segmental stretching the therapist stretches extremity: along its axis or by using the physiological range of movements in the joint. The client must be completely relaxed. During the passive stretching, all soft tissues are affected. The first tissue to be stretched is the skin and connective tissue structures. Only after they are stretched will the muscles start to stretch as well.

The operator has to pay close attention to his or her tactile sensations. Immediately after the beginning of stretching, the operator feels an elastic resistance of connective tissue structures and muscles. With further, slow stretching, the Golgi tendon organ receptors in the tendons are activated and the muscles relax. The therapist feels it as a sudden, small additional give-up of the tissues. Don't go any further, just maintain the same level of stretching for an additional 10-15 seconds.

Also, remember that stretching has to be applied only during the client's exhalation. Slightly decrease pressure during the inhalation. This will help to keep muscles in a relaxed state.

a. Stretching Along Axis of Extremity

To stretch an upper or lower extremity along its axis, the operator must grasp the more distal part (i.e., hand or foot) and gently stretch the entire limb. Fig. 120 illustrates the example of passive stretching of lower extremity along its axis.

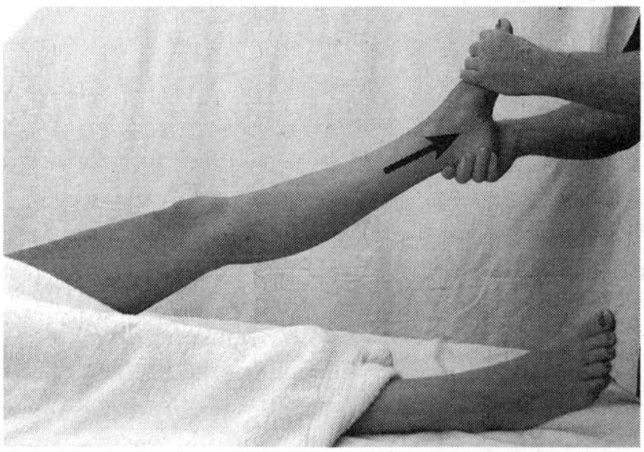

Fig. 120. Passive stretching of lower extremity along its axis

The practitioner can also stretch only the segment of extremity: for example, the forearm and the area of the wrist and elbow joints. To do this, the operator must create counterpressure between the both hands in the direction along the axis of the extremity. The practitioner can maintain the same pressure or apply it in the intermittent regime. Fig. 121 illustrates the example of passive stretching of the forearm muscles, the elbow and wrist joints with oppositely directed pressure.

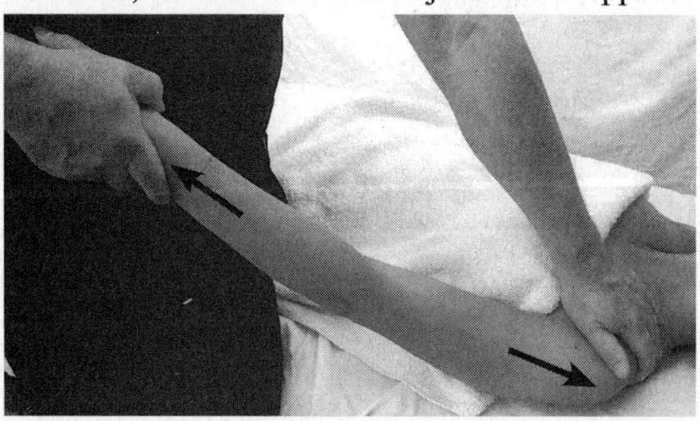

Fig. 121. The passive stretching of forearm muscles and wrist joint

b. Stretching Using Range of Motions

By using the physiological range of movements in the joints and changing the position of the stretched extremity, the operator is able to target a particular muscle or group, or even its part.

For example, the practitioner needs to stretch the hand and finger extensors. He or she can use passive stretching, as shown in Fig. 121. In such case the practitioner will stretch the wrist joint, the fingers' extensors, as well as the flexors. Instead, if the therapist uses passive flexion in the wrist joint, he or she stretches extensors only.

However, even this stretching can be more specific. If the upper extremity is put into position shown in Fig. 122 'a', the stretching will target the proximal part of the extensors. With the upper extremity in the position shown in Fig. 122 'b', the practitioner mostly targets the distal part of the extensors. Such approach to the passive stretching allows precise delivery of the therapeutic impact to the skeletal muscle.

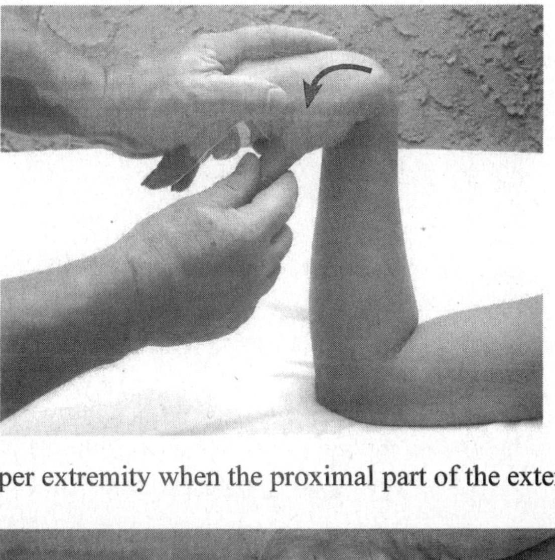

a - position of upper extremity when the proximal part of the extensors is stretched

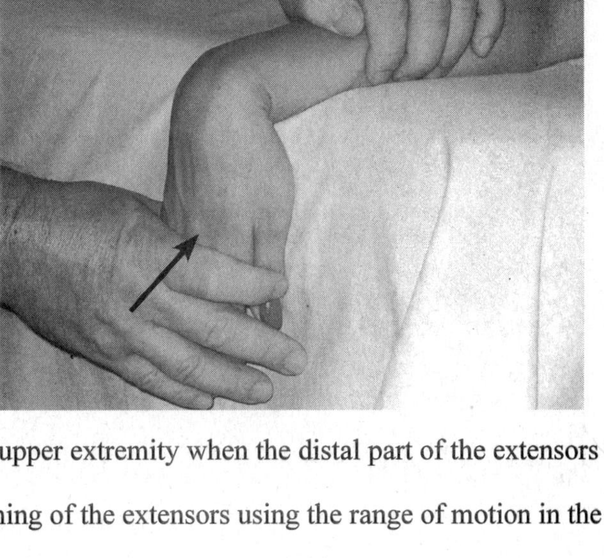

b - position of upper extremity when the distal part of the extensors is stretched

Fig. 122. Stretching of the extensors using the range of motion in the wrist joint

c. Combination of Stretching and Digital Percussion

Another valuable type of passive stretching is a combination of stretching and percussion. As we discussed above, during the contraction of one muscle group its muscle-antagonists are relaxed. This reflex can be used to additionally relax the stretched muscles. Let's discuss the same case of passive stretching of the hand and fingers' extensors.

The operator grasps the client's hand and starts to stretch it. At the same time, he or she applies fast digital percussion to the tendons of the hand's flexors; i.e., muscle-antagonists. As a result, the muscle spindles receptors in the flexor muscles are activated and these muscles contract slightly. This contraction immediately causes the relaxation of the hand's extensors, which is the group the operator stretches. Fig. 123 illustrates a combination of stretching and percussion.

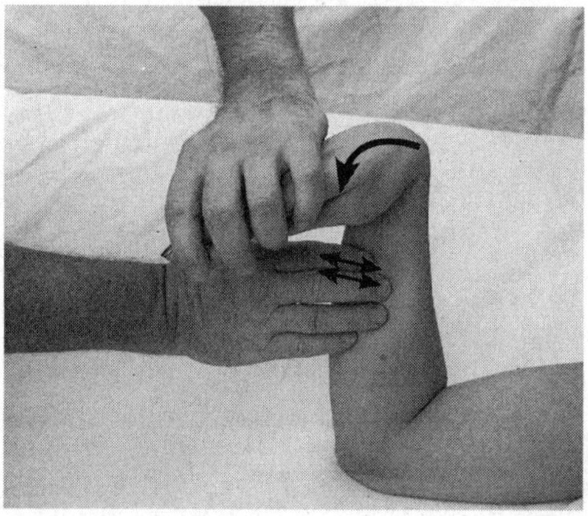

Fig. 123. Combination of passive stretching of the extensors and digital percussion on flexors

The practitioner has to be careful with the amount of applied stretching. It is easy to hurt the client. Thus, the stretching must stop as soon as the client feels even minor pain or uncomfortable sensations in the stretched tissue. Release the stretch, let the client to take one or two deep breaths and again repeat the stretching. Each time you will feel the tissue (especially the skeletal muscles) stretch more easily until the anatomical length is completely restored.

2. LOCAL STRETCHING

Local stretching uses the same rules as segmental stretching. The main difference is in the areas and levels of its application. Local stretching can be applied to the skin (see Fig. 119 'b', to the ligaments (see Fig. 34), to the joint (see Fig. 121-122), and to the skeletal muscles (see Fig. 122). Local stretching can be applied in all possible directions. It depends on the anatomy of the segment and the therapeutic goal of the stretch. The techniques of connective tissue massage are one example of local stretching of the fascia and aponeurosis.

Local stretching affects soft tissue on all levels. This type of passive stretching usually is performed directly on the pathologically changed area; e.g, on the area of trigger points. Before the stretching, always create a fold of skin between both hands and start to stretch slowly (see Fig. 124).

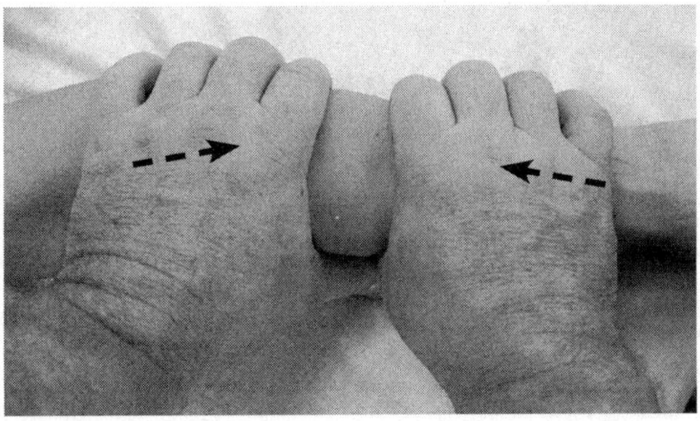

a - starting position of the hands with a fold of skin in between

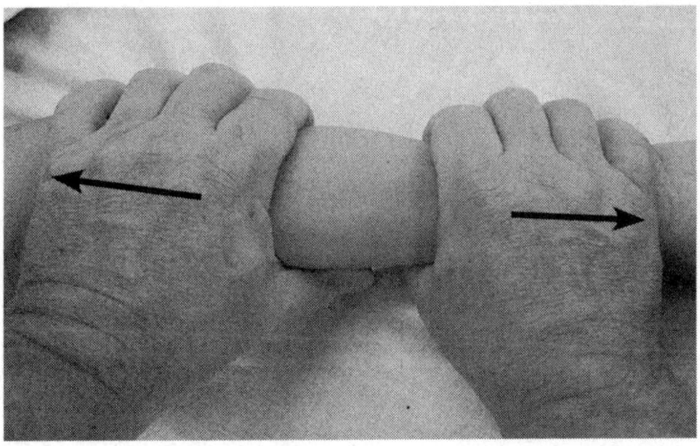

b - local stretching in the opposite directions

Fig. 124. Local stretching of the forearm
Dashed arrows - gentle push to the skin only to create fold between both hands
Solid arrows - local stretching of forearm muscles.

REFERENCES

1. Abrams, S.: *Spondylotherapie*. San Francisco, 1918.
2. Airapetov, S.G.: [Massage as a Part of Complex Treatemnt of Patients with Tromboangiitis Obliterans in the Medical Resort]. In.: *Physical Therapy in Medical Resorts*. "Sochi", 1955.
3. Ahn S, Kim J, Cho J. Effects of breast massage on breast pain, breast-milk sodium, and new born suckling in early postpartum mothers. *J Korean Acad Nurs*. 2011 Aug;41(4):451-9.
4. Akmedzhanov, M.Y., Leshchinskaya, N.P., Arkhangelsky, V.V., Guz, S.Y., Afanasieva, M.S., Sokolov, B.A.: [Pericardic Massage and Its Adaptive Effect in Rehabilitation Therapy with Dosed Physical Exersises in Patients Who had Myocardial Infarction]. *Vopr. Kurortol. Fizioter. Lech. F iz. Kult.*, 4:21-23,1981.
5. Aksenova, A.M.: [New Method of Deep Reflex-Muscular Massage]. *Vopr. Kurortol. Fizioter. Lech Fiz. Kult.*, 4: 30-32, 1997.
6. Aksenova, A.M., Romanova, M.M.: [Influence of Reflex-Muscular Massage on Metabolism of Patients with Complicated Gastric Ulcers]. *Vopr. Kurortol. Fizioter. Lech. Fiz. Kult.*, 6:, 24-26, 1 1998.
7. Aksenova, A.M., Reznikov, K.M., Andreeva, V.V.: [Influence of Deep Massage on Cerebral Circulation in Cases of Cervical Spondylosis]. *Vopr. Kurortol. Fizioter. Lech. Fiz. Kult.*, 3: 19-20, 1997.
8. Anderson, J .C., Eriksson, C.: Electical Properties of Wet Collagen. *Nature*, 218: 166-168, 1968.
9. Antoniev, A.A., Belaya, L.V.: [Physical Therapy, Massage and Self-Massage in Dermatological Practice]. *Vopr. Kurortol. Fizioter. Lech. Fiz. Kult.*, 1: 34-37, 1985.
10. April, E.W.: *Anatomy*. "Narval Publ. Co", Malvern, 1990.
11. Akkro, P.J., Pakarinen, A.J., Kari-Koshinen, 0.: Effect of Whole Body Massage on Serum Protein, Electrolyte and Hormone Concentrations, Enzyme Activities and Hematological Param eters. Int. *J. Sports Med.*, 4: 265-267, 1983.
12. Asdonk, J .: [Physical Lymph Drainage and Therapy of Edema in Chronic Venous Insuficiency]. *Z. Lymphol.*, 5(2): 107-111, 1981.
13. Asdonik, J .: [Myogeloses, Their Pathogenesis and Their Lymph Drainage, Heat and Exercise Therapy]. *Z. Lymphol.*, 9(1): 30-37, 1985. A
14. Avery, M., Van Arsdale, L.: Perineal Massage. Effect on the Incidence of Episotomy and Perineal Laceration in Nullparous Population. *.J. Nurse Midfitery*, 32: 181-184, 1987.
15. Bankov, S.: [Study of the Power of Human Prehensions]. *Orthopeay & T raumatology,* 14(1): 9-16, 1977.
16. Barr, J .S., Taslitz, N.: The Influence of Back Massage on Autonomic Functions. *Phys. Ther.*, 50(12):1679-1691, 1970.
17. Barrett, T.W.: Hyaluronic Acid Salt - A Mechanoelectrical Transducer. *Bioph. Bioch. Acta*, 383: 157, 1975.
18. Bashnyak, V.V.: [*Etiology and Treatment of Gastric Ulcers*]. Vest. Chirurg., 8: 61-63, 1989.
19. Bashnyak, V.V.: [*Manual Therapy of Abdomen*]. "Nadstirya", Lutsk, 1993.
20. Basset, C.A.L.: *Biophysical Principles Affecting Bone Structure. In: The Biochemistry and Phisiology of Bone.* Vol. III. Edited by G.H. Botnne. "Academic Press", New York, 1971.
21. Beal, M.: Viscerosomatic Reflexes: A Review. *J. Am. 0st. Ass.*, 85(12): 786-801, 1985. '
22. Beard, G.: A History of Massage Technic. *Phys. Ther. Rev.*, 32(12): 613-624, 1952.
23. Becker, H., Prysi, M.F.: Quantitive Assessment of Postoperative Breast Massage. *Plastic & Reconstr. Surg.* Aug.: 355-356, 1990.
24. Becker, R.0., Selden, G.: *The Body Electric*. "William Morrow & Co, Inc". New York, 1985.
25. Beeken, J .E., Parks, D., Cory, J ., Montopoli, G.: The Effectiveness of Neuromuscu1ar Release

Massage Therapy in 5 Individuals with Chronic Obstructive Lung Disease. *Clin. Nurs. Res.*, 7(3): 309-325, 1998.
26. Belaya, N.A.: [*Medical Massage Manual*]. "Medicina", Moscow, 1983.
27. Belaya, N.A., Zavadina, K.I., Panina, G.A.: [Various Methods of Massage in Treatment of Patients with Insufficient Cardiac and Cerebral Circulation]. In: *Publications of Central Scien tific Research Institute of Physioptherapy*, V. 40: 32-37, 1978.
28. Bereiter-Halm, J ., Anderson, O.R., Rief, W.E.: *Cytomechanics*. "Springer-Verlag", Berlin, 1987.
29. Berger, M., Cuppers, N.J., Hegner, H., Jorgens, V., Berchtold, P.: Absorption Kinetics and Bio-logic Effects of Subcutaneously Injected Insulin Preparation. *Dibetes Care*, 5(2): 77-91, 1982.
30. Bernhardt, S.: *Neue Erkentnisseuzur F rage der Dosierung bei Segmentmassage*. Heiberufe. 1953.
31. Bemhaupt, M., Gellhom, E., Rasmussen, A.T.: Experimental Contribution to the Problems of Consciosness. *J. Neurophysiol.*, 16; 21-35, 1953.
32. Bierman, W: Influence of Cycloid Vibration Massage on Trunk F lexion. *Am. J. Phys. Med.*, 39: 219-224, 1960.
33. Birukov, A.A.: *Massage. "Fizcultura i Sport"*, Moscow, 1988.
34. Birukov, A.A., Peisachov, N.M.: [Changes of Psycho-Physiological Paramentres after the Application of Different Techniques of Sports Massage]. *Theory & Practice Phys. Exerc.*, 8: 21-24, 1979.
35. Blackman, P.G., Simmons, L.R., Crossley, K.M.: Treatment of Chronic Exertional Anterior Compartment Syndrome with Massage: A Pilot Study. *Clin. J. Sports Med.*, 8(1): 14-17, 1998.
36. Bogorodinsky, D.K., German, D.G., Godovalik, 0.0., Scorometz, A.A.: [*Lumbo-Sacral Radiculi tis Caused by Sponaylosis*]. "Shiintsa", Kishinev, 1975.
37. Boiarsky, N.K.: [*Body Electricity*]. "Medicina", Moscow, 1973.
38. Bologna, M., Vicentini, C., Festuccia, C., Muzi., P., Napolitano, T., Biordi, L., Miano, L.: Early Diagnosis of Prostatic Carcinoma Based on In Vitro Culture of Viable Tumor Cells Harvested by Prostatic Massage. *Eur. Urol.*, 14(6): 474-476, 1988.
39. Bongi SM, Del Rosso A, Passalacqua M, Miccio S, Cerinic MM. Manual lymph drainage im proving upper extremity edema and hand function in patients with systemic sclerosis in edema tous phase. *Arthritis Care Res* (Hoboken). 2011 Aug;63(8):1134-41.
40. Borisov, I: [Stimulation of Skeletal Muscles], *Science & Tech.*, 1: 26-27, 1984.
41. Bork, K., Korting, G.W., Faus, T.G.: Das Verhalten einiger serum-enzyme nach Ganzkorper-Muskelmassage. *Arch. Derm. Forsch.*, 240: 342-438, 1978.
42. Bortfield, S.A., Gorodetskaya, G.F., Rogoleva, E.I.: [*Point Massage for Treatment of Cerebral Palsy Syndrome*]. "Medicina", Moscow, 1979.
43. Brandt, T (Cited in Kamenetz, H.L., 1976): *Nouvelle Methode Gymnastique et Magnetique pour le Traitement des Maladies des Organs du Bassin et en Particular de 1 'Uterus*. Stockholm, 1868.
44. Brocq, L.: *Traite Elementaire de dermatologie Pratique*. Paris, 1907.
45. Brunett, D.M.: Mechanical Stretching Increases the Number of Epithelial Cell Syntesizing DNA in Culture. *J. Cell Sci*, 69: 34-35, 1984.
46. Buhring, M.: Physikalische Therapie bei Patienten mit peripheral arterieller Verschlusskrankheit und Claudicatio intermittens. *Therapiewoche*, 35: 3296-3300, 1985.
47. Bullock, J., Boyle, J ., Wang, M.B., Ajello, R.R.: *Physiology*. "John Wiley and Sons", Pennsyl-vania,1984.
48. Buonocore, M., Manstretta, C., Mazzucchi, G., Casale, R.: [The Clinical Evaluation of Conser vative treatment in Patients with the Thoracic Outlet Syndrome]. *G. Ital. Med. Lav. Ergon.*, 20(4):249-254, 1998.

49. Burovik, A.N., Samtsonova, I.A., Manuilov, I.A.: [An Investigation of the Effect of Individual Variants of Sports Massage on Muscular Blood Circulation]. Soviet Sports Rev., 24: 197-200, 1989.
50. Cafarelli, E., Sim, J ., Carolan, B., Liebesman, J .: Vibratory Massage and Short-Term Recovery from Muscle Fatigue. *Int. J. Sports Med.*, 11: 474-478, 1990.
51. Casley-Smith, J .R., Boris, M., Weindorf, S., Lasinski, B.: Treatment for Lymphedema of the Arm - The Casley-Smith Method. *Cancer,* 83(12): 2843-2860, 1998.
52. Castro-Sánchez AM, Moreno-Lorenzo C, Matarán-Peñarrocha GA, Feriche-Fernández-Castanys B, Granados-Gámez G, Quesada-Rubio JM. Connective Tissue Reflex Massage for Type 2 Diabetic Patients with Peripheral Arterial Disease: Randomized Controlled Trial. *Evid Based Complement Alternat Med.,* Nov 23, 2009.
53. Chaitov, L.: *Muscle Energy Techniques*. "Churchill", Livingstone, 1996.
54. Chaitov, L.: *Soft Tissue Manipulations.* "Healing Arts Press", Rochester, 1988.
55. Chen, B-M., Grinnell, A.D.: Integrins and Modulation of Transmitter Release from Motor Nerve Terminals by Stretch. *Science*, 269: 1578-1580, 1995.
56. Chemigovsky, V.N.: [*Interoreceptors*]. "Medicine", Moscow, 1980.
57. Chopra, S.K., Taplin, G.V., Simmons, D.H., Robinson, G.D., Elam, D., Coulson, A.: Effect of Hydration and Physical Therapy on Tracheal Transport Velocity (TTV). *Am. Rev. Respiratory Dis.*, 15:1009-1014,1977.
58. Ciparet, Y., 1985: Quoted by Dubrovsky, V.I., Dubbrovsky, N.M.: [*Massage Manual*], "Chuvashia", Cheboksari, 1995.
59. Clark, S.M., Cochrane, G.M., Weber, B.: Effect of Sputum on Pulmonary Function. *Thorax*, 28: 262, 1973.
60. Cox, C.A.: *Maternity Massage*. "Stress Less Publishing, Inc.", Scottsdale, 1994.
61. Craig LH, Svircev A, Haber M, Juncos JL. Controlled pilot study of the effects of neuromuscular therapy in patients with Parkinson's disease. *Mov Disord.* 2006 Dec;21(12):2127-33.
62. Cunningham JE, Kelechi T, Sterba K, Barthelemy N, Falkowski P, Chin SH. Case report of a patient with chemotherapy-induced peripheral neuropathy treated with manual therapy (massage). *Support Care Cancer*. 2011 Sep;19(9):1473-6.
63. Curtis, A.S.G., Sheehar, G.M.: The Control of Cell Division by Tension or Diffusion. *Nature*, 274: 52-53, 1978.
64. Curtis, M.: The Use of Massage in Restoring Cardiac Rhythm. *Nurs. Times,* 90(38): 36-37, 1994.
65. Cuthbertson, D.P.: The Effect of Massage on Metabolism. A Survey. *Glasgow Med. J.*, 120: 200-213, 1933.
66. Cyriax, J .: *Theory and Practice of Massage. Textbook of Orthopaedic Medicine*. Vol. 2. Treatment by Manipulation, Massage and Injection. 11th Edition, "Bailliere & Tindall", Toronto.
67. Cyriax, J .: Clinical Application of Massage, pp. 122-145. In: *Massage, Manipulation and Traction*. Edited by: S. Licht. "R.F. Kriger Publ. Co.", New York, 1976.
68. Danchik, J J ., Yochum, T.R., Aspergen, D.D.: Myositis Ossificans traumatica. *J. Manip. Phys. Ther.*, 16(9): 605-614, 1993.
69. Danneskiold-Samsoe, B., Christiansen, E., Lund, B., Andersen, R.B.: Regional Muscle Tension and Pain ("Fibrositis"). *Scand. J. Rehab. Med.*, 15: 17-20, 1982.
70. Davidson, C.J., Ganion, L.R., Gehlsen, G.M., Verhoestra, B., Roepke, J .E., Sevier, T.I.: Rat Tendon Morphologic and Functional Changes Resulting from Soft Tissue Mobilization. *Med. Sci. Sports Exer.*, 29: 313-319, 1997.
71. Deineka, K.: [*Respiration Movements and Health*]. "Zinatne", Vilnius, 1966.

72. Dejerine, J .: *Semiologie des aflections du systeme nerveux*. "Masson et Cie", Paris, 1926.

73. Dembo, A.G.: [Sports Medicine and Physical Therapy]. "*Fizkultura i Sport*", Moscow, 197 3.

74. Dickle, E.: *Meine Bindegewebsmassage*. "Marquardt", Stuttgart, 1953.

75. Dickle, E., Schliack, H., Wolff, A: *Bindegewebsmassage*. "Marquardt", Stuttgart, 1979.

76. Diepgen, T.L., Fartasch, M.: Recent Epidemiological and Genetic Studies in Atopic Dermatitis. *Acta. Derm. Venerol.*, 176: 13, 1992.

77. Dietz, F .R., Mathews, K.D., Montgomery, W.J.: Reflex Sympathetic Dystropy in Children. *Clin.Orthop. Rel. Res.*, 258.(9): 225-213, 1990.

78. Dillon, R.S.: Improved Serum Profiles in Diabetic Individuals Who Massaged Their Insulin Injection Sites. *Diabetes Care*, 6(4): 399-401, 1983.

79. Doering, T.J., Fieguth, H.G., Steuemagel, B., Brix, J ., Konitzer, M., Schneider, B., Fisher, G.C.: External Stimuli in the Form of Vibratory Massage after Heart or Lung Transplantation. *Am. J. Phys. Med. Rehab.*, 78(2): 108-110, 1999.

80. Dolivo, M., Askienazy, E.M.: [Value of Prostatic Massage for Detection of Chlamydia Tracho matis in the Male Urethra]. *Contracept. Fertil. Sex.*, 21(1): 41-44, 1993. '

81. Dossetor, D.R., Couryer, S., Nicol, A.R.: Massage for Very Severe Self_Injurious Behavior in a Girl with Comelia de Lange Syndrome. *Dev. Med. Child. Neurol.*, 33: 636-644, 1991.

82. Drews, T., Kreider, R.B., Drinkard, B., Cotres, C.W., Lester, C., Somma, C.T., Shall, L.M., Woodhouse, M.: Effects of Postevent Massage on Repeated Ultra-Endurance Cycling. *Int. J. Sports Med.*, 112407, 1990.

83. Drinker, C.K., Yoffley, J .M.: *Lymphatics, Lymph and Lymphoid Tissue: Their Physiological and Clinical Significance*. "Harward University Press", Cambridge, 1941.

84. Dubrovsky, V.I.: *[Principles of the Segment Reflex Massage*]. "Fizcultura i Sport", Moscow, 1982.

85. Dubrovsky, V.I.: [*Rehabilitating Massage in Combination with Oxygentherapy*], "Medicine", Moscow, 1990.

86. Dubrovsky, V.I., Dubbrovsky, N.M.: [*Massage Manual*], "Chuvashia", Cheboksari, 1995.

87. Durnev, V.I., Vinnichenko, N.S., Matveev, E.T.: [Influence of Massage on Parameters of White Cells]. *Vopr. Kurort. Physiotherapy & Phys. Ther.*, 1:48-49, 1983.

88. Ebel, A., Wisham, L.H.: Effect of Massage on Muscle Temperature and Radiosodium Clearance. *Arch. Phys. Med.*, July: 399-405, 1952.

89. Ebner, M.: Peripheral Vasculatory Disturbances: Treatment by Massage of Connective Tissue in Reflex Zones. *Br. J Phys. Med.*, 19(8): 176-180, 1956.

90. Ebner, M.: *Connective Tissue Massage and Therapeutic Application*. "Kriger. Huntington". New York, 1975.

91. Eccles, A.S.: *The Practice of Massage: the Physiological Eflects and Therapeutic Uses*. "Wil lam Wood & Co", New York, 1904.

92. Edgecombe, W., Bain, W.: The Effect of Baths, Massage and Exercises on the Blood Pressure. *Lancet*, 1: 1552-1557, 1899.

93. Eisenberg, D.M., Davis, R.B., Ettner, S.L., Appel, S., Wilkey, S., Van Rompay, M., Kessler, R.C.: Trends in Alternative Medicine Use in the United States. 1990-1997. Results of Follow-Up National Survey. *JAMA*, 280(18): 1569-1575, 1998. '

94. Eisenberg, D.M., Kessler, R.C., Foster, C., Norlock, F.E., Calkins, D.R., Delbanco, T.L.: Unconventional Medicine in the United States. Prevance, Costs, and Pattems of Use. *New Eng. J. Med.*, 328 (4):246-252, 1993.

95. Ekici G, Bakar Y, Akbayrak T, Yuksel I. Comparison of manual lymph drainage therapy and connective tissue massage in women with fibromyalgia: a randomized controlled trial. *J Manipulative Physiol Ther*. Feb;32(2):127-33, 2009.

96. Eliska, 0., Eliskova, M.: Are Peripheral Lymphatics Damaged by High Pressure Manual Massage ? Lymphology, 28(10: 21-30, 1995.

97. Elkins, E.c., Herrick, J.F., Gridlay, J.H., Mann, F.C., DeFrost, R.E.: Effect of Various Procedures on the Flow of Lymph. *Arch. Phys. Med. & Reh.*, 1: 31-39, 1953.

98. Emst, E.: Abdominal Massage Therapy for Chronic Constipation: A Systematic Review of Controlled Clinical Trials. *Forsch-Komplementarmed*, 6(3): 149-151, 1999.

99. Emst, E., Matrai, A., Magyarosy, L., Leibermeister, R.G.A., Eck, M., Breu, M.C.: Massage Cause Changes in Blood Fluidity. *Physiotherapy*, 1(73): 43-45, 1987.

100. Ezov, B.B.: [Manual Therapy at the Earliest Steges of Cerebrovascular Disorders]. *Vopr. Ku rortol.Fizioter. Lech. Fiz. Kult.*, 4: 6-9, 1994.

101. Fahmy, 1., Kamal, A., Metwali, M., Rhodes, C., Mansour, R., Serour, G., Aboulghar, M.: Vigorous Prostatic Massage: A Simple Method to Retrieve Spermatozoa for Intracytoplasmic Sperm Injection in Psychogenic Anejaculation: Case Report. *Hum. Reprod.*, 14(8): 2050-2053, 1999.

102. Fakouri, C., Jones, P.: Relaxation: Slow Stroke Back Rub. *J. Gerontol. Nurs.*, 13: 32-35, 1987.

103. Falkenbach, A., Blumental, E., Buhring, M.: Course in Massage Therapy for Medical Students. *Med. Educ.*, 32(5): 514-516, 1998. ,

104. Fassbender, H.G., Wegner, K.: Morphologie und Pathogenese des Weichteilrheumatismus. *Z. Rheumafosch*, 32: 355-374, 1973.

105. Fattah MA, Hamdy B. Pulmonary functions of children with asthma improve following mas sage therapy. *J Altern Complement Med.* 2011 Nov;17(11):1065-8.

106. Fedorovsky, L.S., Menchukov, O.N., Makarenko, O.N., Murashova, N.N.: [Influence of Vibra tion Massage on Pulmonary Ventilation and Gas Exchange after the Abdominal Surgeries]. *Vopr. Kurortol. Fizioter. Lech. Fiz. Kult.*, 5: 45-46, 1982.

107. Fesmire, F.M.: Termination of Intractable Hiccups with Digital Rectal Massage. *Ann. Emerg. Med.*, 17(8): 872, 1988.

108. Field, T.M.: Massage Therapy Effects. *Am. Psych.*, 53(12): 1270-1281, 1988.

109. Field, T.M.: Massage Therapy for Infants and Children. *Devel. & Behav. Pediatrics*, 16(2): 105-111, 1998.

110. Field, T.M., Grizzle, N., Scafidi, F., Abrams, S., Richardson, S.: Massage Therapy for Infants of Depressed Mothers. *Infant Behavior & Dev.*, 19: 109-114, 1996.

111. Field., T.M., Henteleff, T., Hermandez-Reifi M., Martinez, E., Mavimda, K., Kuhn, C., Schanberg, S.: Children with Asthma have Improved Pulmonary Functions after Massage Therapy. *J. Pediatrics*, 132(5): 854-858, 1998.

112. Field. T.M., Hermandez-Reif, M., Seligman, S., Krasnegor, J ., Sunshine, W., Rivas-Chacon, R., Schanberg, S., Kuhn, C.: Juvenile Rheumatoid Arthritis: Benefits from Massage Therapy., *J. Pediatric Psych.*, 22(50): 607-617, 1997.

113. Field, T.M., Ironson, G., Scafidi, F., Nawrocki, T., Goncalves, A., Burman, L., Pickens, J., Fox, N., Schanburg, S., Kuhn, S.: Massage Therapy Reduces Anxiety and Enhances EEG Pattem of Alertness and Math Ciomputations. *Inter. Neuroscience,* 86: 197-205, 1996.

114. Findley, 1., Chamberlain, G.,: ABC of Labor Care. Relif of Pain. *BMJ*, 318(7 1 88): 927-930, 1999.

115. Flerova, S.A.: [*V.A. Manakov's System of Medical Massage*]. “Medgiz”, Moscow, 1956.

116. F okin, V.N.: [*Oriental and European Massage*]. “Fair”, Moscow, 1997.

117. Fukada, E.: *Electrical Phenomena in Biorheology*. Biorheology, 19(1-2): 15-27, 1982.

118. F ukada, E.: Piezoelectricity of Biological Materials. In: *Electronic Conduction and Mechanoelectrical Transduction in Biological Materials*: 125-157. Edited by B. Lipinski. “Marcel Dekker Inc.”, New York, 1982.

119. Fukada, E., Hara, K.: Piezoelectric Effect in Blood Vessel Walls. *J. Phys. Soc. Japan*, 26: 777-780, 1969.

120. Fukada, E., Ueda, H.: Piezoelectric Effect in Muscle. *Japan. J. Appl. Phys.*, 9: 844, 1970. "

121. Fukada, E., Yasuda, 1.: On th e Piezoelectric Effect of Bone. *J. Phys. Soc. Japan*, 12: 1158-1162, 1957.

122. Furukawa, T., Fukada, E.: Piezoelectric Relaxation in Poly-Benzyl-Glutamate. *J. Polym. Sci. Polym. Phys.*, 14: 1979-2110, 1971.

123. Fulton, J .F., Barron., D.H.: *T exbook of Physiology*, "W.B. Sanders, Co", Philadelphia, 1955.

124. Gam, A.N., Warming, S., Larsen, L.H, Jensen, B., Hoydalsmo, 0., Allon, 1., Andersen, B., Gotzsche, N.E., Petersen, M., Mathiesen, B.: Treatment of Myofascial Trigger-Points with Ultrasound Combined with Massage and Exersice. Pain, 77(1): 73-79, 1998.

125. Ganong, W.F.: *Review of Medical Physiology.* "Appleton & Lange", Norwalk, 1993.

126. Garner B, Phillips LJ, Schmidt HM, Markulev C, O'Connor J, Wood SJ, Berger GE, Burnett P, McGorry PD. Pilot study evaluating the effect of massage therapy on stress, anxiety and ag gression in a young adult psychiatric inpatient unit. *Aust NZ J Psychiatry.* 2008 May; 42(5):414-22.

127. Gataulin, R.R., Zripov, A.T.: The Role of Cytoskeleton in Mechanoreceptor Activity of Pacin ian Corpuscles. In: *Mechanoreceptors: Development, Structure and Function*: 209-211. Edited by E.P. Hnik, T. Soukup, R. Vejsada, J . Zelena. "Premium Press", New York, 1988.

128. Gehlsen, G.M., Ganion, L.R., Helllfst, R.: Fibroblast Responses to Variation in Soft Tissue Mobilization Pressure. *Med. Sci. Sports Med.*, 31(4): 531-535, 1999.

129. Geise, S.: Posterior lnterosseus Syndrome Resulting from Deep Tissue Massage. *Plast. Recon str. Surg.*, 102(5): 1778-1779, 1998.

130. Gellhorn, E.: The Physiological Basis of Neuromuscular Relaxation. *AMA. Arch. Internal Med.*, 102(Sept): 392-399, 1958.

131. Geneser, F.: *Texbook Of Histology*. "Munksgaard Lea & Febiger", Philadelphia, 1986.

132. Geranmayeh M, Rezaei Habibabadi Z, Fallahkish B, Farahani MA, Khakbazan Z, Mehran A. Reducing perineal trauma through perineal massage with vaseline in second stage of labor. *Arch Gynecol Obstet.* 2012 Jan;285(1):77-81

133. Glezer, 0., Dalicho, V.A.: *Segmentmassage.* Leipzig, 1955.

134. Goats, C.G.: Connective Tissue Massage. *Br. J. Sports Med.*, 25(3): 131-133, 1991.

135. Goats, C.G.: Massage - the Scientific Base of an Ancient Art: Part 1. The Techniques. *Br. J. Sports Med.*, 28(3): 149-152, 1994.

136. Goldberg, J ., Seaborne, D.E., Sullivan S.J., Leduc, B.E.: The Effect of Therapeutic Massage on H-Reflex Amplitude in Persons with a Spinal Cord Injury. *Phys. Ther.*, 74(8): 728-737, 1994.

137. Goldberg, J ., Sullivan, S.J., Seabome, D.E.: The Effect of Two Intensities of Massage of H-Reflex Amplitude. *Phys. Ther.*, 72(6): 449-457, 1992.

138. Golosova, L.O.: [Local Vibration Massage in the Treatment of Patients with Neurological Manifestations of Cervical Spondylosis]. *Vopr. Kurortol. Fiziother. Lech FIz Kult.*, 6: 14-16, 1983.

139. Granovskaya, P.B.: [*Reactive Changes in Peripheral Nervous System During Massage*]. "Nauka", Dnepropetrovsk, 1960.

140. Groer, M., Mazingo, J ., Droppleman, P., Davis, M., Jolly, M.l., Boyton, M., Davis, K., Key, S.: Measure of Salivary Secretory Immunoglobulin A and State Anxiety afier Nursing Back Rub. *Appl. Nurs. Res.*, 7(1): 2-6, 1994.

141. Gross, D., Williams, W.S.: Streaming Potentials and the Electromechanical Responce of Physiologically-Moist Bone. *J Biomechanics*, 15(4): 277-295, 1982.

142. Gross, D., Williams, W.S., Connor, J.A.: Theory of Electromechanical Effects in Nerve. *Cell. Mol. Neurobiol.*, 3(2): 89-111, 1983.
143. Guan Zheng, Zheng Guiqiu: The Effect of Massage on the Lefi Heart Functions in Patients of Coronary Heart Disease. *J. Trad. Chin. Med.*, 15(1): 59-62, 1995.
144. Gupta, S., Goswami, A., Sadhukhan, A.K., Mathur, D.N.: Comparative Study of Lactate Re moval in Short Term Massage of Extremities, Active Recovery and Passive Recovery Period afler Supramaximal Exercise Sessions, Intern. *J. Sports Med.*, 17: 106-110, 1996.
145. Gusarova, C.A., Kuznetsov, O.F., Gorbunov, F .E., Maslovskaya, S.G.: [Influence of Acupres sure and Classic Therapeutic Massage on Hemodynamic Parameters of patients who Suffered from Cerebral Transitory Ischemic Attaks]. *Vopr. Kurortol. Physiotherapy & Phys.* Ther., 5: 7-9, 1998.
146. Guzelsu, N.: Mechanoelectical Effect in Biological Systems. In: *Electronic Conduction and Mechanoelectrical Transduction in Biological Materials*: 201-281. Edited by B. Lipinski. "Marcel Dekker, Inc.", New York, 1982.
147. Guzzetta A, D'Acunto MG, Carotenuto M, Berardi N, Bancale A, Biagioni E, Boldrini A, Ghirri P, Maffei L, Cioni G. The effects of preterm infant massage on brain electrical activity. *Dev Med Child Neurol.* 2011 Sep;53 Suppl 4:46-51.
148. Hansen, T.l., Kristiansen, J.H.: Effect of Massage. Short-Wave Diathermy and Ultrasound upon 133xe Disapperance Rate from Muscle and Subcutaneous Tissue in the Himan Calf. *Scand. J. Rehab. Med.*, 5: 179-182, 1973.
149. Head, H.: On Disturbances of Sensation with Special Reference to the Pain of Visceral Dis ease. *Brain*, 16: 1-133, 1893.
150. Hedstomi, L.W., Newton, N.: Touch in Labor: A Comparision of Cultures and Eras. **Birth**, 13(3): 181-186,1986.
151. Helleday, U.: On myitis chronical (rheumatica) ett bidgrad till dess diagnostic och behandling. *Nord. Med. Ark.*, 8: 8, 1876.
152. Hennenfent, B.R., Feliciano, A.E.: Changes in White Blood Cell Counts in Men Undergoing Thrice-Weekly Prostatic Massage, Microbial Diagnosis and Antimicrobial Therapy for Genito urinary Complaints. *Br. J. Urol.*, 81(3): 370- 376, 1998. '
153. Herkovitz, S.: Shiatsu Massage-Induced Injury of the Median Recurrent Motor Branch. Muscle *Nerve,* 15(10): 1215, 1992.
154. Hernandez-Reif, M., Field, T., Hart, S.: Smoking Carvings are Reduced by Self-Massage. *Prev. Med.*, 28(1): 28-32, 1999.
155. Hemdl, E., von Mallinckrodt, G., Spilker, G., Schemeer, A.: [Long-Term Results Following Breast Augmentation]. *Handchir. Mikrochir. Plast. Chir.*, 16(2): 188-121, 1984.
156. Hopper, 1., Cohen, M.: Complementary Therapies and the Medical Profession: A Study of Medical Studets' Attitudes. *Alter. Ther. Health Med.*, 4(3): 68-73, 1998.
157. Hsu, C.Y., Huang, L.M., Lee, T.Y., Lin, T.Y., Lee, P.I., Chen, J.M.: Local Massage after Vaccination Enhances the Immunogenicity of Diphteria-Tetanus—Pertussis Vassine. *Pediatr. Infect. Dis. J.*, 14(7): 567-572, 1995.
158. Hudicka, 0., Brown, M.D.: Physical Forces and Angiogenesis. In: *Mechanoreception by Vascu lar Wall.* Edited by Rubanyi, G.M. "Futura Publishing Company Inc.", Mount Kisko, NY, 1983.
159. Iggo, A.: *The Peripheral Nervous System*. "Plenum Press", New York, 1974.
160. Intyre, A.K.: Perception of Vibration. *Australian Ass. Neurologists*, 3: 71-76, Mellboume, 1975.
161. Ironson, C., Field, T., Scafidi, F., Hashimomoto, M., Kumar, M., Kumar, A., Proce, A., Concalves, A., Burman, L., Tetenman, C., Patarca, R., Fletcher, M.A.: Massage Therapy is

Associated with Enhancement of the Immune System's Cytotoxic Capacity. Intern. *J. Neuro science*, 84: 205-217, 1996.

162. Isaev, Y.A.: [*Segment-Reflex and Acupressure Massage in the Clinical Practice*]. "Zdorovie", Kiev, 1993.

163. Jabre JF. "Nerve rubbing" in the symptomatic treatment of ulnar nerve paresthesiae. *Muscle Nerve*. 1994 Oct;17(10):1237

164. Jacobs, M.: Massage for the Relief of Pain: Anatomical and Physiological Considerations. *Phys.Ther. Rev.*, 40: 93-98, 1960.

165. Jacobson, E.: Variation of Blood Pressure with Skeletal Muscle Tension and Relaxation. *Ann. Internal Med.*, 12: 1194—1212,1939.

166. Jacobson, E.: Variation of Blood Pressure with Skeletal Muscle Tension and Relaxation. *Ann. Internal Med.*, 13: 1619-1625, 1940.

167. Jain, M.K., Berg, R.A., Tandon, G.P.: Mechanical Stress and Cellular Metabolism in Living Soft Tissue Composites. *Biomaterials*, 11: 465-471, 1990.

168. Jemmon, J., Magloir, K.: Academic Stress. Social Support and Secretory Immunoglobulin A. *Persp. In Soc. Psych.*, 55: 803-810, 1988.

169. Jemmon, J ., McC1e1land, D.: Secretory IgA as a Measure of Resistance to Infectious Disease. *Behav. Med.*, 15: 63-70, 1989.

170. Jonhagen S., Ackermann P., Eriksson T., Saartok T., Renstrom P.A.F. Sports Massage After Eccentric Exercise. *Am J Sports Med*, September 2004 32:1499-1503; 2004.

171. Jungmann, H.: Untersuchungen zur Direktwirkimg Von Muskel-und Bindegewebsmassagen. *Zeitschrift Physikalische Medizin*, 2: 371, 1971.

172. Kaada, B., Torrsteinbo, 0.: Increase of Plasma Betta-Endorphins in Connective Tissue Mas sage.*General Pharmacology*, 20: 487-489, 1989.

173. Kaaja, R., Tiula, E.: Manual Lymph Drainage in Nephrotic Syndrome during Pregnancy. *Lan cet*, Oct.: 990, 1989.

174. Kallistov, I.P.: [*Sports Massage*]. "Medicina", Leningrad, 1930.

175. Kamenetz, H.L.: History of Masssage: 3-37. In: Massage, *Manipulation and Traction*. Edited by S. Licht. "R.F. Kriger Publ. Co.", New York, 1976. '

176. Kamenetz, H.L. (1985). Quoted in: Field, T.M.: Massage Therapy Effects. *Am. Psych.*, 53(12): 1270-1281,1988.

177. Kametani, H., Sato, A., Sato, Y., Simpson, A.: Neural Mechanisms of Reflex facilitation and Inhibition of Gstric Motility to Stimulation of Various Skin Areas in Rats. *J Physiol*, 294: 407-418, 1979.

178. Kamranov, A.Y., Belaya, N.A.: [Classical and Segment-Reflex Massage in the Complex Treat ment of Patients with Ostheoarthritis]. *Vopr. Kurortol. Fizioter. Lech. Fiz. Kult.*, 1: 17-20, 1985.

179. Kapandji, l.A.: The Physiology of the Joints., "Livingstone, Ltd", London, 1970. -

180. Kellogg, J.: The Home Handbook of Domestic Hygiene and Rational Medicine. "International Pract. Society", London, 1900.

181. Kerr, H.D.: Ureteral Stent Displacement Associated with Deep Massage., *WMJ,* 96(12): 57-58, 1997.

182. Kim SJ, Kwon OY, Yi CH. Effects of manual lymph drainage on cardiac autonomic tone in healthy subjects. *Int J Neurosci*. 2009;119(8):1105-17.

183. Kimura Y, Ge HY, Zhang Y, Kimura M, Sumikura H, Arendt-Nielsen L. Evaluation of sympa thetic vasoconstrictor response following nociceptive stimulation of latent myofascial trigger points in humans. *Acta Physiol (Oxf)*. 2009 Aug;196(4):411-7

184. Kirchberg, F.: *Handbuch der Massage und Heilgymnastik*. Leipzig, 1926.

185. Kiss, F., Szentagothai, J.: *Atlas Anatomiae Corporis Humani*. "Medicina", Budapest, 1960.

186. Kohlrausch, H.: *Reflexzonen massage in Muskulatur und Bindegewebe.* "Hippokrates Verl.", Stuttgart, 1955.

187. Koizumi, K., Sato, A., Terui, N.: Role of Somatic Afferents in Autonomic System Control of the Intestinal Motility. *Brain Research,* 182: 85-97, 1980.

188. Komuro, 1., Katoh, Y., Kaida, T., Shibazaki, Y., Kurabayashi, M., Hoh, E., Takaku, F., Yazaki, Y.: Mechanical Loading Stimulates Cell Hypertrophy and Specific Gene Expression in Cultured Rat Cardiac Myocytes. *J. Biol. Chem.*, 266(2): 1265-1268.

189. Kordez, I.K., Uibe, P., Idabich, B.: *Massage.* "Medicina", Moscow, 1983.

190. Kotwica, S., Split, W., Rog-Malinowski, M., Gredziak, B.: [Spa Treatment of Shoulder Pain at Swieradow]. *Neurol. Neurochir. Pol.*, 10(5): 715-717, 1976.

191. Kovacs, R.: *Electrotherapy and Light Therapy with Essentials of Hydrotherapy and Mechanotherapy.* "Lea & Febiger", Philadelphia, 1945.

192. Kovanov, V.V., Travin, A.A.: [*Surgical Anatomy of Human Extremities*]. "Medicina", Moscow, 1983.

193. Kramarenko, V.K.: [*Sports Massage*]. "Gosmedizdat", Kiev, 1953.

194. Kreymer, A.Y.: [*Vibration Massage at Diseases of the Nervous System*]. "Tomsk University", Tomsk, 1987.

195. Krilov, V.N., talishev, F.M., Burovik, A.N.: [The Use of Restorative Massage in the Training of High Level Bsketball Players]. *Soviet Sports Rev.*, 20: 7-9, 1985.

196. Krogh, A.: *The Anatomy and Physiology of Caplillaries.* "Yale University Press", New Haven, 1929.

197. Krusen, F.N., Kottke, F.J., Ellwood, P.M.: *Handbook of Physical Medicine and Rehabilitation,* "WB. Saunders Co.", Philadelphia, 1965.

198. Kuhn, C.M., Schanberg, S.M., Field, T., Symansky, R., Zimmerman, E., Scafidi, F., Roberts, J.: Tactile-Kinesthetic Stimulation Effects on Sympathetic and Adrenocortical Function in Pretenn Infants., *J. of Pediatr.*, 119(3): 434-440, 1991.

199. Kuhnke, E.: Die physiologischen Grundlagen der mannuellen lymphdrainage. *Physiotherapie,* 66: 12, 1975.

200. Kukulka, C.G., Beckman, S.M., Holte, J.B., Hoppenwoith, P.K.: Effect of Intermittent Tendon Pressure on Alpha Motoneuron Excitability. *Phys. Ther.*, 66(7): 1091-1094, 1986.

201. Kukulka, C.G., Fellows, W.A., Oehlertz, J .E., Vanderwilt, S.G.: Effect of Tendon Pressure on Alpa-Motoneuron Excitability. *Phys. Ther.*, 65(5): 595-600, 1985.

202. Kunichev, L.A.: [*Massage Therapy*], "Medicina", Leningrad, 1985.

203. Kuprivan, W.: *Physical Therapy for Sports.* "W.B. Sanders Co", Philadelphia, 1995.

204. Kurosawa, M., Lundenberg, T., Agren, G., Lund., 1., Uvas-Meberg, K.: Massage-Like Stroking of the Abdomen Lowers Blood Pressure in Anesthetized Rats: Influence of Oxytocin. *J. Autonomic. Nerv. Syst.*, 56: 26-30, 1995. '

205. Kurtz, I.: *Textbook of Dr. Vodder 's Manual Lymph Drainage.* Vol. 3. "HAUG", Heidenberg, 1990.

206. Kutz, W., Wittlinger, B.S., Limanovitch, Y.L., Romanoff, H., Preifer,tY., Tal, E., Sulman, F.G.: Elfect of Manual Lymph Drainage Massage on Urinary Excretion of Neurohormones and Minerals in Chronic Lymphedema. *Angiology*, 29: 764-772, 1978.

207. Kuznetsov, O.F.: [*Effectiveness of New Intensive Methods of Massage and Physical Therapy in the Rehabilitation Patients with Chronic Pulmonary Disorders*]. "Medicina", Moscow, 1987 .

208. Kuznetsov, O.F.: [Massage in the Treatment Patients with Chronic Pneumonia]. *Vopr. Kurortol. Fizioter. Lech. Fiz. Kult.*, 1: 40-42, 1978.

208. Kuznetsov, O.F., Kuznetsova, B.A.: [Mechanism of Therapeutic Effects of Classical and

Assymetric Reflex Massage in Cases of Chronic Pulmonary Disorders]. *Vopr. Kurortol. Fiziother. Lech. Fiz. Kult.*, 3: 52-54, 1981.

209. Kuznetsov, O.F., Makarova, M.P., Markina, L.P.: [Therapeutic Influence of Classical Massage on Patients with Chronic Salpingo-Oophoritis]. *Vopr. Kurortol. Fizioter. Lech Fiz. Cult.*, 2: 20-23, 1998.

210. Kuznetsov, O.F., Tsarkava, L.N., Popkovskaya, E.I., Yakubson, I.M.: [Effect of Massage on the Acid-Base Balance in Patients with Chronic Pneumonia]. *Vopr. Kurortol. Fizioter. Lech. Fiz. Kult.*,4: 15-20, 1979.

211. Kuznik, B.I., Vasiliev, N.B., Tsibnikov, N.N.: [*Immunogenesis, Metabolism and Immunity*]. "Medicina", Moscow, 1989.

212. Labrecque, M., Eason, E., Marcoux, S., Lemiex, F., Pinault, J.J ., Feldma, P., Laperriere, L.: Randomized Controlled Trial of Prevention of Perineal Trauma by Perineal Massage During Pregnancy. *Am. J. Obstet. Gynecol.*, 180(3 Pt 1): 593-600, 1999.

213. Ladd., M.P., Kooke, F.J., Blanchard, R.S.: Studies of the Effect of Massage on the Flow of Lymph from the Foreleg of the Dog. *Arch. Phys. Med.*, 33: 604-612, 1952.

214. Lather, 1., Bevan, J .A.: Stretch-Dependence Myogenic Tone in Isolated Blood Vessel. In: *Mechanoreception by Vascular Wall*. Edited by Rubanyi, G.M. "Futura Publishing Company, Inc." Mount Kisko, NY, 1983.

215. Lakin, G.F.: *Biomatria*, "Medicina", Moscow, 1990.

216. Lämås K, Lindholm L, Stenlund H, Engström B, Jacobsson C. Effects of abdominal massage in management of constipation--a randomized controlled trial. *Int J Nurs Stud*. 2009 Jun; 46(6):759-67.

217. Lapinski, B.: Biological Significance of Piezoelectricity in Relation to Acupuncture, Hatha Yoga, Osteopathic Medicine and Action of Air Ions. *Med. Hypotheses*, 3(1): 9-12, 1977.

218. Larsen, J-H.: Infants' Colic and Belly Massage. *The Practitioner*, 234(l487): 396-397, 1990.

219. Lassar, 0.: Ueber Oedem und lymphostrom bei der Entzuendung. *Virch. Arch.*, 69: 518, 1877.

220. Lee, R.C., Grodzinsky, A.J., Glimcher, N.J.: The Electromechanics of Normal and Chemically Modified Articular Cartilage. In: *Electrical Properties of Bone and Cartilage*. Edited by: Brighton, C.T., Black, J . and Pollack, S.R. " Gnme & Stratton", New York, 1979.

221. Leone, J .A., Kukulka, C.G.: Elfect of Tendon Pressure on Alpha Motoneuron Exitability in Patients with Stroke. *Phys. Ther.*, 68(4): 475-480, 1988.

222. LeRoy, R.: Le vie du tissu conjonctif et sa defense par le massage. *Rev. de Me. Paris.*, 58: 212, 1941.

223. Leung, D.Y.M., Gladov, S., Mathews, M.B.: Cyclic Stretching Stimulates Synthesis of Martix Components by Arterial Smooth Muscle in Vitro. *Science*, 191: 475-477, 1976.

224. Limansky Y.P., Macheret, E.L., Vashenko, E.A., Chebotareva, L.L., Samosyuk, I.Z.: [*Neuro surgical Syndromes of Sponaylosis*]. "Zdorovie", Kiev, 1988.

225. Linde, B.: Dissotiation of Insuline Absorption and Blood Flow During Massage of a Subcuta neous Injection Site. *Diabetes Care.*, 9(6): 570-574, 1986.

226. Li, Z.M.: 235 Cases of Frozen Shoulder Treated by Manipulation and Massage. *.J Tradit. Chin. Med.*, 4: 213-215, 1884.

227. Liu, B.: Extracranial Intemal Carotid Artery Dissection Secondary to Neck Massage. Vizual ization of Mural Hematoma by MRI. *Kao Hsiung I Hsueh Ko Hsueh Tsa Chin.*, 9(5): 322- 327, 1993.

228. Livingston, W.K.: The Vicious Cicle of Causalgia. *Ann. N Y Acad. Sci.*, 50: 247-258, 1948.

229. Longworth, J.C.D.: Psychophysiological effects of Slow Stroke Massage in Norrnotensive Females. *Advan. in Nurs. Scien.*, July: 44-61, 1982.

230. Lucas-Championniere, J.: *Traitement des Fractures par le Massage et la Mobilization*. Paris.

1985.
231. Mackenzie, C.L., Iberall, T.: *The Grasping Hand.* "North Holland", Amsterdam, 1994.
232. Makarova, M.P., Kuznetsov, O.F., Markina, L.P., Gusarova, S.A., Styajkina, E.M.: [Influence of Massage Treatment on Muscular System and Blood Coagulative System of patients with Salpingo-Oophoritis]. *Vopr. Kurortol., Fiziother. Lech Fiz. Kult.*, 6: 45-48, 1998.
233. Malaquin-Pavan, E.: [Therapeutic Benefits of Touch-Massage in the Overall Management of Demented Eldery]. *Rech-Soins Infirm*, Jun(49): 11-66, 1977.
234. Manella C, Backus D. Gait characteristics, range of motion, and spasticity changes in response to massage in a person with incomplete spinal cord injury: case report. *Int J Ther Massage Bodywork.* 2011 Mar 30;4(1):28-39.
235. Maniotis, A.J., Chen, C.s., Ingber, D.E.: Demonstration of Mechanical Connections Between lntegrins, Cytoskeletal Filaments, and Nucleoplasm that Stabilize Nuclear Structure. *Proc. Natl. Acad. Sci. USA*, 94(3): 849-854, 1997.
236. Marin, I, Lepresle, C., Mechet, M.A., Debesse, B.: [Postoperative Pain after Thoracotomy. A Study of 116 patients]. *Rev. Mal. Respir.*, 8(2): 213-218, 1991.
237. Matev, I., Bankov, S.: *Rehabilitation of the Injuried Hand.* "Medcina e Fizcultura", Sofia, 1981.
238. Mattem, A.V.: Gastro-Duodenal ULcer and Its Non-Surgical Treatmen. *JAOA*, Jan: 188-191, 1937.
239. Matveeva, L.A., Kuzmenko, O.V., Kirilova, G.N.: [Thermal Vibromassage in the Threatment of Dyskinesia of the Biliary Tract]. *Vopr. Kurortol. Fizioter. Lech. Fiz.. Kult.*, 1: 12-14, 1997.
240. Majakovsky, D.N.: [*Chronic Inflammation*]. "Medicina", Moscow, 1991.
241. McKechnie, A.A., Wilson, F., Wanson, N., Scott, D.: Anxiety States: A Preliminary Report on the Value of Connective Tissue Massage. *J. Psychosom. Res.*, 27(2): 125-129, 1983.
242. McKeon, F.D., Krischner, M.W., Caput, D.: Homologies in Both Primary and Secondary Struc ture Between Nuclear Envelope and Intermediate Filament Proteins. *Nature*, 319: 463-468, 1986.
243. Medvedev, E.A.: [Case of Acute Unilateral Neurosensory Hearing Loss Caused by Massage of Trapezius Muscle]. *Vestn. 0torinolaringol.*, 3: 38-39, 1994.
244. Mennell, J .B.: *Physical treatment by Movement, Manipulation and Massage.* "The Blakiston Co."Philadelphia, 1945.
245. *Merck Manual.* "Merck & co", Rahway, 1992.
246. Mezlack, R., Schecter, B.: *Itch and Vibration. Science*, 147(Feb): 1047-1048, 1965.
247. Mezlack, R., Wall, P.: *Pain Mechanism: A New Theory. Science*, 150(Nov): 971-979, 1965.
248. Mezlack, R., Wall, P.: *The Chalange of Pain.* "Penguin", NY, 1989.
249. Mikhail, A.: Renal Artery Embolization Alter Back Massage in a Patient with Aortic Occlu sion. *Nephrol. Dial. Transpl.*, 12(4): 797-798, 1997.
250. Mislin, H.: *Lymphgefassmotorik. Materials of the Congress of the Society for Dr. Vodder 's Manual Lymph Drainage.* Hamburg, 1972.
251. Mitz, V.: [Fasciitis Following Face Lift]. Ann. Chir. Plast. Esthet., 42(6): 603-607, 1997.
252. Moberg, E.: Objective Methods for Determining the Functional Value of Sensibility in the Hand. *J. Bone Joint Surg.*, 40-B: 454-476, 1958.
253. Mogutaev, Y.B.: [Treatment Sciatica Injuries by Vibration Massage]: 15-20. In: [*Vibration Massage in Experimental and Clinical Practice*]. "Tomsk University", Tomsk, 1980.
254. Moraska A., Chandler C. Changes in Psychological Parameters in Patients with Tension-type Headache Following Massage Therapy: A Pilot Study. *J Man Manip Ther.* 2009; 17(2): 86–94.
255. Morelli, M., Seabome, D.E., Sullivan S.J.: H—Reflex Modulation during Manual Muscle Mas sage of Human Triceps Surae. *Arch. Phys. Med. Rehab.* 72: 915-919, 1991.

256. Mortazavi SH, Khaki S, Moradi R, Heidari K, Vasegh Rahimparvar SF. Effects of massage therapy and presence of attendant on pain, anxiety and satisfaction during labor. *Arch Gynecol Obstet.* 2012 Jan 21.

257. Mortimer, P.S., Simmonds, R., Rezvani, M., Robbins, M., Hopewell, J .W., Ryan, T.J.: The Measurement of Skin Lymph Flow by Isotope Clearance-Reliability, Reproductibility, Injec tion Dynamics, and the Effect of Massage. *J. Invest. Dermatol.*, 95(6): 677-682, 1990.

258. Mosengel, V.: Beeinflussung der corenaren Durchblungsstorung von der headschen zone. *Arch. Clin. Chir.*, 551: 19-20, 1876.

259. Moshkov, V.N.: [*Physical Therapy for the Treatment of Hypertension*]. "Medicina", Moscow, 1950.

260. Moshkov, V.K.: [*Physical Therapy for the Inner Organs Disorders*]. "Medicina", Moscow, 1982.

261. Mumm, A.N.: Zoster afier Shiatsu-Massage. *Lancet*, 341(8842): 447, 1993.

262. Myamoto, S., Okamoto, M ., Hopi, G.: Clinical Application of Tonia Vibration Reflex Stimuli. *Tonia Vibr. Reflex.*, 121-137, 1975.

263. Myers, E.R., Armstrong, C.G., Mow, V.C.: Swelling Pressure and Collegen Tension. In: *Connective Tissue Matrix*. Edited by D.W. Hukins. "Verlag Chemie", Florida, 1984.

264. Nagrale AV, Herd CR, Ganvir S, Ramteke G. Cyriax physiotherapy versus phonophoresis with supervised exercise in subjects with lateral epicondylalgia: a randomized clinical trial. *J Man Manip Ther.* 2009;17(3):171-8.

265. Nordshow, M., Bierman, W.: The Influence of Manual Massage on Muscle Relaxation: Effect on Trunk Flexion *J. Am. Phys. Ther. Assoc.*, 42910): 653-657, 1962.

266. Odeh, M., Bassan, H., Oliven, A.: Termination of Intractable Hiccups with Digital Rectal Massage. *J. Intern. Med.*, 227(2): 145-146, 1990.

267. Oliveira DS, Hachul H, Goto V, Tufik S, Bittencourt LR. Effect of therapeutic massage on insomnia and climacteric symptoms in postmenopausal women. *Climacteric*. 2012 Feb; 15(1):21-9.

268. Ouchi Y, Kanno T, Okada H, Yoshikawa E, Shinke T, Nagasawa S, Minoda K, Doi H. Changes in cerebral blood flow under the prone condition with and without massage. *Neurosci Lett.* 2006 Oct 23; 407(2):131-5.

269. Palastanga, N., Field, D., Soames, R.: *Anatomy of Human Movements*. "Heinemann Medical Books", Oxford, 1989.

270. Patino, O., Novick, C., Merlo, A., Benaim, F.: Massage in Hypertrophic Scars. *J. Burn. Care Rehabil.*, 20(3): 268-271, 1999.

271. Pedini, G., Zaietta, P.: [On some Aspects of Activation of Tissue Lypolysis by Mechanical Fac tors]. *Minerva Med.*, 66(7): 318-323, 1975.

272. Perlman AI, Ali A, Njike VY, Hom D, Davidi A, Gould-Fogerite S, Milak C, Katz DL. Massage therapy for osteoarthritis of the knee: a randomized dose-finding trial. *PLoS One.* 2012;7(2):e30248.

273. Peterrnans, J., Zicot, M: [Musculo-Venous Pump in the Elderly]. *J. Ma. Vasc.*, 19(2): 115-118, 1994.

274. Petrov, P.V., Khaitov, P.M., Manko, V.M., Michailova, A.A.: [*Control and Regulation of Immune Response*]. "Nauka", Leningrad, 1981.

275. Pham, Q.T., Peslin, R., Puchelle, E., Salmon, D., Caraux, G., Benis, A.M.: Respiratory Function and Reological Status of Bronchial Secretions Collected by Spontaneous Expectoration and afier Physiotherapy. *Bull. Physiopathol Respir.*, 9: 292, 1973.

276. Pick, F.: *Verhandlungen des Kongressesfuer Innere Medizine. XX*, Weibaden.

277. Popelansky, Y.Y., Ivanichev, G.: [*Manual Therapy of Local Muscular Hypertonuses. PIR Meth od*]. "Kazan Medical School", Kazan, 1984.
278. Popelansky, Y.Y., Zaslavsky, E.S., Veselovsky, V.P.: [Medico-Social Significance, Etiology, Pathogenesis, and Diagnosis of Extra-Articular Afiections of the Extremities and Dorsum Soft Tissues]. *Vopr. Reumatologii*, 3: 38-43, 1976.
279. Posadzki P, Parekh-Bhurke S. Incorporation of massage into psychotherapy: an integrative and conjoint approach. *Chin J Integr Med*. 2011 Feb;17(2):154-8
280. Potapov, I.A., Avishev, T.M.: [Influence of Massage on Formation and Transport of Lymph]. *Vopr.Kurortol. Fizioter. Lech. Fiz. Kult.*, 5: 44-47, 1989.
281. Predel, K.: Physical Therapy in Gastoenterology. *Z. Gesamte. Inn. Med.*, 42(4): 112-114, 1987.
282. Pruden, B.: *Pain Erasure: The Bonnie Pruden Way*. "M. Evans & Co", New York, 1980. '
283. Pugachev, I.V.: [*Physiological Explanation of Vibration Massage*], Perm, 1965.
284. Putt, S.C., Weinsteinl, L., Dzindolet, M.T.: A Case Study: Massage, Relaxation and Reward for Treatment of Alopecia Areata. *Psychological Reports,* 74: 1315-1318, 1994.
285. Rabischong, P.: L'Innervation propprioceptive des muscles lumbricaux de la main chez l'homme.. *Rev. Chir. Orthop.*, 48: 234-246, 1967.
286. Raviv G, Shefi S, Nizani D, Achiron A. Effect of craniosacral therapy on lower urinary tract signs and symptoms in multiple sclerosis. *Complement Ther Clin Pract*. 2009 May;15(2):72-5.
287. Richards, A.: Hands on Help. *Nurs. Times*, 94(32): 69-75, 1998.
288. Richards, K.C.: Effect of a Back Massage and Relaxation Intervention on Sleep in Critically Ill Patients. *Am. J. Critical Care,* 7(4): 288-299, 1998.
289. Rodenburg, J.B., Steenbeek, D., Schiereck, P., Bar, P.R.: Warm-up, Stretching and Massage Diminish Harmful Effects of Eccentric Exercises. *Intern. J. Sports Med*, 15: 414-419, 1994.
290. Roh YS, Cho H, Oh JO, Yoon CJ. Effects of skin rehabilitation massage therapy on pruritus, skin status, and depression in burn survivors.*Taehan Kanho Hakhoe Chi*.2007 Mar:37(2):221-226.
291. Rothman, S.: *Physiology and Biochemistry of the Skin*. "University of Chicago Press", Chi cago, 1954.
292. Sarkisov-Sirasini, I.M.: [*Sports Massage*], "Fizcultura i Sport", Moscow, 1957.
293. Sato, A., Sato, Y., Shimada, F., Torigeta, Y.: Changes in Gastric Motility Produced by Nocicep tive Stimulation of the Skin in Rats. *Brain Research,* 87, 151-159, 1975.
294. Sato, Y., Terui, N.: Changes in Duodenal Motility Produced by Noxious Mechanical Stimula tion of the Skin in Rats. *Neuroscience*, 2: 189-193, 1976.
295. Schachner, L., Field, T., Hemandez-Raif, M., Duarte, A.M., Krasnegor, J .: Atopic Dermatitis Symptom Decreased in Children Following Massage Therapy. *Pediatric Dermatology*, 15(5): 390-395, 1998.
296. Schlesinger, G.: *Der mechanische Aufban der kiinstlichen Glieder. Ersatzylieder und Arbeit shilfen*. "Spriger Verlag", Berlin, 1919.
297. Sherbak, A.E.: [Further Experimental Studies of Physiological Effects of Mechnical Oscilla tions]. *Psychology Review*, 9: 641-649 and 10: 722-733, 1903. 1
298. Sherbak, A.E.: [*Questions of the Physiological Eflect of Reflex Massage*]. 'Medicina", Mos cow, 1936.
299. Shor-Posner G, Hernandez-Reif M, Miguez MJ, Fletcher M, Quintero N, Baez J, Perez-Then E, Soto S, Mendoza R, Castillo R, Zhang G. Impact of a massage therapy clinical trial on im mune status in young Dominican children infected with HIV-1. *J Altern Complement Med*. 2006 Jul-Aug;12(6):511-6.

300. Shipman, M.K., Boniface, D.R., Teffi, M.E., McCloghry, F.: Antenatal Perineal Massage and Subsequent Perineal Outcomes: A Randomised Controlled Trial. *Br. J. Obstet. Gynecol.*, 104(Jul): 787-791, 1997.
331. Shirinsky, V.P., Antonov, A.S., Birukov, K.G., Sobolevsky, A.V., Romanov, Y.A., Kabaeva, N.V., Antonova, G.N., Smirnov, V.N.: Mechano-Chemical Control of Human Endothelium Orientationand Size. *J. Cell Biol.*, 109, 331-339, 1989.
332. Shamos, M.H., Lavine, L.S.: Piezoelecticity as a Fundamental Property of Biological Tissues. *Nature*, 213: 267-269, 1967.
333. Shtemgertz, A.E.: [*Physical Therapy and Massage at Traumas and Disorders of Peripheral Nervous System of Children*]. "Zdorovie", Kiev, 1989.
334. Shtemgertz, A.E., Belaya, N.A.: [*Massage for Adults and Children*]. "Zdorovie", Kiev, 1992.
335. Sirotkina, A.V.: [*Eflect of Massage at Traumas and palsy of Dififerent Etiology*]. 'Medicina", Moscow, 1964.
336. Sister Angela, Miller, L.E.: Helping the Breast-Feeding Mother. *Am. J. Nurs.*, 72(8): 1420-1423, 1972.
337. Sister Elizabeth: Sensory Stimulation Techniques. *Am. J. Nursing*, 6692): 281-286, 1966.
338. Scholtz, H.G.: *Physikalish-diatetische Therapie*. "George Thieme", Leipzig, 1951. ~
339. Scott, M.G.: *Analysis of Human Motion*. "Appleton-Century-Crotts", New York, 1963.
340. Sahin, A., Ozen, H., Balbay, D., Bircan, K., Koray, Z., Karaagaoglu, E.., Remzi, D.: [Effect of Prostatic Massage on Serum levels of Prostatic Acid Phosphatase and Specific Antigen]. *Bull. Cancer*, 79(11): 1097-1100, 1992.
341. Smith, L.K., Weiss, E.L., Donlehmkuhl, L.: *Clinical Kinesiology.* "F.A. Davis Company", Philadelphia, 1996.
342. Smith, L.L., Keating, M.N., I-Iolbert, D., Spratt, D.S., McCammon, M.R., Smith, S.S., Israel, R.G.: The Effect of Athletic Massage of Delaed Onset Muscle Soreness. Creatine Kinase and Neutrophil Count: Preliminary report. *J. Orthp. Sports Phys. Ther.*, 19(2): 93-99, 1994.
343. Snow, M.L.: *Mechanical Vibration. Its Physiological Application in Therapeutics*. New York, 1917.
344. Sommer, J .: Zur Frage der Einwirkimg von mechanischen Schwingungen auf den Eigereflexapparat des menschen. *Luftjhart Med.*, 4: 292-293, 1940.
345. Somjen, D., Binderman, I., Berger, E., Harell, A.: Bone Remodeling Induced by Physical Stress in Protoglandin E2 Mediated. *Biochim. Biophys. Acta.*, 627: 91-100, 1980.
346. Starling, E.H.: The Influence of Mechanical Factors on Lymph Production. *J. Physiology*, 16: 224,1894.
347. Steindler, A.: *Kinesiology of the Human Hand*. "Ch. Thomas", Springfield, 1964.
348. Stillerman, E.: *Mother Massage*. "Delta Book Rublishing", New York, 1992.
349. Stoma, M.F.: [Vibration massage as a Test for the Defmition of Different Degree Muscles Endurance]. In: *Publications of Leningrad Medical Institute*, 78: 151-156, 1964.
350. Straborsky, N.K., 1887. Quoted fiom: Shtemgertz, A.E., Belaya, N.A.: *[Massage for Adults and Children*]. "Zdorovie", Kiev, 1992.
351. Sucharev, V.I., Etingen, B.Z., Zastenker, F.S., lofma, O.S., Bogdanovich, L.I., Krilov, N.P., Sultaton, A.A.: *Physiotherapy, Massage and Physical Therapy.* "Medicina", Moscow, 1965.
352. Sullivan, S.J., Blumberg, J ., Lachowicz, C., Raymond, D.: Does Massage Decrease Laryngeal Tension in a Subject with Complete Tetraplegia. *Perception & Motor Skills,* 64: 169-170, 1997.
353. Sullivan, S.J., Williams, R.T., Seaborne, D.E., Morelli, M.: Effects of Massage on Alpha Motoneurons Excitability. *Phys. Ther.*, 71(8): 555-560, 1991.

354. Sunderland, S.: The Nerve Lesion of the Carpal Tunnel Syndrome. *J. Neurol. Neurosurg. Psychiatry*, 39: 615-626, 1976.
355. Swedborg, 1.: Effectiveness of Combined Methods of Physiotherapy for Post-Mastectomy Lymphedema. Scana'. *J. Rehab. Med.*, 12(2): 77-85, 1980.
356. Tachi, J ., Amino, N., Myai, K.: Massage Therapy on Neck: A Contributing Factor for Destructive Thyrotoxycosis ? *Thyrology*, 2(1): 25-27, 1990.
357. Teirich-Lebe, H.: *Grundriss der Bindegewebsmassage*. "Fischer", Stutgart, 1960.
358. Thomsen, J .R., Koltai, P.J.: Sternomastoid Tumor of Infancy. *Ann. Otol Rhinol. Laryngol*, 98 (12 Pt 1): 955-959, 1989.
359. Tichy, H., Seide, K.: *Beitrage Zur Rheumatologie*. Berlin, 1969.
360. Tiidus, P.M., Shoemaker, J.K.: Etfeleurage Massage, Muscle Blood Flow and Long Term Postexercise Strength Recovery. *Intern. J Sports Med*, 16: 475-483, 1995.
361. Travell, J .G., Simons, D.G.: *Myofascial Pain and Dysfunction. The Trigger Points Manual*. "Williams & Wilkins, Baltimore, 1983.
362. Troisier, 0.: [Tennis Elbow]. *Rev. Prat.*, 41(18): 1651-1655, 1991.
363. Trubetskoy, V.S., Whiteman, K.R., Torchilin, V.P., Wolf, G.L.: Massage-Induced Release of Subcutaneously Injected Liposome-Encapsulated Drugs to the Blood. *J. Controlled Release*, 50:13-19, 1998.
364. Turchaninov, R..: *Medical Massage*. "Aesculapius Books", Phoenix, 1998.
365. Turin, A.M.: [*Traditional and Nontraditional Massage*]. "Iscusstvo-CPB", St. Petersburg, 1992.
366. Tumer, G.: [Percussion as a Method of Stimulation of fracture and Pseudoarthrosis Healing]. *Russki Vrach*, 15: 8-13, 1908.
367. Tumer, R.A., Altemus, M., Enos, T., Cooper, B., McGuinness, T.: Preliminary Research on Plasma Oxytocin in Normal Cycling Women: Investigating Emotion and Interpersonal Distress. *Psychiatry*, 62(2): 97-113, 1999.
368. Ueda, W., Katatoka, Y., Sagara, Y.: Effect of Gentle Massage on Regression of Sensory Analgesia During Epidural Block. *Anesth. Analog.*, 76(4): 783-785, 1993.
369. Valculenko, L.A.: [The Use of Deep Reflex-Muscular massage in Combined Treatment of Neurological Disorders in Cervical Spondylosis]. *Vopr. Kurortol. Fizioter.Lech Fiz. Kult.*, 5: 26-29, 1980.
370. Valiani M, Ghasemi N, Bahadoran P, Heshmat R. The effects of massage therapy on dysmenorrhea caused by endometriosis. *Iran J Nurs Midwifery Res*. 2010 Fall;15(4):167-71.
371. Van Hove, E.: Prevention of Trombophlebitis in Spinal Injury Patients. *Paraplegia*, 1693): 332-335, 1978.
372. Vasichkin, V.I.: *[Massage Manual*]. "Medicina", Leningrad, 1991.
373. Vasilescu, D., Comillon, R., Mallet, G.: Piezoelectric Resonances in Aminoacids. *Nature*, 225: 635, 1970.
374. Vega J.A., García-Suárez O., Montaño J.A., Pardo B., Cobo J.M. The Meissner and Pacinian sensory corpuscles revisited new data from the last decade. *Microsc Res Tech.* 2009 Apr;72(4):299-309.
375. Verbov, A.F.: [*Basic Principles of Medical Massage*]. "Medicina", Moscow, 1966.
376. Verhoef, M.J., Page, S.A.: Physician' Perspectives of Massage Therapy. *Canadian Fam. Physician*, 44: 1018-1024, 1998.
377. Vodder, E.: *Le drainage lymphtique, une npovelle methods therapeutique*. "Sante pour tous", 1936.
378. Vogler, P., Krauss, H.: *Periostbehandlung*. Leipzig, 1953.
379. Vogler, P., Krauss, H.: *Periostbehandlung, Kolonbehandlung*. Leipzig, 1975.

380. Von Mosengeil: Uber Massage, deren Technik Wirkung und Indikationen. *Arch. Klin. Chirurgie*, 19: 2-4, 1876.
381. Wakim, K.G., Martin, G.M., Terrier, J .C., Elkins, E.C., Krusen, F.N.: The Effect of Massage on the Circulation in Normal and Paralized Extremities. *Arch. Phys. Med.*, Mar: 135-144, 1949.
382. Wall, P.D., Crowly-Dillon, J .R.: Pain, Itch and Vibration. *A.MA. Arch. Neurol.*, 2: 19-29, 1960.
383. Walton, W.J.: *Texbook of Ostepathic Diagnosis and Technique Procedures.* 2nd Edition. "Mathewa Book C.", St. Louis, 1972.
384. Wang, N., Butler, J .P., Ingber, D.E.: Mechanotransduction Across the Cell Surface and Through the Cytoskeleton. *Science*, 260: 1124-1127, 1993.
385. Watson, .1 .: Pain Mechanisms: A Review. Endogenous Pain Mechanisms. *Austr. J. Physiotherapy*, 28(2): 38-45, 1982.
386. Weinberg, R., Jackson, A., Kolodny, K.: The Relationship of Massage and Exercise to Mood Enhancement. *Sports Psychologists,* 2: 202-211, 1988.
387. Weinrich, S.p., Weinrich, M.C.: The Effect of Massage on Pain in Cancer Patients. *Appl Nurs. Res*, 3(4): 140-145, 1990.
388. Weiss, J .M.: Discussion. In: Ebel, A., Wisham, L.H.: Effect of Massage on Muscle Temperature and Radiosodium Clearance. *Arch. Phys. Med.*, July: 399-405, 1952.
389. Weiss, J .M.: Treatment of Leg Edema and Wounds in patients with Severe Musculoskeletal Injuries. *Phys. Ther.*, 78(10): 1104-1113, 1998.
390. Wells, K.T., Luttgens, S.K.: *Kinesiology*. "W.B. Sanders Co", Philadelphia, 1976.
391. Wendt, L.: *Krankheiten verminderter Kapillarmembranpermeabilitat.* "E. Koch-Verlag", 1973.
392. Wenous, J .Z., Brilla, L.R., Morrison, M.D.: Effect of Massage on Delayed Onset Muscle Soreness. *Med. Sci. Sports Exer.*, 22: S34, 1990.
393. White-Traut, R.C., Goldman, M.B.C.: Premature Infant Massage. Is it Safe ? *Pea. Nurs.*, 14(4): 285-289, 1988.
394. Williams, W.S.: Sources of Piezoelectricity in Tendon and Bone. CRC Critic. *Rev. Bioengineer.*, 2(1): 95-118, 1974.
395. Williams, H.L., Elkins, E.C.: Myalgia of the Head. *Arch Phys. Ther.*, 23: 14-22, 1942.
396. Wirtz, H.R.W., Dobbs, L.G.: Calcium Mobilization and Exocytosis afler One Mechanical Stretch of Lung Epithelial Cells. *Science*, 250: 1266-1273, 1990.
397. Wiltshire EV, Poitras V, Pak M, Hong T, Rayner J, Tschakovsky ME. Massage impairs postexercise muscle blood flow and "lactic acid" removal. *Med Sci Sports Exerc*, 2010 Jun; 42(6):1062-71.
398. Witort, M.: *Tap Into Your Future*. Unpublished Article, 1999.
399. Wittlinger, H., Wittlinger, G.: *Textbook of Dr. Vodder 's Manual Lymph Drainage.* Vol. I. "HAUG", Brussels, 1992.
400. Wood, E.C.: *Massage Principles and Techniques*. "W.B. Saunders Co", Philadelphia, 1974.
401. Wood, E., Becker, P.D.: *Klassische Massagemethoden*. "Grimd-Wirkung-Technik der Ganz", Stuttgart, 1984.
402. Yang W, Chen J, Zhou L. Effects of shear stress on intracellular calcium change and histamine release in rat basophilic leukemia (RBL-2H3) cells. *Environ Pathol Toxicol Oncol*, 28(3):223-30, 2009
403. Yeo, T.C., Choo, M.H., Tay, M.B.: Massive Hematome from Digital Massage in Anticoagu lated Patient: A case Report. *Singapore Med. J.*, 35(3): 319-320, 1994.
404. Yumashev, G.S., Funnan, M.I.: *Spondylosis*. "Medicina", Moscow, 1984.
405. Zabludovsky, I.V.: [*Massage Techniques*]. St Petersburg, 1913.
406. Zanolla, R., Monzeglio, C., Balzarimi, A., Martino, G.: Evaluation of the Results of Three Dif

ferent Methods of Postmastectomy Lymphedema Treatment. *J. Surg. Oncol.*, 26(3): 210-213, 1984.

407. Zavadina, K.I.: [Clinical and physiological Foundation of Usage the Classical and Segment-Reflex Massage at Lumbo-Sacral Spondylosis]. *Vopr. Kurortol. Fizioter. Lech. Fiz. Kult.*, 6: 35-38, 1978.

408. Zelenkin, E.M., Prozorovskaia, K.N., Mirkin, A.S., Zavgorodniaia, E.G., Kandaurova, A.N.: [Low-Frequency Vibrations in the Treatment of Patients with Acute Maxillary Sinusitis and Ethmoiditis. Non-Specific Resistance and Immunity]. *Vestn. 0torinolaringol.*, 3: 41-43, 1998.

409. Zotterman, Y.: Touch, Pain and Tickling: an Electrophysiological Investigation on Cutaneous Sensory Nerves. *J. Physiology*, 95: 1-28, 1939.

INDEX

A

B

C

D

E

F

G

H

I

K

L

M

N

O

P

R

S

T

U

V

W

ABOUT THE AUTHOR

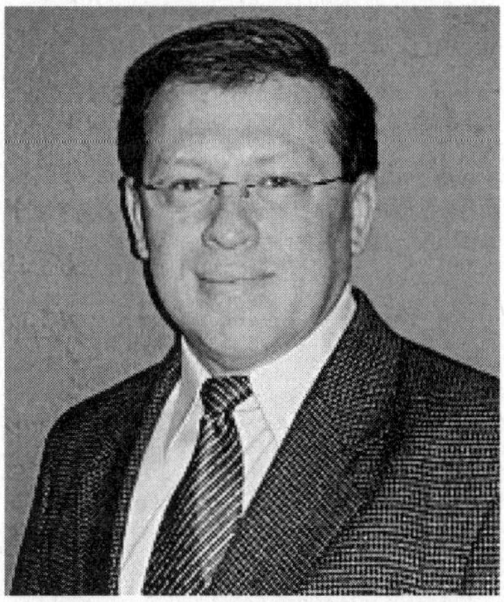

In 1983 Dr. Turchaninov graduated from the Odessa Medical University in Ukraine with honors and was then selected for resedency program in the Kiev Orthopedic Institute for Scientific Research. In 1985 he finished a two-year program at this institute with a specialization in trauma surgery and posttraumatic rehabilitation under the supervision of Academician K.S.Temovoy, M.D. At the same time Dr. Turchaninov began his scientific dissertation "Surgical and Rehabilitation Treatment of Patients with Bone Defects." He obtained his PhD degree in 1989.

During his residency, Dr. Turchaninov also studied electric acupuncture under the supervision of O. Leonenko, M.D.

Between 1985-1988 he worked as the chief supervisor of the rehabilitation program at the Ministry of Public Health of Ukraine. In 1990 Dr. Turchaninov graduated from a chiropractic and medical massage program designed for medical doctors at the Orthopedic Institute of Kiev.

In 1988-1991 he worked as a senior scientific researcher in the Clinic of Trauma Complications in the same institute in cooperation with Professor N.K.Ternovoy.

Dr.Turchaninov moved to the USA in 1992 due to consequences of the Chernobyl disaster and is now living in Phoenix, Arizona.

Dr. Turchaninov is actively involved in several education and research projects on the subject of somatic rehabilitation and pain management. He has presented the results of his work and research at the Annual Conference of the American Academy of Pain Management in Las Vegas, the International Congress of Beauty Medicine in Moscow, the Massage Therapy Foundation in Seattle, etc. He actively lectures in hospitals and colleges across the nation and is the editor of the *Journal of Massage Science* (**www.scienceofmassage.com**).

Dr. Turchaninov is the author of 31 scientific articles published in the former Soviet Union, Russia, Ukraine; Germany, and the USA. He holds two patents in the former Soviet Union. Dr. Turcahninov is the author of two volumes textbook *Medical Massage*.